TAOIST SEXUAL MEDITATION

MEDITATION

Connecting Love, Energy and Spirit

BRUCE FRANTZIS

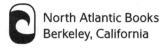

North Atlantic Books
Berkeley, California

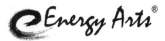

Published by Energy Arts, Inc., P.O. Box 99, Fairfax, California 94978-0099
415-454-5243 www.energyarts.com
Distributed by North Atlantic Books, P.O. Box 12327, Berkeley, California 94712
800-733-3000 www.northatlanticbooks.com

The following trademarks are used under license by Energy Arts, Inc., from Bruce Frantzis:
Frantzis Energy Arts® system, Mastery Without Mystery®, Longevity Breathing® program, Opening the Energy Gates of Your Body™ Qigong, Marriage of Heaven and Earth™ Qigong, Bend the Bow™ Spinal Qigong, Spiraling Energy Body™ Qigong, Gods Playing in the Clouds™ Qigong, Taoist Neigong Yoga™, Living Taoism™ Collection, Chi Rev Workout™, *Energy Arts* and HeartChi®.

Taoist Sexual Meditation: Connecting Love, Energy and Spirit is sponsored by the Society for the Study of Native Arts and Sciences, a nonprofit educational corporation whose goals are to develop an educational and cross-cultural perspective linking various scientific, social and artistic fields; to nurture a holistic view of arts, sciences, humanities and healing; and to publish and distribute literature on the relationship of mind, body and nature. North Atlantic Books is part of this organization.

Editing: Geralyn Gendreau; Diane Rapaport, Jerome Headlands Press; Caroline Frantzis; Jessica Moll, North Atlantic Books.
Cover Design: Thomas Herington, Angger Aristo
Interior Design: Heidi Helyard, Bluewood Studio; Veronica Sosa; Lisa Petty, GirlVibe, Inc.
Illustrations: Emmeralda Yang, Michael McKee
Photography: Caroline Frantzis, Bruce Frantzis, Mark Thayer, Danny Connor, Audrey Fontanilla
Printed in the United States of America

PLEASE NOTE: The creators, publishers and distributors of this book disclaim any liabilities for loss in connection with following any of the practices, exercises, and advice contained herein, and implementation is at the discretion, decision and risk of the reader. To reduce the chance of injury or any other harm, the reader should consult a professional before undertaking this or any other martial arts, movement, meditative arts, health or exercise program. Any physical or other distress experienced during or after any exercise should not be ignored and should be brought to the attention of a healthcare professional. The instructions and advice printed in this book are not in any way intended as a substitute for medical, psychological or emotional counseling with a licensed physician or healthcare provider.

Library of Congress Cataloging-in-Publication Data

Frantzis, Bruce Kumar.
  Taoist sexual meditation : connecting love, energy and spirit / Bruce Frantzis.
    pages cm
  Includes bibliographical references and index.
    ISBN 978-1-58394-495-0 (pbk.)
1. Sex instruction--Religious aspects--Taoism. 2. Sex--Religious aspects--Taoism. 3. Taoism. I. Title.
  HQ64.F73 2012
  299.5'14--dc23

                                2012038322

1 2 3 4 5 6 7 8 9 Peter Schultz Printing 17 16 15 14 13 12

This book is dedicated to yin and yang—woman and man—and what they can achieve together in sexual union.

You are invited to join
Bruce Frantzis' email list to receive
a special audio recording about
Taoist Sexual Meditation at:
www.energyarts.com/sexmeditation

Contents

Acknowledgments

Acknowledgments usually are tedious lists that nobody wants to read, but I felt that this book merited something different. Bringing it into existence was an intense process for all concerned. The Energy Arts book production team worked 24/7 to complete the manuscript and get it to the printer in time for the Random House distribution deadline. It's my sincere hope that you, the reader, find everyone's hard work worthwhile.

My grateful thanks to the Energy Arts team (and their partners too, who were in effect sex book widows and widowers while this project was going on). Now that the book is out, I hope everyone has a bit of time to lie back and enjoy some of the material in it. My special thanks go to:

Accomplished illustrator Emmeralda Yang, who, artistically speaking, bared her breasts and threw her bra out of the window to create the beautiful, tasteful yet sexy line drawings in this book. Our two main models were very impressed with her renditions. No complaints about penis or boob sizes, always a touchy issue. They were actually photographed modestly wearing swimsuits, and Emmeralda used her artistry to remove the clothing (ironically, clothing had to be drawn back onto the drawings for article submissions). Many of our models preferred to remain anonymous, so many thanks to them and anyone else who helped with this book but chose not to be named.

San Francisco Bay Area sex maven Geralyn Gendreau, for extensive editorial work, including developmental editing, and her wonderful Preface. She added a more feminine perspective to the language of this book. Keep that qi flowing through your Microcosmic Orbit, GG!

Diane Rapaport of Jerome Headlands Press, who, true to her name, has developed a great rapp(ap)ort with me over many years of collaborating on my book projects together. An experienced editor and long-time Energy Arts Certified Instructor, she worked on conceptual and developmental editing. She read the original rough draft back in the mid-nineties, so she's one of the few people who really knows exactly how much work it took to take the manuscript from there to here.

Mountain Livingston, who is truly as stable as a Mountain. He was in charge of organizing the illustrations for this book. He kept his cool amid all the chaos, managing and coordinating countless things to do with the production of this book. He was also one of our Taoist Neigong Yoga models—fully clothed, of course.

Energy Arts' resident digital media expert, Thomas Herington, who worked on cover design, photos, illustrations, and video and audio recordings of various seminars and retreats I have taught, transcriptions from which some of the material in this book is derived. Although posing nude is not really part of his job description, drawings of his naked body adorn many pages of this book. In fact he was very adept at digitally clothing some of the naked drawings for those articles.

Lisa Petty of GirlVibe, Inc., who has already typeset the interior layout for several of my previous titles and knows how to make countless illustrations flow well on the pages. My Dragon and Tiger Medical Qigong book was her biggest challenge, with more than 650 illustrations, but this is the first time she's been moving a lot of naked bodies around.

Heidi Helyard of Bluewood Studio in Australia for interior design, and Veronica Sosa in Spain for interior design consulting, who were both very gracious about dealing with some brutal differences in time zones. Angger Aristo helped with the cover design. Michael McKee created the hand drawings.

Footnote and bibliography queen Kaualani Pereira, for editorial and administrative assistance as well as being one of our Taoist Neigong Yoga models. She has the most attractive name of anyone involved in this project. Kaualani means Heavenly Rain in Hawaiian. It sounds very Taoist.

Editor Jessica Moll and Art Director Paula Morrison at North Atlantic Books. They both very graciously handled being given all kinds of changes to deal with at the very last minute.

I also want to thank our indefatigable project manager and editor who worked tirelessly and paid close attention to all aspects of creating the final text; indexer Ken DellaPenta, who did his most rushing of rushes for this book; photographers Mark Thayer and Audrey Fontanilla; and Camille Coates for editing assistance.

Finally my deepest thanks are reserved for the woman I love most dearly in my life, my wife Caroline, even though she doesn't think I'm much of an Adonis (maybe that's why nobody asked me to model for the drawings). A former BBC journalist, not only was she heavily involved in the editing and production process, but also, despite being an extremely private person, she was willing to write from the heart to create a very personal Foreword to this book.

Foreword

He was no Adonis, yet the sexual chemistry between us was unmistakable. We were walking hand in hand beside the Yangtze River in South China on a warm evening in 1984. My time as a university student in 1970s England had been a golden age for promiscuity—sexual freedom, no AIDS, no herpes, free contraception—absolutely nothing to fear in any encounter, whether short- or long-term. I considered myself quite sexually experienced, even though until meeting this seriously unconventional fellow, the big O—orgasm—had eluded me.

From the very first time we made love, it was as if he were telepathic. My body was an open book to him, and he knew exactly how to turn me on. Unable to even comprehend what it was that he was doing, I realized how ignorant I really was about my body and sex in general. At the time, I could not grasp the fact that it was as much my energy—my qi—as my physical body that he was working with.

Now, having been married to Bruce for more than twenty-five years, I can understand a little more of that all-encompassing qi matrix that underlies not only sex, but also health and spirituality. I have been practicing qigong and tai chi for many years, but still remain very much a novice. Our sex life, after a quarter of a century, is more exhilarating than ever, particularly as I grow ever more aware of the subtle currents of energy in both our bodies. Sure, like most couples, there have been ups and downs. Raising children can be the most effective contraceptive out there, and during periods when either of us has gone through insane work schedules, illness or injury, sex can be the last thing on our minds.

Nevertheless, many other older couples we know that have been married as long as we have seem to have settled into celibacy. They say it takes too much energy, that it's become boring, their lives have just become too stressful and busy or that health problems stop sex being fun anymore. I'm grateful that, after all these years, I'm still finding sex with my husband to be exquisitely satisfying and fulfilling. There is no doubt in my mind that it allows us to connect on a higher plane, clichéd as that may sound.

This book has taken almost two decades to come to fruition. Bruce wrote the original manuscript for *Taoist Sexual Meditation* back in the mid-1990s. It was put on the back burner for a long time. One of the reasons for this was that he did not want to release it while our children were still small. Now that they are grown and have trained in qigong and meditation, they are in a good position to begin to understand what their father is writing about. More importantly, over those two decades, Bruce has written several seminal books on qigong, Taoist meditation and internal martial arts that provide the foundation for the sexual qigong and sexual meditation described in this book.

Someone with no experience at all in these subjects can read this book and discover all kinds of ways to take the sensual experience of sex to a new level of exhilaration. However, incorporating qigong and meditation into the process leads you on the path of making lovemaking something incredible that is beyond words to describe.

Until I read this book, I did not realize exactly how considerate my husband was as a lover, and the degree of artistry and skill he displayed in the bedroom. He spent more than fifteen years in Asia, mostly in China, studying martial arts, Oriental healing techniques, qigong and meditation, including Taoist sexual practices, as intensively as a world-class Olympic athlete trains in his sport. This training was not lecture- or book-based—it was extremely practical and hands-on. To fully understand the sexual techniques, male students were expected to have sex with one thousand women, and female students with a hundred men. Western sensitivities and morals as regards sex were simply not part of the package. You might think this would make the student nothing more than an arrogant Lothario, incapable of making any long-term loving relationships. I can attest to the fact that this is not the case. After more than twenty-five years, I remain an appreciative beneficiary of all that training, although I'm glad it was more or less complete before we got together.

My hope is that you use this book to start new and exhilarating chapters in your own sex life. Whatever your age, Taoist sexual practices can enable you to take the relationship with your partner, both inside and outside the bedroom, from the mundane to the sublime. Enjoy your research!

Caroline Frantzis
Marin County, California
September 2012

Preface

In the early days of television when everything on the tube was black and white, all three of the existing channels completed their programming by midnight. People who watched TV simply enjoyed what they had. Only a rare dreamer would have bothered to imagine what it might be like to see a full-color picture on the small, grainy screen. And yet here we are, a mere sixty years later, enjoying high-definition color, and round-the-clock programming on a ridiculous number of channels. That much variety, depth and color—even more, in fact—can be brought into your sex life.

Like so many of my women friends, I'd been led to believe that I should be able to tell a man—even "train" him—how to please me in bed. This purportedly enlightened, liberated approach often left me feeling more like a drill sergeant than a sex kitten. By the age of forty, I was deeply frustrated. I kept thinking, "There has to be more to it than this!" I knew I hadn't fulfilled my sexual potential and feared that I never would. Then I met someone unusual. Here was a man who knew more about what my body wanted than I did. Sweet surrender. I could finally get out of my head and into my body. He was a natural—so brilliant in bed that I could let go of being in control and allow our mutual arousal to take me into unknown territory. No more following a predictable routine, making love became a sensual adventure. Everything that happened was fresh and new, unpredictable in the most delightful way. This wasn't just chemistry; this was a special type of genius. I began to refer to it as *sexual intelligence.*

As a marriage and family therapist, I began to wonder if this type of sexual intelligence could be learned. I wasn't willing to accept that a person was either born with the gift or not, but I knew of no comprehensive training to increase a person's sex IQ. Even in the San Francisco Bay Area, the Tantric sex capital of the Western world, very few people could grasp that sex isn't something you do—it's a place you go.

Try as I might to describe my experience and develop a curriculum, I couldn't find the words for what my special lover just seemed to know. Then I received an early copy of this manuscript. After I finished reading it, I felt encouraged: here was an author who could teach men how to read the intricate signals that tell them what a woman's body wants. The manuscript also contained crucial information women should have about what gets a man turned on. Even more exciting, the author himself wasn't born with the gift.

Bruce Frantzis was once as oblivious to the secrets of a woman's body as the average man on the street. At the age of eighteen, he left his home in New York City to study martial arts in the Far East. Initially in Japan and then in China, Frantzis trained intensively, studying under renowned masters of qigong, tai chi, hsing-i, bagua and Taoist meditation for fifteen-plus years. Early in his training, he had the rare opportunity to be invited into a secret Taoist community that practiced sexual meditation as an accelerated spiritual path. This marked the beginning of a radical departure as Frantzis shifted his allegiance from pure martial arts training to the ancient three-fold path of the warrior-healer-priest.

Since his return to the West in 1987, Frantzis has taught over twenty thousand students and certified hundreds of tai chi and qigong teachers around the world. He has written more than ten books—including the groundbreaking *Opening the Energy Gates of Your Body,* which details core principles of qigong, and *The Power of Internal Martial Arts and Chi,* a fascinating read and consummate guide—that have established him as a definitive authority in the field.

In any given area of study, certain individuals stand out for their mastery and expertise. In the best-selling book *Outliers,* Malcolm Gladwell examines what makes these people unique. One factor he identifies is having undergone at least ten thousand hours of training. By conservative estimate, Frantzis has trained and taught for fifty thousand hours in various subtle arts of energy, or what the Chinese call *qi* or *chi.* This puts him in a unique position to teach us about energy sex and, beyond that, the more advanced practices of Taoist sexual meditation.

Truth be told, information alone cannot possibly usher us across the divide that separates us from our slumbering sexual intelligence. Nor can this type of crossing be accomplished in a Tantra weekend. In a world where self-proclaimed "sexperts" flood the Internet with advice, finding your way through the maze of information is no simple task. At first I asked myself, "Why another book on Taoist sexuality?" What I discovered is that Frantzis' perspective and teachings are distinct from those of other authors in two very significant ways.

First of all, most of what has been written about Taoist sexual practices has been primarily limited to sexual qigong; the deeper subject of sexual meditation has not yet been brought to the West. Secondly, most if not all authors who write about Taoist sex are describing the perspective of the Fire tradition of Taoism, a specific approach that emphasizes the use of force and pushing through limits that may result in injury. The Water tradition is relatively unknown in the Western world. Nearly lost to antiquity, this approach focuses on letting go and relaxing into a natural state of pure Being. Frantzis was able to study under such a master—the Taoist sage Liu Hung Chieh—on a full-time basis for three solid years. Liu took the unprecedented step of adopting Frantzis and passing on the lineage.

The story of Frantzis joining a secret Taoist group and being adopted by an old Taoist sage initially struck me as far-fetched, even unbelievable. However, once I got to know Frantzis and witnessed him teaching qigong and other energy arts, I could feel the veracity of what he carries in terms of a pure Taoist lineage. Clearly, this man is a master of qi, exceptional in his command of subtle energies that most of us in the West barely know exist. He is uniquely positioned to deliver this esoteric tradition to Westerners in digestible form. The aim of this book is really that—to give readers unparalleled access to sexual meditation as a blissful, transformative process. No flowery metaphors—just substantive information, demystified in down-to-earth, contemporary terms.

The Taoists have harnessed sexual intelligence as an essential part of their religion. When an ancient tradition that has actualized the spiritual potential of sex cross-pollinates in the Western world through a master teacher like Bruce Frantzis, we get a truly important breakthrough. In Silicon Valley, advances of this magnitude are often referred to as "disruptive technologies" simply because they disrupt the status quo. With the sexual status quo of so many people locked onto a setting that reads "dissatisfied," this is one disruption that is long overdue. Change can be challenging, of course. Whether we're adapting to new technology or increasing our sex IQ, we progress through a natural learning curve. Once we achieve a higher baseline, all sorts of possibilities that were previously unimaginable are ours to enjoy. In the sexual realm, the terrain is infinite—literally—and that's the Tao.

What I've seen of where this information leads has given me tremendous respect for the Taoists' expertise. Theirs is an intricate, exacting system for unearthing the true nature of human beings. This is the ultimate aim and destiny of every sentient being: to achieve an extraordinary degree of body-mind integration and ecstatic union with the Tao.

I recommend that you approach this book with curiosity and suspend any expectation that simply reading it should result in complete comprehension right away. The content has a vibrational quality that will not translate to your linear mind. Instead of trying to comprehend everything you read, consciously intend that your deeper self will be affected. You cannot understand what you have not yet experienced, so let go and surrender to an instinctive encounter. This book is designed to plant seeds in your mind, seeds that will be watered subliminally by the Tao out of which your very thoughts arise. In time, you may well find that the information in this book becomes personal, direct knowledge when the reality that words can only point to reveals itself in the field of your awareness.

This has happened for me a number of times since I first read the manuscript. Detailed instructions I don't even remember reading suddenly just transpire, revealing new terrain. For example, one evening I found myself focusing on my lover's upper body rather than responding to what was going on below his waist. According to Taoist theory, this allows his yang energy to build. I worked on my man's head, neck and shoulders while he pressed into me with his yearning. I could feel his essential yang more tangibly than ever before, which gave my yin nature a new of level of permission to open, receive, and be nourished by his masculine energy.

On another occasion, a surprising revelation occurred with respect to the Microcosmic Orbit, the energy current that flows through the human body. Many times over the years, I'd seen intriguing drawings of lovers whose bio-electric circuitry had become intertwined, but the actual existence of this inner current remained conceptual—little more than a lovely idea. Then, shortly after I completed a qigong instructor training with Frantzis, my lover and I were in the throes when, out of nowhere, the Microcosmic Orbit became a tangible reality. It was as if a river of energy was running through my body. Once I began to feel and sense the movement of this river, I was able to connect with that flow through *his* body as well. This gave me a glimpse of who and what he might be beyond the conventional idea of a "person." That made me very excited to learn more about both of us beyond the ordinary construct of "man and woman."

Inside every one of us there is a seed that has never left the Tao. Let that part of you be stirred by the words in this book. Read, not as though the information is foreign, but as though it is native. Somewhere, in the multiplex of universes, an old Taoist has just sent you an invitation to discover the truth of who you are.

Geralyn Gendreau, MS, MFT
Coauthor and editor, *The Marriage of Sex and Spirit: Relationship at the Heart of Conscious Evolution*
Marin County, California
August 2012

Author's Introduction

I was a nineteen-year-old hotshot martial arts champion. It was the 1960s, and I had managed to get myself introduced to the legendary tai chi, hsing-i and bagua master Wang Shu Jin. Amazingly, he was willing to take me on as a student. On a hot and humid afternoon, we were sitting together in his living room in Taichung, Taiwan. Bald-headed, big-bellied, with arms and legs like tree-trunks, the old man, speaking in Chinese, proceeded to lay into me. "I can fight better than you. I can eat more than you," and then, hitting me way below the belt, at least metaphorically, he added, "and I can fuck better than you. There's more to being strong than youth. It's all to do with how much qi you have."

Later, in the middle of sparring practice, Wang took the idea further: "You look like a sexually high-spirited young man," he said, "but do you really know how to do it?" I didn't like where the conversation was going. Here was a man in his sixties, carrying three hundred pounds on a 5 foot 8 inch, rotund frame—not the body type you might commonly associate with the buff, macho sexuality paraded about in the West. Who was he to challenge my youthful enthusiasm and what I thought of as natural prowess?

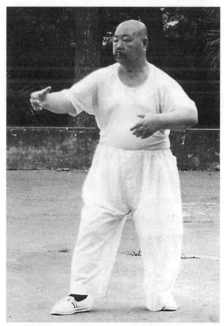

Photo by the author

In fact, I knew full well who he was—one of the best fighters in all of China. When I realized that his intent was not to insult me but to open my mind, I began to get curious about what he might know. I'd already experienced the remarkable power of Master Wang's qi firsthand when he had first invited me to spar with him. Even though I had black belts in judo, karate, jujitsu and aikido, I couldn't get near him. When he asked me to punch him in the gut as hard as I could, he bounced me right off his big belly like a rubber ball. As

The late Wang Shu Jin demonstrates standing qigong in a park in Taichung, Taiwan.

a martial artist, he was matchless. That much was abundantly clear. Equally remarkable were his older students, some in their sixties and seventies, including women, who could spar with me and hold their own. Without a doubt, Wang was an extraordinary teacher, skilled at teaching people how to use qi.

Although he never discussed the matter with me directly, I also knew that the venerable Master Wang lived with nine women, only one of whom was his servant and housekeeper. The other eight, loosely speaking, were his concubines. Clearly there was something about the old man that made them want to stay with him.

Wang talked to me about a secret Taoist group with a comprehensive knowledge of sex and meditation far beyond what I could imagine. He gave me a personal introduction to this group that trained adepts to become Taoist priests.

TAOIST PRIESTHOOD TRAINING

Although I had practiced Zen Buddhist meditation in my youth, my primary interest was in experiencing the world rather than retreating from it. I grew up in New York City, where the word "priest" evokes strong images: the black and white collar, the man at the altar with an offering raised overhead. Like most of my generation, I associated priests with the Catholic Church, the tight confines of a confessional and vows of celibacy. I did not in any way aspire to become a priest. In fact, I wasn't even interested in spirituality at that point in my life. As a martial artist and a healthy, sexually-active young man, celibacy was the furthest thing from my mind.

Wang, to my astonishment, completely demolished my cultural stereotypes. I was ushered into a world where priests were not encouraged to renounce their sexual nature—quite the opposite.

Through Master Wang's personal introduction to this Taoist community, I quickly came to realize that my youthful enthusiasm for sex was largely an automatic, unconscious activity, driven by instinct. As a lover, I was on autopilot, unaware and out of touch, not only with whoever was my partner, but also with my own body, mind and heart. I could not yet recognize that sexual attraction and fulfillment was beyond looks, personality and thinking. Rather sexual joy and satisfaction were determined by how well the invisible energy flowed between lovers and on how many levels those energetic flows were compatible (for more on this subject, see Chapter 6). I was completely oblivious to the multidimensional experience everyone can access by consciously engaging sexuality.

Moreover, this unconsciousness and almost naïve lack of awareness of my inner Being also, at the time, extended into my personal relationships. Perhaps this more than anything else persuaded me to embark on a seven-year course of study to be ordained as a Taoist priest.

The word "priest" is used completely differently in the East than in the West. In China, training to be a *tao shi* (literally "spiritual teacher," the Taoist word for "priest"), involves total immersion in multiple Taoist energy arts. A *tao shi* is, first and foremost, a master of internal energy or qi. At each stage of development, an initiate is required to undergo practical, in-depth training, during which he or she must embody and demonstrate the ability to work with qi within his or her body and later with the qi of others. An elaborate sequence of spiritual rituals and vows is involved.

The course of study, utterly foreign in the West, includes a complex array of subjects:

1. Comprehension of the classic Taoist texts, especially the *I Ching*, which is studied in depth, much as a Christian studies the Bible.

2. Qigong (energy work) for mastering the energy circuits and flows in the body and becoming healthy.

3. Meditation methods for health and vitality, releasing karma, and developing psychic capacities to move toward enlightenment and the Tao.

4. Healing arts such as herbs, acupuncture and my particular specialty, *qigong tui na* (bodywork that uses both physical and qi techniques), one of the eight branches of Traditional Chinese Medicine.

5. Spiritual martial arts—tai chi, hsing-i and bagua, with their physical, martial, psychic and healing skills, and then the entire meditation process that leads toward the Tao.

6. Performing or assisting with exorcisms.

7. Spiritual midwifery—ushering sentient beings into the world by working with women during pregnancy and delivery, to enable the soul to fully enter in the healthiest possible spiritual condition.

8. Death and dying practices—to guide people through the pre-dying process and help them cross over to the other side—and, if appropriate, teach them what happens and what to do when consciousness permanently leaves the body.

9. Rites and rituals that minister to the spiritual needs of the community.

10. All aspects of sexuality, from improving relationships to resolving physical, mental, emotional and spiritual blockages, and opening the door to higher levels of consciousness through solo and sexual meditation practices.

In this particular Taoist priesthood group, an initiate was required to engage in sex as a vehicle for personal transformation. This particular training was not exclusively for men; women were also allowed to train as a *tao shi*. Understanding sexual energy and all that goes with it was a vital part of the training. In fact, the vows of the *tao shi* placed initiates under a mandate to be sexual in many circumstances even when they felt disinclined.

This training also involved total secrecy. The methods were to be shared only with initiates of an exclusive, nonpublic group. Outside my group of initiates, I was not permitted to mention my membership in the group or any of my activities to anyone, including my family and closest friends, sexual or not. Likewise, I was never allowed to elaborate what transpired in the priesthood except in the broadest terms.

It was considered a great honor and privilege to gain access to this sacred knowledge. Receiving the teachings generated an unprecedented level of personal responsibility, because the subject matter dealt with the core of each person's inner life. The teachings were not a matter for casual consideration or gossip. Only after I became ordained was I able to share the Taoist work, not to fulfill anyone's idle curiosity, but only to help alleviate deeper human and spiritual needs.

It was while training to become a *tao shi* that I learned the depth of knowledge that the Taoists hold about sexuality. Here in the West, it was the advent of birth control that sparked the free-love movement. Contrast this with ancient Taoist communities, which didn't need modern medicine and "the pill" to prevent pregnancy. Having perfected the techniques of semen retention, the Taoists have had reliable birth control for thousands of years. That's two thousand years of uninterrupted sexual exploration. Far from a fad or new innovation, Taoist sexual qigong and sexual meditation is grounded within one of the world's great religious traditions.

Before I lead you further into this unusual and fascinating realm, I want to offer an important point of clarification. I want to state, right here at the start, that while the Taoists may appear unrestrained in sexual matters, the behavior prescribed for priesthood training does not involve selfish indulgence or sexual exploitation at all. Its primary purpose is spiritual acceleration and advancement with consenting partners. An exalted understanding of human sexuality is what makes this possible.

LIU HUNG CHIEH AND THE TAOIST WATER TRADITION

After seven years of priesthood training, studying a wide range of energy practices, including martial arts, qigong, meditation and healing modalities with Wang

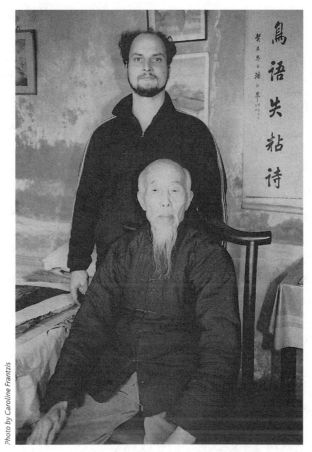

Photo by Caroline Frantzis

The author was a disciple of the late Taoist Lineage Master
Liu Hung Chieh, of Beijing, China.

Shu Jin and other masters, I met Liu Hung Chieh. He was a master of a different Taoist lineage who was considered a Spiritual Immortal, or what is often termed "a fully realized Being."

With the exception of one Chinese student, Liu had not been teaching, much less taking on new students, since the Communists rose to power in 1949. However, shortly before we met, he had a prophetic dream in which a big foreigner arrived at his doorstep to study with him. Because of this dream and a personal letter of introduction I had brought with me, Liu agreed to take me on as a student.

Just as in Tibetan Buddhism, within the Taoist arts, a lineage is a line of teaching that runs from one master through successive generations of worthy students, who become masters in their own right and pass on the knowledge. As Sogyal Rinpoche writes in *The Tibetan Book of Living and Dying:* [1]

"Lineage serves as a crucial safeguard: It maintains the authenticity and purity of the teaching...It is not a question of preserving some fossilized ritualistic knowledge, but of transmitting from heart to heart, from mind to mind, an essential and living wisdom and its skillful and powerful methods."

Liu would fully teach me yet another Taoist tradition unknown in the West—the Water method, based on two classic Taoist texts, the *Tao Te Ching* by Laozi, who is also known as Lao Tse or Lao Tzu (see Appendix D, "The Spelling of Chinese Words in English") and the *I Ching.* Liu would also complete my education in the Fire methods of Taoism that I had learned during my Taoist priesthood training and from other masters.

Liu Hung Chieh took my learning to extraordinary levels, for which I have deep gratitude. From Liu I received authentic lineages in bagua, tai chi and hsing-i (the three internal martial arts of China), as well as in qigong and Taoist meditation. One of the responsibilities of my lineage was to teach and carry the knowledge forward to this and future generations, if I so chose.

I have written this book for the same reason as my previous ones—to ensure that even if I should die tomorrow, important parts of the Taoist lineage to which I belong will be not be lost but instead will be available to people in the West. My aim is for this profoundly transformative material to continue to benefit future generations over multiple lifetimes.

SEXUAL MEDITATION: THE WAY OF LOVE, ENERGY AND SPIRIT

Taoism has a well-worn phrase, "If there is the real, then there is the false." In this book I have attempted to write only about the "real," as my lineage and personal sense of integrity require. This book introduces the Taoist view on sexual meditation as a direct method to the highest attainments of Eastern spirituality. More than just another sex manual, it is an entry point into the largely untapped potential of human sexuality.

Sexual energy is the single most powerful, natural internal force that is readily available to a human being to foster his or her spiritual development. For thousands of years, Taoists have harnessed that supercharged energy using precise and very pragmatic methods. By introducing these multidimensional methods, I hope to

---

1. Sogyal Rinpoche, *The Tibetan Book of Living and Dying* (New York: Harper, San Francisco, 1994), 128.

help people become comfortable talking about sex and engaging in it, a subject that is both natural and profound. Then couples can begin to see and actualize the dormant possibilities sex offers as a method to reach their highest human and spiritual potentials.

Becoming a better lover is not just about physical techniques. It is mostly about becoming energetically aware of and sensitive to increasingly deeper dimensions within you and your partner. As this occurs, sex not only becomes increasingly pleasurable and emotionally satisfying, but it also becomes a method to broaden intimacy between you and your partner, both in the bedroom and in your day-to-day relationship. Each chapter explores the context and theory of sex from the Taoist tradition. As you move through the book, you may be surprised by Taoism's pragmatic approaches to solving some of the sexual hang-ups and conditioning that get in the way not only of pleasure but also of having a relaxed and satisfying relationship with your partner. You may also be intrigued by the Taoist view of morality in the larger context of karma and of sexuality as a means to achieve enlightenment.

Learning Taoist sexual practices is a multilevel process. The beginning level can be called "ordinary sex" or "the way of love." The intermediate level is what Taoists refer to as "sexual qigong" or "the way of energy." This involves intentional engagement with the subtle energy dimension of sexuality. The advanced level is "sexual meditation" or "the way of Spirit," an accelerated path to full enlightenment. Most of what Westerners have come to know as "Tantra," in Taoism falls under the category of energy sex or sexual qigong rather than sexual meditation.

Although the practices in this book are not necessarily easy, they are not too difficult to consider trying, even if certain aspects may seem way out of your reach. Many normal human beings, just like you, have successfully engaged in these methods for millennia. Most began working with ordinary sex and progressed step-by-step over time. Rather than thinking sexual qigong and meditation were impossible, they adopted the attitude that "if others have done it, I, too, may get there in time." They recognized that "not yet" is quite different from "never" or "impossible."

According to an old Taoist saying, "If time is limited, don't ask a master whys or wherefores. Rather, ask how to do what is being proposed." In other words, focus on the practices that give you the direct experience rather than only explanations. Only by doing what is suggested can you discover what the practice is meant to reveal. To this purpose, the sexual practices in this book are sequentially numbered to give you the ideal order in which to experiment with the material. Nevertheless, I leave it to your judgment to decide how to proceed.

Many specific exercises will provide you with an understanding of Taoist sexual arts and how to learn them. Each exercise is categorized according to its level of practice:

 Ordinary sex, symbolized by the Chinese character *jing* (sperm/ovary generative energy that governs the physical body).

 Energy sex or sexual qigong, represented by the Chinese word *qi* (vital energy, including thoughts, emotions and psychic energy).

 Spiritual sex or sexual meditation, denoted by the Chinese character *shen* (Spirit or karmic and essence energy).

The techniques within these practice sections form the essence of the book. Each new level includes methods of the previous ones. In order to reach the higher levels of practice, some degree of skill and competence at the earlier levels is required. In the transition phase between two levels, the methods tend to mix and match before they become more complete and stable at the next level.

Although ordinary Taoist sexual practices can be learned by almost everyone, this may not be the case for advanced methods of sexual qigong and meditation. These require a higher level of commitment to learn the subtle energy skills that provide a pathway to success. The necessary foundation is commonly gained in such preliminary practices as qigong, tai chi and tai chi push hands, explained in more detail in Chapter 10. For Taoist sexual meditation work, it is necessary to have had significant training and practice in both the Taoist methods of meditation and the energetic techniques of *neigong,* the Taoist art and science of how to consciously move energy through the body, which consists of sixteen components (see Chapter 10, "The Art and Science of Neigong").

The Taoist Water tradition is not rigid, however, and fully recognizes that readers are likely to experiment with methods from different levels to satisfy their natural curiosity. Nonetheless, it must be stated that reading about Taoist sexual practices from a book does not have the same power or subtlety as learning under the guidance of an experienced master. It does, however, allow for a worthwhile start, as actual masters of this material are difficult to find. At the very least, it may inspire you to learn some of the other energy practices, such as qigong, that can not only dramatically improve your sex life but also help you become extremely healthy and vibrant.

THE RELEVANCE OF TAOISM AND SEXUAL MEDITATION TO MODERN LIFE

This book introduces Taoist spirituality through the lens of Taoist sexuality, a subject little known about, much less taught. Developing and strengthening life-force energy through sexuality is one of the Taoist paths toward spiritual awakening.

During the final years of my Taoist studies in Beijing, I once asked Liu Hung Chieh why he didn't teach more people meditation. His answer was, "Not many want to learn." Today, Liu's words reach across to Eastern and Western cultures that are deeply mired in a malaise of anxieties and fears. Modern life for many feels out of balance and continually stressful. Few people set aside the time for a regular spiritual practice, meditation or otherwise.

For many couples, sex has become just another task or chore for which they can't seem to find the time or energy.

Imagine how much better the world would be if everyone was having thoroughly satisfying sex. In their daily lives, both inside and outside the bedroom, people would feel happier and more relaxed, as well as less prone to negative emotions such as depression, fear and anger.

Prolonged, sustained commitment to a spiritual path is never easy. However, Taoist sexual practices can allow you and your partner to work together and gain accelerated access to that path. Using Taoist meditation, as you release that which energetically binds you, pure states of awareness, joy and love can begin to arise naturally. This becomes your new baseline. The goal is to explore who you are at the level of your soul or Being.

This book gives you a systematic way to improve the quality of your lovemaking on a variety of different levels, and, if you so choose, to begin working toward becoming more spiritually awake. More fulfilling sex is just a tiny fraction of what Taoism, one of the world's great religious traditions, has to offer. Its potent, transformative techniques can benefit you in all kinds of ways, from the everyday to the esoteric.

I wish you well on your journey towards the Tao.

Bruce Frantzis
Marin County, California
September 2012

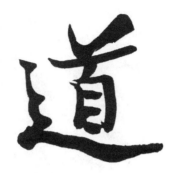

SECTION 1

THE TAOIST CONTEXT

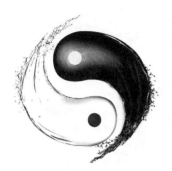

CHAPTER 1

Ordinary Sex, Energy Sex and Spiritual Sex

Within the Taoist tradition, lovemaking is viewed as not only a learnable skill but also an art. Anyone who puts in the time and effort to study the Taoist sexual arts and stays the course can expect to learn to improve at it, just as with any other activity, such as sports, academics, cooking or playing a musical instrument. At its deeper levels, sexual training can be a doorway to the higher possibilities of your own soul.

Taoists see sexuality as essential to who and what we are—an aspect of our nature that can be cultivated, rather than repressed or denied. Instead of attempting to conquer our "lower nature" and suppress what are essentially healthy impulses, Taoists encourage living in harmony with that which is natural to a human being.

Indeed, traditionally in China, the bedroom arts were taught in an atmosphere that was very open and direct—nothing like what might be presented in a class on sexuality at a Western university. A hallmark of the training was a frank and unabashed exploration of sexuality from many perspectives, ranging from the pragmatic to the sacred.

In the classic method of "from the mouth of a master to the ear of a disciple," the intellectual information and energetic subtext were not only verbally explained but also silently taught in a profound spiritual manner, using what is called "energetic transmission." Once a transmission was passed on, it would remain a seed that would only grow through practice. Students were expected to practice what was taught or give up any expectation of receiving greater detail and deeper teachings. The practice sessions were expected to be pleasurable, or at the very least, interesting. If sex became a chore, the student was clearly missing something.

At the beginning, students were taught basic techniques that increased sensitivity, pleasure and the connection with their partners. This could be called "ordinary sex" or "the way of conventional love." Only then were students taught the higher potential of sex as both an energetic force and spiritual path—termed "sexual qigong" and finally "sexual meditation."

ORDINARY SEX

Ordinary sex is about having more pleasure, emotional satisfaction and peace during lovemaking and in the course of your normal life. The base practices at this level include learning how to navigate and activate all the body's erogenous zones to best effect and utilizing every part of your body to accomplish the task. Ordinary sex also addresses the whys and wherefores of sexual positions, and how often and under what conditions to have sex or not.

You learn an array of specific physical skills to enable and release more pleasurable orgasms. These include all aspects of foreplay, such as kissing, rubbing, nuzzling, blowing on, biting or scratching any part of the body; varieties of oral sex; and copulation techniques, such as how to move during intercourse and how to change positions and rhythms.

As important as the physical techniques, you also learn how to become aware of what gets in the way of being a good lover emotionally or mentally, and you study the pragmatic Taoist techniques for dealing with those obstacles. The more sex releases the emotional barriers inside you and inside your partner, the easier it is to apply all the physical techniques that enhance pleasure.

Learning and using the Taoist techniques of ordinary sex will help you and your partner develop a more loving emotional and mental connection, both in and out of bed, deepening the relationship between you. This can ease the strains of daily life and calm the storms that arise between you and your partner, breaking down some of the barriers between you. Every once in a while, lovers can experience a type of supernatural ecstasy and bliss through lovemaking.

In addition, ordinary sex techniques smooth out the hormonal system and release internal pressure. They can help you relax and release your nerves so that sex can become enjoyable. Feeling frustrated and irritable after a long workday? Having sex can release stress and make everything feel fine, or at least more bearable. Along with the feel-good experience that makes both people happy, sex regulates the natural sexual urge that, if left unfulfilled, can make a person edgy and irritable. Sex helps to sustain people through life's pressures, miseries and hardships. It gets the pleasure endorphins going. Sexual activity helps to regulate the flow of bodily fluids, improve mood and balance hormones.

The techniques for ordinary sex presented in this book are suitable for average people who are interested in enhancing their sex life. The only requirement is being willing to give it a go. No specialized esoteric training is needed. If you are capable of having sex, you are also capable of trying out these very practical methods.

The overwhelming majority of sex books address this ordinary level only. Within Taoist sexuality, however, these ordinary practices enhance normal sex to the point where partners are sufficiently developed to undertake more advanced levels of sexual qigong or meditation with relative ease.

Becoming a Better Lover

The percentage of people who will naturally be sexually satisfying, good lovers, also referred to as "magic lovers," only make up a minority—likely under twenty percent of the population. The other eighty percent or so will be split into the categories of "mediocre to a bit above the norm" with a smaller percentage in the category of "downright terrible."

For anyone in the eighty-percent group, or the statistical average, all hope is not lost. Some simple training and the desire to be better can enable most to become much better lovers over time.

Back in the 1970s in Asia, when I was originally told that this rough breakdown of great, average and terrible lovers was the consistent Taoist experience over several millennia, I didn't quite know what to make of it or if it were true. However after many years, I have come to the same conclusion based not only on my own experience and but also after having discussed the matter with both Chinese and Western women and men with similar or greater experience than my own.

SEX AND TENSION

Sadly, many couples in our modern times don't even enjoy an ordinary sex life because their nervous systems are regularly overloaded. Uncomfortable in their bodies, tired and anxiety ridden, many people in our age have lost interest in sex because it requires too much energy. Without any energy left at the end of the day, many resort to passive entertainment such as TV, Internet and movies instead of directly experiencing life and the opposite sex.

In many preindustrial societies, tired farmers or physical laborers who had worked a twelve-hour day could still come home and make love late into the night. Why was this so? Although their muscles were tired, their nerves were not.

Nerve fatigue—a common event in our overwhelmed, overscheduled, fear-driven, technology-dependent lives—greatly impairs sexual functioning. Nervous exhaustion diminishes the sex drive by dulling the central nervous system in general and the sexual nerves in particular, rendering them incapable of feeling and responding. This is why people say "my nerves are shot" after a day of excessive visual and other stimulation. The nerves actually get temporarily burned out through overuse of the mind and volatile emotional swings. This is more than the nerves can handle and often directly lowers a person's sex drive.

At the very least, Taoist ordinary sex practices can help resolve many of the avoidable tensions that get in the way of enjoying sex. Over thousands of years, Taoists have developed and honed precise and very practical methods to relax and release the nerves.

Relaxation helps a man prolong the sex act, maintain erections longer and climax without ejaculating. Relaxation can enable a woman to achieve orgasm more easily or become multi-orgasmic, and she can learn to expand her orgasm so that it ripples in waves through her entire body. The two beginning practices below are easy ways to help partners relax and restore tired nerves.

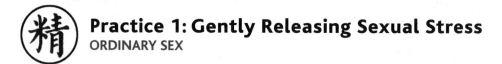 ## Practice 1: Gently Releasing Sexual Stress
ORDINARY SEX

Part 1: Merge Your Breathing

The simplest way to rejuvenate tired nerves is for you and your partner to breathe together. It is helpful to breathe just loudly enough that you can hear one another. Simply hold each other in a comfortable position and continue until your breaths gradually begin to synchronize. Slowly allow each breath to become deeper and quieter, until both of you grow very quiet inside and breathe as one person. This is a wonderfully simple way to create a loving connection, deepen emotional bonding and reawaken sexual desire.

Part 2: Pulsing

Another way partners can calm their exhausted nerves is by holding and gently pulsing each other's hands, which involves gently opening and closing the hand and wrist joint in a smooth rhythm (see Chapter 13, "Opening and Closing: The Pulse of the Universe" for more details on pulsing). Begin with light squeezes and then gradually add more intensity as your sexual contractions begin to awaken. Eventually, you will be pulsing together in unison. Keep the pulsing synchronized while the mind and nervous system slows down and begins to relax.

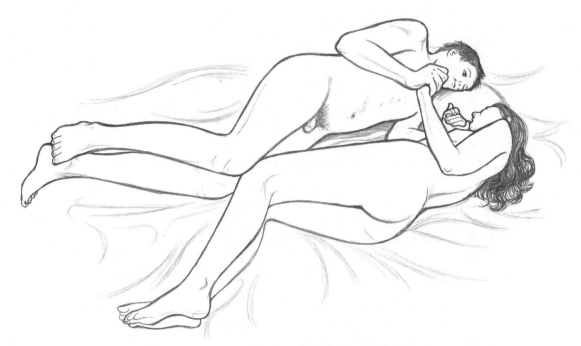

Figure 1-1: Partner Breathing, Handholding and Pulsing

You can also use both of these methods simultaneously: breathe and pulse hands in unison. Eventually, you and your partner will become quiet and calm, aware of the simple pleasure you are generating in each other's bodies as one rhythmic whole. Let nervous exhaustion fade away as you both relax into and feel the loving interplay of each other's yin and yang energy.

Pulsing is the body's basic condition during lovemaking. Pulsation occurs naturally in your genitals during pleasurable writhing and sexual contractions. The basic question is, "Can you relax your nerves sufficiently so that you and your partner can pulse together during sex?" Pulsing with your partner helps put you on that path.

Commonly, one partner is so exhausted that he or she simply closes down and becomes numb in the prelude to sex or during sex. A verbal or nonverbal signal says "No thank you," and that's where it ends. When you are tired, just breathe and pulse in unison with your partner to develop mutual relaxation. Sexual rapport and increased desire will often be reignited.

It is important to allow your partner the time he or she needs to release nervous exhaustion before moving onto the sexual act. After a few minutes of pulsing, as accumulated nervous system tension releases, your partner might just be in the mood. If he or she falls asleep, or prefers to rest, simply allow it. When he or she wakes up, the deep state of relaxation that your pulsing has induced will often lead to renewed sexual interest. ●

Choice of Sexual Position

This book's illustrations show only a few, relatively ordinary sex positions. There are more than a hundred sexual positions in total, many of which people find too difficult, because they do not have the sufficient flexibility, or because the positions work well only for a relatively small number of people whose bodies fit together just right.

This is not the 1950s anymore, and you can find all the positions on the Internet and in other sex books. Often, within ordinary sex, certain positions are touted for their health and healing value. From the author's experience these benefits are commonly overstated. The argument behind claiming the health benefits (which may or may not be the case in reality) of a specific ordinary sex position is typically threefold. First, some positions naturally activate certain acupuncture meridians. Second, they create specific biomechanical pressures on internal organs and glands. Finally, they stretch and bring better blood circulation to various parts of the body, especially the joints and muscles.

The primary purpose of this book is not ordinary sex but rather sexual qigong and sexual meditation. For these more advanced practices, any sexual position will do, so long as there is a point of contact through which either person, or both, can send, receive and dissolve qi. The main points of contact are the lips, fingers, tongue or genitals. An electrical data port or wireless internet connection that receives data must have a connection point that stays stable and sensitive to transfer information. This is also true for the connection point between lovers. Some genital contact positions are easier to maintain for some people than others and often it comes down to personal preferences. Most will find their natural preferences are based upon relative flexibility, previous injuries in the body, how tired they are and how easy it is to hold specific positions for varying lengths of time. Just remember that the key point is to maintain the flow of energy rather than to achieve specific physical positions.

SEXUAL QIGONG: ENERGY SEX

Sexual qigong, or energy sex, goes beyond ordinary sex by working directly with the subtle energy—the *qi*—that flows through a human being. This next level of sex works with deeper physical, energetic, emotional, mental and psychological dimensions and, potentially, with the psychic energy realm.

The sexual act itself causes your energy to naturally become vibrantly apparent and accessible to you. This makes it possible to increase the sensitivity and awareness of qi flows in you and your partner. When sex becomes about subtle energy, or qi, it really comes alive.

> *When sex becomes about subtle energy, it really comes alive.*

Sexual qigong involves consciously engaging, activating and directing the flow of qi within and between sexual partners. The same physical techniques learned in ordinary sex become vehicles for accessing the energy flow between you and your lover.

DIRECTING QI INTO THE BODY

Once you can feel and access the flow of qi, then you learn the techniques for directing qi through the body's physical and emotional energy pathways, including the various energy channels, centers and transference points. Emitting or receiving energy from the genitals, mouth, tongue or fingers can cause orgasms to become more possible and powerful than from just physical rubbing alone.

For example, a man can project energy from his palms and fingers into his lover's vagina and from there to the bottom of her feet or beyond to energize the yin energy of her lower body. He can do this with or without touching his lover (Figure 1-2 A).

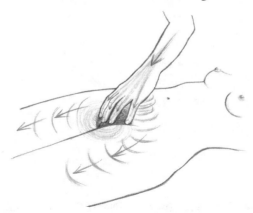

Figure 1-2 A: Projecting Energy into the Vagina and Lower Body

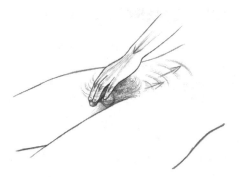

Figure 1-2 B: Projecting Energy into the Penis and Upper Body

Likewise, a woman can project energy from her palms and fingers into her lover's penis, and from there, up his body to the crown of his head or beyond to energize the yang energy of his upper body (Figure 1-2 B). She can do this with or without touching his penis. She can also project energy from her vagina into her man in this way while being penetrated by him.

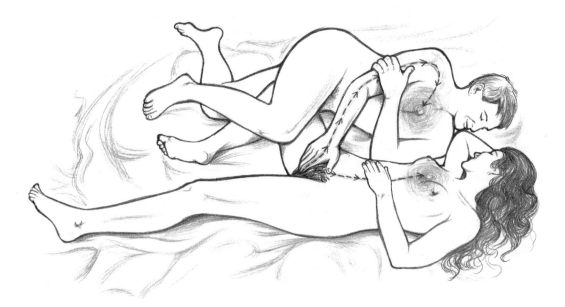

Figure 1-3: Connecting Energy to Lovers' Heart Centers through Fingers and Genitals

The man can also project energy from his hand to his lover's heart center through her vagina, and at the same time she can project energy from her vagina up his arm to his heart center (Figure 1-3).

In Figure 1-3 the man physically inserts his fingers into her vagina, just as she could hold and move his genitals. Energetically this corresponds to the way two computers network information with each other with data ports on both ends and a connecting cable in between. For example his finger, through projecting, can transfer energy to her heart center or anywhere else within her body. The transference of qi can make orgasms stronger and more pleasurable.

The Meaning of Qi or Chi

Qi and chi are the same Chinese word, just transliterated or spelled differently. The fundamental meaning of qi is "life force," that which gives life to all living matter. It flows like a river inside you. The stronger and more balanced the flow, the more alive and alert you feel. A weak flow results in sluggishness and fatigue.

Qi is a universal concept, as Cyndi Dale points out in her work *The Subtle Body:* "In Japan, it is called *ki*. To East Indians, *prana*. The ancient Picts of northern England called it *maucht*…More recent researchers might call it bioenergy, biomagnetism, electrochemical energy, subtle energy or just plain energy."[1]

Thousands of years ago, Taoists mapped the qi flows through human beings along precise energetic pathways. Acupuncturists use some of these pathways to balance the flow of qi for therapeutic purposes. Through practice, these energetic pathways can be made as tangible and accessible as other circulatory systems in your body, such as the vascular system.

BENEFITS OF SEXUAL QIGONG

Learning the energy dimensions of sex builds on ordinary sex but takes it to the next level. This can help you to:

- Increase the pleasure that both the body and the mind can experience
- Awaken the psychic potential within either or both lovers
- Heal illness and give you more vitality
- Make you physically stronger
- Create a depth of intimate contact and direct communication with your lover that goes far beyond the reach of ordinary sex.

---

1. Dale, Cyndi, *The Subtle Body: An Encyclopedia of Your Energetic Anatomy* (Boulder: Sounds True, 2009), 166.

Over time, men and women who may initially be mediocre or even lousy in bed can use sexual qigong to become excellent lovers. Not only does sexual qigong increase a man's ability to maintain his erection, it affords him skill in directing energy to specific areas in a woman's body. He can make sex last longer and can control his ejaculations, thus helping his lover attain more and/or better orgasms. When a man becomes more energetically sensitive, he can even increase his lover's arousal by not moving at all—dropping into a state of stillness and establishing a holding pattern, while energy moves through her in ripples and waves.

When a woman learns to receive a man's qi and respond to the subtler energy movements in her own body, both her sexual desire and sensitivity will increase. Women can also learn to direct energy to specific areas in a man's body. The difference is that with her orgasm she cannot send yang (male) energy into the man. A woman's orgasm does not energize a man, whereas a man's orgasm energizes a woman. In terms of qi, usually a woman gains and a man loses. However, there are advanced semen retention techniques that involve the man receiving energy from the woman when she has an orgasm. Such practices are outside the scope of this book.

WORKING WITH SUBTLE ENERGY

Sexual qigong also allows you to begin working with subtle energies of emotion. It helps you let go of negative emotions so that positive emotions such as happiness and compassion can flourish. With increased skill, you can shift from being unduly influenced by your feelings—where you identify with whatever is blasting your body and mind in the moment—to actually being able to reduce or increase the intensity of emotions, just like a dimmer switch. Once you learn to work with your energy to balance and harmonize it in your body, by choice you can bring suppressed emotions to the surface to deal with them or you can tone down the emotions that tend to flare up and wreak havoc in your life and relationships. Learning to work with subtle energy is a powerful tool to master.

In addition to helping you become emotionally healthier, sexual qigong has several other benefits. It energizes your mental and creative processes, and combined with the technique of Outer Dissolving (see Chapter 11), sexual qigong can release the energetic blockages that diminish your capacity to experience sexual pleasure. In all of these ways, sexual qigong has dramatic psychological implications and value.

The primary purpose of sexual qigong is to use a systematic and reliable approach to open, balance and strengthen the flow of energy in your body and that of your partner. The complete intricate network of energy points and channels—some four or five thousand of which have been identified—are more extensive than those utilized within acupuncture. Many are deep inside the body.

Sexual qigong is essentially a methodology to supercharge the subtle energy anatomy of human beings above and beyond what is possible in an ordinary sexual encounter. Over time, energy channels with weak functioning are strengthened and can eventually become super-strong. Because one or both sex partners are independently moving their energy, this allows them to work directly with their body's subtle energy channels, activating them to improve functioning.

In the Eastern traditions that harness subtle energies in a sexual context, the price of admission is to develop the ability to feel and work with energy—not something most can do without significant training. This is often achieved by studying energetic practices such as Indian or Taoist yoga, qigong, or the push hands practices of tai chi. These mind-body methods train you to become sensitive to where energy flows smoothly and where it feels stagnant. Sexual qigong, in turn, is the bridge to Taoist sexual meditation, a sophisticated method of channeling your subtle energy for spiritual purposes.

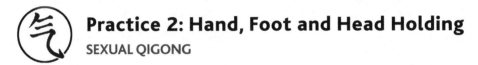 # Practice 2: Hand, Foot and Head Holding
SEXUAL QIGONG

This is a basic sexual qigong partner exercise that uses Outer Dissolving, a practice described in more detail in Chapter 11.

Part 1: Hand Holding

This exercise starts with the hands, because they are easy to feel, and eventually extends to each body part. Hold hands with your partner. One or both hands may be used.

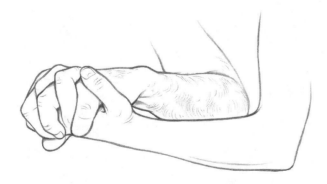

Figure 1-4: Lovers Holding Hands

1. From the wrist and ending at the fingertips, each of you should completely dissolve any blockages in your own hands, releasing any tightness you find there. Outer Dissolving methods should be used initially in sexual qigong and later only for primarily physical issues in the earlier stages of sexual meditation.

2. One common result of the Outer Dissolving process is that you may start feeling your blood pumping more strongly. Try to notice what is happening inside you. Can you feel the sensations of your physical tissues, or the more subtle sensations of your qi, emotions or combinations thereof? Feel for the subtle sensations that are precursors of a full-body emotional experience. Trust yourself. Allow everything to be easygoing and relaxed.

3. After you have dissolved your own hand, dissolve the energy of your partner's hand. Let your mind and whole body relax as much as you can as you energetically sink into (that is, feel and engage what is below the surface of the skin) the other person's hand. Gradually let your mind recognize something deeper than the physical body. See if you can feel the bio-energy of your partner and, afterward, his or her emotions. Take a rest whenever you need to. Make this an adventure rather than a chore.

Now, each of you dissolve your own and your partner's hand simultaneously.

Part 2: Foot Holding

This procedure is described from the point of view of the man holding the woman's foot (thereby activating her yin energy). Certainly the reverse could be described.

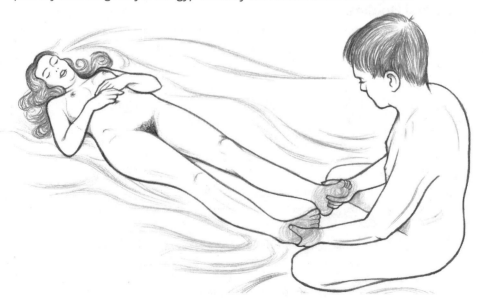

Figure 1-5: Foot Holding and Dissolving

Several hand and foot permutations are possible, but for simplicity, let's focus on only one hand holding one foot.

1. The man and woman each respectively dissolve any or, ideally, all the blockages in their own hands and feet, beginning from their wrists and ankles and finishing at the tips of their fingers or toes.

2. The man then dissolves his hand and the woman's foot as she dissolves her foot and his hand, with both people gaining a sense of mutual hand and foot merging.

After this initial stage is complete, the next level of this practice is for partners to dissolve up the leg and arm. The partners should be capable of dissolving their own hands and feet before they moving on to dissolving the entire arm or leg of the other person. Dissolving up and through a partner is the next more subtle level of the dissolving process. Your consciousness and awareness must now focus through your own body part into another's energy field, requiring a much higher level of sensitivity and energetic training.

Part 3: Head Holding

Next shift the focus to the woman holding the man's head and activating his yang energy. This practice can also be used when either partner has a headache.

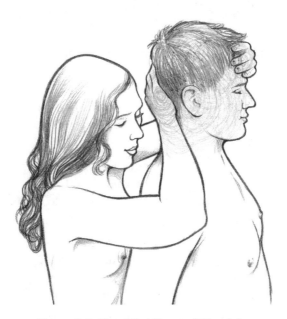

Figure 1-6: Head Holding and Dissolving

1. The woman holds the man's head as shown in Figure 1-6. Moving from the crown of the head to the bottom of the occiput (at the back lower part of the head), the man

dissolves the energy in his head. At the same time, the woman dissolves the energy in her hands.

2. The woman dissolves her hand and the man's head, and the man dissolves his head and the woman's hand, with both people gaining a sense of mutual hand and head merging. ●

THE NATURE OF ENERGY BLOCKAGES

Part of life is to recognize and work through any issues that get in the way of having healthy relationships with our partners, families and even coworkers. With our intimate lovers, any energetic hang-ups inevitably inhibit relaxed lovemaking. Taoists call the subliminal source of these imbalances energy blockages. At the level of sexual qigong, blockages commonly exist on physical, emotional and mental levels. Tense muscles and headaches are examples of a physical blockage. Negative emotions, mood swings and road rage are examples of emotional blockages. Mental churning and over thinking are examples of mental blockages.

Blockages don't exist independently of one another. For example, negative emotions or obsessive thoughts can make your body clench up and cause physical blockages to become more intense, and vice versa. A rigid belly or tight shoulders can cause you to have negative thoughts and emotions.

In mapping the energy pathways, Taoists discovered that qi flows at successively deeper and more subtle vibrational levels in the body, mind and spirit through eight distinct energy bodies (see Chapter 3, "Eight Energy Bodies").

One of the major purposes of qigong is to help you recognize and access blockages in your eight energy bodies and then "dissolve" or let go of them. The result is that your energy flows more cleanly. Your nerves relax and you feel less tense. You become more open and vibrant.

At the level of sexual qigong, Taoists refer specifically to dissolving as "Outer Dissolving," because the blockages are dispersed and released to the outside of your body. The metaphor the Taoists use is "ice to water to gas." When you discover a blockage, it will often feel frozen and tight inside you.

Releasing blockages can revitalize, heal and strengthen your body. This process can also dissipate stress-induced negative emotions caused by one or more of your internal organs being energetically jammed up. For example, anger might be produced by the liver, fear from the kidneys, and anxiety and joylessness from the heart.

Outer Dissolving within sexual qigong is the necessary first step to start working with the eight energy bodies. Then, as you advance, you learn the Taoist sexual meditation method of Inner Dissolving[2] to let go of the deepest energetic blockages.

---

2. For in-depth Inner Dissolving exercises, see Frantzis, Bruce, *Tao of Letting Go* (Berkeley, CA: North Atlantic Books, 2009) and accompanying CD set.

As you release deeper and deeper blockages, you will move toward finding new levels of peace, joy and happiness inside yourself—a place where you have the energy of life and the love that actually moves through it. You can become deeply connected to and nourished by a wellspring of bliss that allows you to be rooted and present with everything. This state of being does not come about because of an external cause but rather through the ongoing inner experience of being fully alive.

As powerful and life-changing as sexual qigong can be, from a Taoist perspective, the extreme pleasure of sexual qigong alone cannot bring someone into the extremely subtle realms of the Tao, Universal Consciousness and enlightenment. Sexual qigong is a bridge to sexual meditation, not the destination. The Taoist experience has been that an overemphasis on energetic sexual techniques can easily disconnect people from their humanity and future spiritual development. As you progress and get more proficient at sexual qigong, the natural progression is to then begin sexual meditation practices, which lead you into extraordinary higher dimensions, profound beyond measure.

AFFECTION, UNATTACHED LOVE AND UNIVERSAL LOVE

The Water tradition of Taoism, which at its core is more yin than many other spiritual groups, maintains that the most important ingredients for loving relationships and great sex are generosity and kindness, as well as the willingness to fully let someone in with complete openness. These ingredients can seed a relationship so it has the potential to grow and develop into genuine, non-attached love.

Non-attachment means love going toward and coming from another person without any expectation, desire of bonding or implication of possession. When this is not the case, although the animal side may be satisfied, the softer and more human part of both partners may be left greatly unfulfilled.

Love typically grows in three stages. In the first stage, in ordinary sex, affection, kindness and the generosity of giving yourself and being willing to energetically accept and let the other into your whole energy system is a necessary prerequisite to great physical sex. Yin gives birth to yang, and yang to yin. For sexuality to reach its full potential in a relationship, a strong yin energy catalyzes the yang energy, which can then provoke and maximize extreme pleasure. Ordinary sexuality with this flavor is an easy place to personally understand this magnetic dynamic. The felt expression of love through the physical body is what enables sex to go as far as it can.

In the second stage, within sexual qigong, you aim to reach a place of unattached love, expressing or receiving loving energy without the demand that it be repaid in any way. This enables you to be as present, sensitive and nurturing as much as possible in each and every moment. Attached love makes this less than so. In the best of worlds, unattached love is reciprocated by your partner, however, this is not necessary. The quality of possessive love that is often found in many ordinary sex relationships prevents the more enriching quality of unattached love from arising. The more that you want to possess love or determine what future it leads to besides that moment in time, you are shutting down your system and creating karma.

Unattached love can be equally present for those who are in long-term committed relationships as for two people who have only met an hour ago, but who express this inner quality. As much as possible, if a couple has this kind of love, they can both give and receive it at the same time. Even though this is a significantly higher vibration of love than just a strong physical connection, this type of love is still one person to one person.

Sexual meditation, the third stage, takes love even further. Kindness, nurturing and generosity of spirit become fused into ordinary emotional and spiritual affection. Non-attached love morphs into a higher level of universal love and compassion, not just for your lover and yourself, but to everything that your mind, heart and spirit can contact. In this way, sexuality becomes a powerful opportunity to catalyze your capacity to lovingly contact another and dissolve any blockage, regardless of where you encounter it. This love extends beyond one person to all and everything in the universe. It is love contacting love without any reason except for love.

SEXUAL MEDITATION

For many, the word "meditation" conjures up a person sitting on a cushion in an upright posture with eyes closed, quietly communing with a higher power. We don't generally associate meditation with making love. Yet the Taoists found combining sex and meditation to be one of the fastest methods to accelerate a practitioner's spiritual advancement. Going beyond physical and energetic techniques into unconditional and unattached love is also what makes sex human.

It's important to make two distinctions here. First, there is a world of difference between what is often called "sacred sex" or "sacred sexuality" with authentic Taoist sexual meditation. Real sexual meditation is not related to the spiritualization of sex that comes with creating a sacred container, building an altar or performing a *puja* (the ceremonial invocation of the god and goddess within that is part of Indian Tantra). All of those practices offer certain benefits, and have their appropriate place in certain traditions. Sexual meditation is of another order altogether.

The other key distinction is when people begin to perceive energy and start moving it, they sometimes get trapped into thinking that they are practicing meditation.

This is not the case. Running energy is just running energy. Through sexual meditation, you build on the foundation of ordinary sex and sexual qigong, then take it to a much higher level of refinement.

ACCELERATED MEDITATION METHODS

The Taoists discovered that through sexual meditation, one can gain access to up to four times the energy that would normally be available within ordinary solo meditation practices to dissolve spiritual blockages (see Chapter 15, "Accessing Four Times the Energy for Meditation"). Turning on and accessing this energy could be likened to going from a steam engine to nuclear power.

With sexual meditation you build on and move beyond Outer Dissolving to use the more advanced method of Inner Dissolving to:

- Consciously enter and merge with your partner's consciousness and have your partner do likewise with yours.
- Consciously dissolve the energetic blockages within all of your own and your partner's eight energy bodies (see Chapter 3) and have your partner simultaneously do likewise.
- Go beyond the limitations of corporeal form or having some kind of condensed physical body rather than a totally non-physical form.

In the Taoist world, sexual meditation is first and foremost a vehicle for spiritual development and practice. The goal is to work toward what is commonly called enlightenment. It is considered a direct and accelerated path that enables lovers to start engaging with spirituality by harnessing sexual energy, a naturally powerful energy readily available to human beings.

Sexual meditation is based on resolving an individual's spiritual blockages into emptiness. While sexual qigong typically activates and frees up the first (physical), second (qi) and to some extent the third (emotional) energy bodies, sexual meditation methods go well beyond this. While making love, these practices enable you to access and activate the third, fourth, fifth, sixth, seventh and eighth energy bodies (emotional, mental, psychic, karmic, essence and body of the Tao).

At these levels, sex refines and increases your ability to release the deepest spiritual blockages that prevent the full flowering and emergence of your soul. Sex becomes a means to open a direct path to uncovering the possibilities of Spirit[3] and releasing your full human potential.

---

3. In this book, the word "Spirit" with an initial capital denotes what is known in Chinese as *shen*, one of the three treasures of Taoism. *Shen* encompasses psychic, karmic and essence energy.

A LIVING SPIRITUAL PATH

Everyone has their own idea of what it means to be on a true spiritual path. Some want to be one with God or the Divine. Others may want to leave their isolated state to be relieved of countless forms of suffering, or they might want to relieve the suffering of all sentient beings. Others just want to live from a place of compassion and love in the world.

Regardless of your interpretation of the meaning of the word "spirituality," an underlying theme runs throughout. "Spirituality" implies feeling that you are engaged in or saturated with something of a subtle nature that is much larger than your personality alone. This could be described as the universal connection, that which connects all and everything, whether you call it God, the Great Spirit, the Divine, Universal Consciousness or the Tao.

Taoist meditation is a living spiritual path that can take you there. It can help you attain states of profound levels of consciousness that exist only in the inner stillness of pure awareness, but not at the level of calculated thought. You can travel into the deepest recesses of your unconscious mind and bodily cells, or out of earth's orbit, where you can move beyond your consciousness out toward the stars, to connect with the energy of the universe.

Through meditation you move beyond the promise of any given mental belief into the land of living experience. Once you have the experience of higher states of consciousness, you can then embody those states at a personal level. Ultimately, the potential reality represented by the belief becomes a concrete, knowable reality, actualized in your daily life.

DISSOLVING ENERGY BLOCKAGES

Once you start to recognize the blocks and conditioning within you, then what? The next step is to start to do something with what you find. It bears repeating that the one constant thread running through all Taoist Water tradition practices is that the burdens of conditioning present in your inner life are recognized as energetic blockages in all of the first seven of your energy bodies. These are resolved through awareness practices and the various dissolving methods—Outer Dissolving for qigong, including sexual qigong, and Inner Dissolving for all meditation, including sexual.

These practices enable you to let go of the spiritual muck and grime inside you and your partner, layer by layer. It can be hard going, as you'll encounter the dark side that is inside every unenlightened soul. Working toward being potentially free of emotional and mental blockages is difficult, but even more so is the full spiritual journey toward enlightenment as you encounter deeper and more significant blockages in the higher energy bodies.

The essential difference between solo qigong and meditation practices to dissolve energy blockages is that using solo practices can often be very hard going, accompanied by considerable internal resistance. For example, denial causes many to avoid or even flee from what's inside them, which defeats the purpose of meditation. Often people think, "As long as it's over there—out of sight, out of mind—I'm safe not dealing with it." The result of this avoidance strategy is that the person becomes stuck on his or her spiritual journey.

Taoist sexual practices done in committed relationships can provide faster antidotes to free you from what binds you externally and internally. The dissolving methods can initially release positive repressed energies, which can give both partners access to considerable pleasure, joy and bliss. This often creates enough counterforce to empower you to become strong enough to deal with your darker sides. The grim stuff and the bliss start to balance out, making it less difficult to engage that which you might reflexively avoid. The candy helps the bitter medicine go down. In Taoist sexual practices there will always be both the light and dark to work with.

THE SUPERIOR MAN OR WOMAN OF THE *I CHING*

The *I Ching—Book of Changes* refers to the superior man or woman, and it also mentions the inferior man or woman. Almost everything that transpires in conventional society is from the reference point of the inferior man or woman. All the craziness of politics and corruption are nothing more than the actions of the inferior man or woman. The majority of people in the world simply don't have access to the subtle dimension of their soul. They remain impoverished of Spirit, even though their insides contain an immense amount of untapped wealth. It's as if they have a million dollars in the bank, but have lost the access code and account number.

If you want to become a superior man or woman, you have to let go of all of your blockages—the obstacles that prevent your conscious mind from recognizing what the rest of you truly is. If you don't recognize who and what you are—if you don't "gain your soul," as Gnostic Christians would say—you are left to fixate, moment by moment and time after time, on whatever piece of you appears to be a big deal.

The distraction, upset or fascination of the moment becomes your whole world. There are trillions and trillions of fixations that your mental and emotional body could make important, but none of this will make you smooth inside. Nothing you gain on the outside leads to freedom from all the nonsense; it just perpetuates your fixations. What drives you crazy and maintains your fixations remains. Freeing your bound energy is what sexual meditation and, in fact, all Taoist meditation is about. You want to release that energy so it can be free to do what it's supposed to do rather than remain stuck and churning inside, causing no end of upset, tension and unresolved expectations.

Taoist meditation, sexual and otherwise, leads you on the path of becoming the superior man or woman of the *I Ching*. It allows you to become extraordinary, to go beyond what Buddhists refer to as "obstacles," Indian yogis call "sanskaras" and the Taoists call "blockages." These are the blocked impressions, the energies within you that prevent your conscious mind from recognizing what you truly are.

Highly refined practice methods enable you to arrive at a state of freedom. In Christian terms, the aim is to literally know God's mind. In Taoist meditation, it's to gain your Being,[4] to be inside the mind of the universe. To attain this ultimate realization is the reason that the wide spectrum of spiritual practices using qi work originally came into existence within Taoism.

Once you have become familiar with the reality of your mind and Spirit by traveling inside yourself and gaining your soul, sooner or later the time will come when you realize you are at the next stage. This requires that each individual engage with the world, explore how the world and the soul are connected and how each can fulfill or block each other. This is the mutually reinforcing circle of life that carries us through many stages of spiritual evolution.

---

4. The word "being" means a person or sentient entity whether corporeal or noncorporeal. In this book, a "Being" with an initial capital refers to the essence or soul of a being.

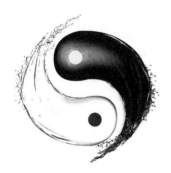

CHAPTER 2

Laozi's Tradition of Taoism

Although Taoism is one of the great religions of the world, it is not widely understood by Westerners. Many have been introduced to Taoism through three ancient literary works—the *Tao Te Ching* (also transliterated as *Dao De Jing*) by Laozi (also spelled as Lao Tse or Lao Tzu), the *I Ching* and the *Book of Zhuangzi* (also known as Chuang Tse or Chuang Tzu), which have been translated and analyzed by scholars and studied in academic circles.

Unfortunately, many scholars miss the point that Taoism is a living religion, actively practiced by many millions of people in China, rather than just a literary philosophy. A popularization and coadaptation of concepts from Taoism has occurred in the West that would create disharmony and outrage if done with other religious traditions. Taoism is a living spiritual tradition or religion in the same manner as Buddhism, Christianity, Hinduism, Islam and Judaism.

At its core, the essence of Taoism is about pragmatic practices that make it possible to live well in the world. It is very much about how to make something work rather than how to think about a subject or analyze it. What are the steps to becoming vibrantly healthy? How do you best work out emotional issues that have plagued you since childhood? How do you become a better and more sensitive lover? How do you train to become a more effective fighter? What is the best way to deal with fear or change? How do you access your past lives and work through your karma?

The ancient Taoist perspective is based entirely on the practical application of methods that integrate body, mind and spirit. Taoists approached these issues as a science. Nothing within Taoism is taken on belief alone. One learns through direct experience. The arts that they developed are among the most effective and sophisticated in the world, honed over millennia and tested by many hundreds of millions of people.

The religious canon of Taoism is known as the *Tao Tsang* and has over 1,600 volumes. It is both deep and extensive beyond being purely intellectual, including topics such as:

- Medical arts: acupuncture, qigong, sexual qigong, qigong tui na, herbs
- Fighting arts: tai chi chuan, bagua, hsing-i
- Sexual arts: ordinary sex, sexual qigong, sexual meditation
- Spiritual arts: solo Taoist meditation, sexual meditation
- Spiritual martial arts: transcending violence, aggression, fear and many other negative characteristics of the material world

All religions have spiritual beliefs, but most do not include medical, martial and sexual arts in their religious canon. Taoism is unusual in that it does. Nor do many religions aside from Taoism have a living sexual meditation tradition that guides you step-by-step on the path of spiritual awakening.

The principles and some core practices of these pragmatic arts are embedded in ancient religious texts. These techniques nourish the deepest needs of the human intellect, heart and soul. All Taoist practices are based on the principles of how energy works and flows through everything. At the end of the day, Taoism is about recognizing the qi of the entire universe, with nothing excluded.

> *At the end of the day, Taoism is about recognizing the qi of the entire universe, with nothing excluded.*

TAOISM AND RELIGION

Taoism as a living spiritual force is not yet very well known in the West. In the West, the term "religion" is often used solely to mean a spiritual, philosophical and moral system that bases its authority and beliefs on a higher power or "God."

Although fully respectful of this position, neither Buddhism nor Taoism affirm or deny the existence of God. They neither base their authority on this kind of higher power, nor do they think that a moral and spiritual framework suitable for human beings requires it.

WATER AND FIRE TRADITIONS: TWO BRANCHES OF TAOISM

Within Taoism there are two major branches, the Water and the Fire traditions, just as Buddhism has different schools and as Christianity has various denominations. Both Water and Fire Taoist branches have practices that teach you how to feel, master and control qi, but how they go about it is radically different. This book explains Taoist sexual meditation from the perspective and approach of the Water tradition, which is much less well-known than the Fire tradition in the West.

More than 2,500 years old, the Water tradition descends directly from Laozi and Zhuangzi. The Fire tradition emerged 1,500 years later and was influenced by Buddhist thought, yoga and Buddist Tantra. In academic literature, the Fire tradition is often referred to as neo-Taoism.

In many Eastern meditation traditions such as Taoism, practitioners are not just asked to believe; they are given practices to actualize their beliefs. Coming to know the Divine is not purely a matter of faith, but rather faith combined with highly refined methodologies practiced consistently over time. It is similar to musicians who might "believe" they can play an instrument brilliantly, but who must practice, practice, practice if they want to perform at Carnegie Hall. The serious student of meditation accepts that discipline is par for the course.

Taoism gives you the direct means and practices to resolve the deepest physical, emotional, mental and karmic issues inside you. Often these are the very issues that make people abandon serious commitment to their spiritual journey.

> *Taoism gives you the direct means to resolve the deepest physical, emotional, mental and karmic issues inside you.*

Why Buddhism Is Mentioned in a Book about Taoism

This book is about Eastern spirituality rather than the religious traditions of the West. Both Buddhism and Taoism are primary Eastern religions, comprising spiritual and philosophical systems. Before becoming a Taoist master, my main Taoist teacher, Liu Hung Chieh, was also declared enlightened by the head of the Tian Tai Buddhist sect.

Historically Taoism and Buddhism were separate traditions in China, however, in the popular Chinese mind they are often combined as one. Buddhism and Taoism share many important philosophical tenets and, although they explain them using different language, the meaning is more or less the same. Since Buddhist practices are fairly well known in the West while those of Taoism are not, explaining the similar positions may make it easier for readers to understand some of the finer points of this book.

WHY TAOISM IS LESS WELL KNOWN
THAN BUDDHISM AND HINDUISM

In the West, there has always been more access to India's spiritual knowledge than that of China. Since India was a former British colony, it is common for the leading spiritual lights of Hinduism and Buddhism to speak or write in English, or at least to have good translators. Moreover, many Buddhist and Hindu teachers have been willing to come to the West to spread their knowledge.

The Chinese have always been somewhat insular. Even today, they exert little or no effort to share their cultural or spiritual knowledge with outsiders, and their language forms a largely impenetrable barrier to learning.

CONTRASTING THE TAOIST FIRE AND WATER SEXUAL PRACTICES

Within both the Fire and Water traditions there is an incredible variety of sexual knowledge and practical methods regarding ordinary and energetic sex, far beyond what might normally be found in sex manuals. Although both traditions come from the same source—Taoism—the approach they take often is quite different.

Similarities

Both the Fire and Water traditions of Taoism include techniques to do the following, albeit often in quite different ways:

- Release and resolve blockages that prevent the soul or consciousness from evolving to full spiritual potential.
- Move qi through the human energetic anatomy, including channels, energy centers and points. However, different schools and masters may have greater or lesser knowledge as to the number of channels, points and so on that they know how to skillfully utilize.
- Use the qi and the functions of the five elements and three *tantiens*—lower, middle and upper (for the locations of these energy centers see Chapter 3, Figure 3-4).
- Work with internal alchemy,[1] although both traditions define the term differently.
- Ensure that men are not damaged by physical ejaculation.
- Enable nonorgasmic women to become orgasmic and orgasmic women to become more so.
- Work with generating and using internal orgasms.

---

1. For more about internal alchemy, see Frantzis, Bruce, *The Great Stillness* (Berkeley, CA: North Atlantic Books, 2001), 189–208.

Differences

Water and Fire methods diverge in many areas. As previously stated, this book's emphasis is on sharing the Water methods, as they have rarely been publicly available in the West or even in China.

Fire Practices

In the early stages of Fire methods, visualization, combined with intent, is commonly used to activate, open up and move energy through the body's energetic anatomy and qi channels. One is instructed on how to direct qi to where one wishes to use it for various specific purposes.

To resolve internal blockages, the Fire method initially uses practices centered on the transformation of energy within a person. More advanced Fire practices work with the ball of light, commonly called *nei dan* in Chinese and "inner cosmic egg" in English.

The Fire school primarily advocates ejaculation control to prevent semen from being emitted. This is done to protect men from perceived damage that can occur from too many ejaculations.

Water Practices

The heart of Laozi's Water tradition primarily uses Inner and Outer Dissolving, explained in later chapters. These two dissolving meditation methods are *not* part of the Fire tradition.

Outer Dissolving activates and opens the body's energetic anatomy and qi pathways. The Outer Dissolving practice of sexual qigong is used to mitigate or heal illness as well as to release the body's energetic resistance to having more pleasure. It can also be used to bring out greater physical abilities, for example to help an athlete perform better in competition or to give a mountain climber more stamina.

The Inner Dissolving of sexual meditation is used to release and resolve one or, ideally, both sexual partners' deeper energetic blockages at the higher energy bodies so that they can evolve spiritually all the way to enlightenment.

There are three progressive stages of dissolving practices:

1. The preliminary stage initially involves qigong and sexual qigong techniques based on Outer Dissolving.

2. The second stage, based on Inner Dissolving, is used in solo and sexual meditation.

3. The third stage fuses Inner and Outer Dissolving by taking dissolving to its

higher potential in order to transcend the limitations of being corporeal (that is, having a physical body).

Another difference in Water and Fire schools is their position on men's ejaculation. Although Water schools share some parallels with the Fire tradition regarding methods to control ejaculation, they also take into consideration normal family or singles lifestyles. In Fire schools, non-ejaculation is considered very important and essential for a man. In contrast, Water schools have developed an alternative solution to the issue of ejaculation draining male energy to ill effect. Rather than solely seeking to control semen emission, they also advocate total relaxation ejaculations (see Chapter 8).

Why I Teach the Water Tradition

I am often asked why I prefer the Water tradition over the Fire tradition. My reason is fairly straightforward: I field-tested both and found the Water method took me to a dramatically deeper level.

In my experience, the Fire tradition can create a false ceiling that limits what an individual—a Westerner, especially—can experience and move through in the course of his or her spiritual development. These same barriers can be transcended by practices that are fundamental to the Water tradition. The Western mind tends to have an extreme Fire mentality. We are in a phase in our cultural development that burns through everything using undue force and strain. Given the increasing and observable stress we experience in a technological society, we are already driven by the often stress-creating Fire energy in more ways than we can process.

The Fire tradition emphasizes force and pushing forward. Fire pushes and easily creates stress. It cannot help but exert control. Fire wants to make something happen—now! It excites the nervous system, pushing you to give one hundred percent and more. Practitioners in this tradition at times forcefully hold their breath, and push past physical mental and psychic discomfort to complete a practice. They believe pushing forward is necessary to get results.

These traits are readily understood in our Western culture. Whatever effort you put in is never enough. You are driven to do more, have more, be more and consume more. People are fired up and passionate about their work or cause.

In modern society, however, the overdevelopment of Fire characteristics has led to tension, anxiety and stress, the diseases of our age. The minute you try to be in control, you begin to live in a continuous state of tension. Many people are workaholics as a result of becoming addicted to the adrenaline produced by stress and the need to control. This leads to a cascade of negative effects that over time downgrades the nervous system, potentially causing chronic health problems.

Conversely, Water allows. The Water approach knows about prudent reserves. When Water dominates your system, you only do things at seventy or eighty percent of your capacity. You relax your nervous system. You don't push. This eliminates the backwash of stress, along with the harm it does to your body, both immediately and down the line. It eliminates the "two steps forward, one step back" tendency that slows down progress. For these reasons the sexual qigong and sexual meditation practices in this book emphasize the Taoist Water method.

Most of my knowledge in both the Taoist Fire and Water sexual practices is derived from direct instruction by living masters of both lineages through verbal discussion and practicum in the bedroom. I first learned the sexual meditation Fire tradition during my Taoist priest training in Taiwan and Hong Kong, then later the Water tradition in Beijing through my primary teacher, Taoist Lineage Master Liu Hung Chieh. Through him, I received all the relevant technical information and transmissions regarding sexual meditation in both the Water and Fire traditions. I also received the practicum bedroom knowledge of the Water tradition from Liu's female associates, who were different masters in the lineage.

EIGHT PRINCIPLES OF LAOZI'S WATER TRADITION

The following eight principles are fundamental to Taoist sexual qigong and meditation; they lie at the core of Laozi's Water tradition. A complete treatise on these and other important relevant principles would take a whole volume, not just a chapter, but you will find all of these principles flow through the knowledge and practices presented in this book.

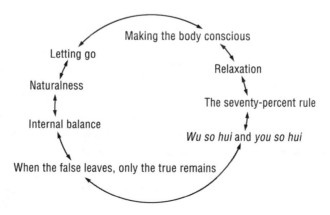

1. NATURALNESS

The Chinese word *zi ran* has many meanings, but most commonly refers to nature or naturalness. Da zi ran, or great nature, is another expression for " Tao." Rather than let sex be natural, it is tempting to frame it as something that is either sacred or profane. To Taoists, sex may be either, neither or both. In fact, from the viewpoint of spiritual evolution, neither an abundance of sexual need and desire nor a complete lack of it is relevant. Sex is a natural part of human nature.

In the chapters that follow, sexuality is discussed in energetic terms, always moving in the direction of harnessing it as a vehicle for pure spirituality. Spirituality, in this sense, goes beyond rigid belief or rejection of belief and instead seeks to release, resolve and transcend the blocked and limited forces in an individual. Taoism asserts neither that there is nor that there is not an absolute and proper way of doing anything.

Natural Breath

When ordinary sex continues over a long time and two people begin to bond, something special begins to emerge during sex that Taoists refer to as natural breath. Natural breath enables energy channels to open naturally and easily, without conscious attempt. This happens spontaneously when the connection between two people has developed sufficiently.

As couples grow more and more in synch with each other, they can calibrate to this natural breath with a light kiss, by holding hands, or simply being in each other's presence. Primal and instinctive, natural breath is one of the principal bonding mechanisms that keeps a couple together for thirty, forty or fifty years and more. Through all of life's trials and tribulations, through periods where sex is exciting, frustrating or altogether absent, the natural breath is a consistent bonding agent.

Natural breath does not necessarily mean that the lovers have synchronized breathing, just that there is a subtle connection on various levels. Nothing is more soothing when you are in a ragged, unsettling mood than climbing into your partner's arms. At the physical level, this is due, in part, to the calming effect of natural breath. This is a gift that people can bring to one another: a rock-solid sense of stability. The more natural breath is activated, the more the energy channels remember the smooth, connected feeling. When this happens it is easier to remember and maintain this connection. Sexual qigong allows natural breath to be turned on more quickly between couples than does ordinary sex.

Naturalness is the goal. With regard to sexuality, this means being natural, comfortable and at ease in all phases of sexuality. Let the flow be natural from the initial meeting of a lover to foreplay and all the way to orgasm. In this spirit, neither attempt nor engage in games to manipulate the other. Leave aside any cookbook approaches. Instead, focus on what arises naturally from the energy that spontaneously is present between friends and lovers.

2. INTERNAL BALANCE

The cornerstone of Taoist sexuality is the ability to attain internal balance—something often desperately sought in today's frenetic world. Internal balance is an essential factor to living a satisfying life. Sex should make a couple feel smooth inside, both in the midst of sexual play and more importantly for a lingering period afterward. Developing internal balance is the key for being able to have longer and more stable relationships. When sex does not create internal balance, the erratic, jangled afterglow diminishes the possibility of both partners wanting to stay bonded either as platonic friends or lovers.

3. RELAXATION

The entire Water tradition emphasizes relaxation at all levels of human experience. Beyond relaxing your muscles and nerves, its methods help you relax into the deepest substructures of your anatomy. Energetically, Laozi's Water tradition systematically teaches you to relax the energy that allows your physical body, emotions, thoughts and hidden psychic capacities to smoothly function. Relaxing your Being or soul is also exceptionally important in the Water tradition. Spiritual relaxation initially results from letting go of both your own and your partner's energetic blockages in all seven energy bodies, something that is infinitely easier if both lovers do the practices together.

In each moment, the Outer and Inner Dissolving practices enable you and your partner to energetically let go so that both become more natural and relaxed. The more relaxed you are on every level, from the physical to the psychic, the better the sex you can have. Integrate relaxation in all stages of sex. Relax ever more deeply as foreplay continues. Let the ever-increasing relaxation of sexual, emotional or mental foreplay lead you gradually into intercourse. During and after orgasm, continue to melt into even greater states of relaxation.

4. MAKING YOUR BODY CONSCIOUS

The Taoist tradition is one of the few that truly brings people fully into their body. Relaxation is prerequisite to make a body fully conscious. Full consciousness is not possible when the body is tense. Practices like Taoist breathing, qigong and tai chi are meant to strengthen the human nervous system and prepare the body for higher spiritual work. Taoist practices teach you how to focus your full attention inside your body until it wakes up and feels alive, not as an imagined visualization, but as a felt reality.

In *Slow Sex*,[2] Nicole Daedone advocates that "we learn to shift our focus from thinking to feeling, from a goal orientation to an experience orientation" and replace the idea of a fast and hard approach to sex with being slower and more connected. To make your body conscious you have to drop your mental energy lower into your body. Only then can you fully connect with your body and heart.

The Taoist methods that develop internal feeling, derived from the Water tradition of Laozi, concentrate on allowing, following and working with the energies that already exist in your body in each instant of time. The practices teach you to think less and feel more. To feel good, it is necessary to activate your feeling part first. When you feel an exciting physical or emotional sensation, peel away the many layers. Savor the moment, linger, feel deeper and consciously experience all that you can with each step of the sexual journey. By taking the time for your awareness to penetrate your own body and receive the sensations from your partner, feeling good can take on meanings you have never even imagined.

5. SEVENTY PERCENT: DO NEITHER TOO MUCH NOR TOO LITTLE

All Taoist qi practices from the original Water tradition of Laozi incorporate the principle of moderation, which can be described as the "seventy-percent rule." Lacking the seventy-percent rule you can never fully relax.

The rule states that you should only do a practice or technique to seventy percent of your capacity. Striving for one hundred percent produces excess tension and stress that causes the body to tense up or shut down, without you necessarily being consciously aware that this is happening. You can apply the seventy-percent rule to all your practices, comfortably using your full effort without strain.

In his classic book, *Introduction to Tantra*,[3] Lama Yeshe emphasizes the importance of moderation and abandoning unreasonable expectations, "Realize that expectations are a hindrance and let go of them as soon as they arise." He adds, "Sometimes we put too much energy into our practice...thinking that this will bring us more quickly to our realizations. But too much effort often has the opposite effect; it prevents our progress instead of helping it."

---

2. Daedone, Nicole, *Slow Sex: The Art and Craft of the Female Orgasm* (New York: Grand Central Life and Style, 2011), 12.

3. Lama Yeshe, *Introduction to Tantra: A Vision of Totality* (Boston: Wisdom Publications, 1987), 136.

In this modern era, people are led to believe that by straining, they will progress faster and further. Most people do not want moderation; they want excess. However, if you always push your energy to one hundred percent, you will never allow your nerves, muscles and mind to relax, which is necessary for you to be able to progress efficiently, without producing unnecessary stress or burnout. The seventy-percent rule and relaxation are inexorably linked.

This is especially true when sexual practices are involved, because they create a high energetic output that can result in a large amount of internal resistance within one or both partners. Moreover, one of the partners may be sexually less responsive, a sign of internal weakness at some energetic level.

The seventy-percent limit can differ widely from one person to another. For this reason both partners need to be very aware of where the thresholds and boundaries are in themselves and their partners, so that the stronger partner never pushes beyond seventy percent of the limits of the weaker partner. For best effect, gear the seventy percent limit to the sexually less-responsive partner or the partner who gets overexcited significantly more rapidly. When your partner is in pain or injured, whether physically or emotionally, he or she should not be pushed to more than fifty percent of his or her capacity.

At any stage of foreplay or intercourse, the human capacity to experience extreme sensation has a limit, call it one hundred percent. When this limit is reached or exceeded then it reverses. In the middle of the sexual act when this happens, one or both partners may begin to lose sensation, become overloaded, go numb, begin to drift or turn off, without necessarily knowing why. When you reach seventy percent on the way toward the hundred-percent limit, regardless of the potential to lead into the sheer pleasure of orgasm, retreat from what you are doing, shift your sexual attention, or just take a rest and hug until your nervous systems recover. Then begin again. This takes time to learn because most people in the West lack sensitivity to know when they are at seventy-percent and have been trained since childhood to always push their limits.

After both partners have trained sufficiently and are smooth, natural and relaxed at the seventy-percent level, they can then adjust to use an eighty-percent boundary.

6. LETTING GO

There are two primary ways of implementing any philosophy, energetic or spiritual, to influence the forces of nature within you—either through exerting control or by letting go. A metaphor for this is the way that a great statue can emerge from a huge piece of marble. In *the way of control,* the artist creates a vision of what he wants it to look like in the end. The artist draws up clear plans with all desired specifications according to his vision. Next the plans are precisely executed; each detail is controlled perfectly; and from this you get a statue. This is the way of Fire and control.

The Water tradition takes a different approach, *the way of letting go*. The artist places the big piece of marble in the studio, looks at it and observes it while letting go of any idea of what the rock should become. The artist waits and merges his or her energy field with the rock's energy field. The rock then tells the artist what has to be let go of and chiseled away. The statue thus emerges from the nature of the combined energy of the rock and the artist. The artist becomes the agent through which the flow of manifestation moves.

In the end, the artist is delighted and surprised at the content of the art that emerges. The outcome required that the artist get out of the way and let go of any need to control the process. He or she just had to choose to be a part of it.

As Sogyal Rinpoche so eloquently explains in *The Tibetan Book of Living and Dying,*[4] "Although we have been made to believe that if we let go we will end up with nothing, life itself reveals again and again the opposite: that letting go is the path to real freedom."

The Inner and Outer Dissolving meditation methods are the primary methods by which letting go is accomplished within the Taoist Water tradition. You recognize what is tense or dysfunctional inside and then let it go.

7. *WU SO HUI* AND *YOU SO HUI*

Two commonly used Chinese phrases central to the Taoist approach to morality are *wu so hui* and *you so hui*. These two phrases lie at the core of how Taoists decide to implement any moral or philosophical principle in life.

Wu so hui means "the small stuff"; "it's neither here nor there"; "it's okay if you do or don't." Often these are the thousands of small decisions a person makes each day. *You so hui* considers what is critically important, essential to living. This is the big stuff that really matters.

Taoists generally view most of the choices we make about life's daily events as *wu so hui*. If you use "no harm, no foul" as a general principle, your choices probably won't carry a lot of moral implications. On the level of ordinary sex between consenting adults, the choices generally can be called *wu so hui*. Likewise, if you have three or four things you feel, want or need to practice and there is no compelling reason to especially focus on one or the other, it's probably *wu so hui*, really not so important.

---

4. Sogyal Rinpoche, *The Tibetan Book of Living and Dying* (New York: HarperSanFrancisco, 1994), 35.

From the Taoist spiritual perspective generally, that which positively or negatively affects the events of your life on this earth, but will not create karma nor follow and potentially control you in future lives, is spiritually *wu so hui*. This is important to address with care, but not critical.

Often what causes stress in many people's lives is that their mind becomes filled with things that don't matter much creating discord and disharmony. It is wise to look at all you hold in your mind to sort between what matters and what does not. Then you can consciously direct your attention to the things that matter and that you can influence.

When something is deeply gnawing your guts, has repetitively gotten in the way of health, emotional or sexual relationships, it's *you so hui*. If it can damage you and negatively condition your spirit not only in this life but potentially afterward, then it's *you so hui*. Likewise, compassion is generally *you so hui*, but how it's implemented and taken on the road is generally *wu so hui* and to be determined by the confluence of real time variables surrounding the point, the object of the compassion.

Whatever your culture or religion, looking at your choices in life from the perspective of these two phrases is an interesting and practical method for consciously examining them, particularly in terms of sexuality. It's another tool for accessing your awareness.

8. WHEN THE FALSE LEAVES, ONLY THE TRUE REMAINS

As you make your body more conscious, you become more able to see what is inside. This brings us to the principle of "When the False Leaves, Only the True Remains." Once you start to see what is inside you and apply dissolving meditation practices, then, as your blockages resolve, you will be left only with what is true.

Dissolving blockages will enable you to let go of layer after layer of falsehoods. These layers are what Taoists call "red dust" and what Buddhists call "samsara" or "clouds that obscure the sky." Without these false layers, it becomes much easier to see what is true in all times and places. By ridding yourself of all that is false, you will arrive at your true nature and the Tao. Likewise, if you arrive at your nature there can be nothing that is false.

These eight principles have no hierarchy. All Taoist practices and principles each flow into the other. Like life itself, each principle or qi practice in Taoism should seamlessly flow into and integrate with the others.

LAOZI'S MEDITATION TRADITION

There are many different methods of meditation. The Taoist meditation path from the Water tradition of Laozi is one of feeling, using energy, letting go and openness. Many have read the words of this tradition in books like the *Tao Te Ching,* the *Book of Zhuangzi* and the *I Ching*. Although the words ring true, the practical meditation methods behind the words in these books may seem vague and hidden. However, the author's training as a Taoist priest and with Lineage Master Liu enabled him to understand the living meditation tradition described in those texts.

FOUR PRACTICE AREAS IN TAOIST MEDITATION

Laozi's Water method of meditation includes four key areas of focus.

1. Making Your Body Conscious

The first emphasis is to become conscious in your body and the energies inside you and, most importantly, to become present to the awareness of awareness itself which can enable you to recognize the subtleties of your deeper levels of energy. Most people are unaware of the deeper levels within, but these energies are always simultaneously very alive and active inside you, whether you recognize them or not. Taoist breathing, qigong and tai chi are meant to bring your consciousness fully into your body so you can then work with what you discover inside yourself during meditation. These practices also naturally make your body healthy and strong so you develop the stamina required to practice Taoist meditation.

2. Understanding Your Conditioning and Morality

The second area of practice is to understand your conditioning and morality. Without understanding morality, virtually everyone will be controlled by his or her karma. Taoism holds that every meditator needs to delve inside and personally discover the roots of the morality he or she is willing to live life by. You do this by looking at aspects of any conceivable kind of moral and ethical issue that could happen to you or to anyone else, in terms of how to pursue a course of action, the potential ways the issue can affect your deepest unconscious mechanisms, how it will color the experience of all that transpires in life and how it might affect others.

Most importantly, truly understanding morality and ethics means you can observe how all the little moral pieces join and interconnect—including you, others and various situations taking into account both content and context. In Taoist meditation, developing your own authentic moral and ethical bedrock can spring only from heightened awareness.

Central to all this is the guiding principle that there are no absolutes, because what seems simple on the surface may or may not be extremely complex underneath. Thus, what may initially seem to be kind or cruel may, when seen from a larger, free and uncontracted space, be quite different.

To truly engage with this significant task of investigating morality requires developing a larger amount of awareness and clarity. To do this and embody enough of both, the meditator first ponders and looks at a wide variety of moral issues from multiple levels. Then you sit, meditate and release some or all of your personal conflicts and conditioning that prevent you from recognizing and releasing your internal numbness. The goal is that in the end you can be truly morally present in whatever situation life gives you.

3. Recognizing and Resolving Your Blockages

The third emphasis of practice is to recognize where you are currently stuck or blocked, then let go of those blockages and become free. You let what is closed, paralyzed and contracted become internally open and spacious. This is the road of emptiness, resolving your own personal blockages at every level of your being and in all your energy bodies. This task is accomplished in Laozi's branch of Taoism by using the Outer and Inner Dissolving methods described in Chapters 11 and 15.

4. Finding the Unchanging Still Point

Lastly, the meditator's aim is to find the vibrant, still point beyond time and change. You engage with it on all levels, both in quiet meditation and during all the active roles played in life in all its infinite variations. You do this until you find your true essence—the energy body of individuality that is beyond your personality, personal history and all intellectual knowledge.

When you reach this stage, the work of Taoist inner alchemy begins. Internal alchemy seeks through advanced meditation and certain mind-body-spirit practices to:

- Work with the consciousness of an individual in order to become aware of the cellular vibratory energetic level of the body to heal every form of disease.
- Raise, bring out, and change normally hidden qualities and capacities of the body-mind.
- Elevate ordinary consciousness to higher and more refined levels of super-consciousness until the mind expands to encompass the whole of the universe.

Through Taoist inner alchemy, you take your essence and continuously transform its vibratory essence as you experience many, if not most, of the ways essence can manifest in the universe. When you have enough experience you realize the Tao and become what is referred to in Taoism as a Spiritual Immortal. This is the culmination of all Taoist meditation practices.

Taoist and Tantric Sexual Traditions

The use of the word "Tantra" in today's Western culture can be loaded with misconceptions, vague definitions and promises of ecstatic sex. Phrases such as "loving deeply," "sacred sexuality" or "sexual bliss" are used but often have little connection to the very old, esoteric Hindu and Buddhist traditions that Tantra derived from. In many cases, few of the spiritual goals of Tantra have been retained. This does not necessarily mean that the pure spiritual tradition no longer exists, only that teachers who know the complete tradition are difficult to find.

In the West, the Tantric emphasis in popular culture is often to enhance skills related to sexual pleasure, things that the Taoist tradition addresses mostly within ordinary sex and sometimes through sexual qigong. If having an enriching, orgasmically good time with sex is the goal, however, the Taoist viewpoint is that there is no need to gloss it with any kind of spiritual overlay. Nor does anyone need spiritual permission to do what Taoists consider natural sexual urges. The old traditions never promoted sexual entertainment games primarily to create fun and interesting experiences.

Many people teaching "Tantra," or "Neo-Tantra," freely combine techniques from India's Tantra and yoga, Taoist Fire traditions, Cherokee or other Native American traditions, and/or anything else that is deemed sexually useful or that creates a happy, sexual experience. For example, to raise a group's sexual energy, some modern Tantra practices may have people sitting in a circle holding hands and breathing in specific ways while someone in the middle masturbates. It's no wonder that some people are confused about Tantra and what, if anything, the word has to do with the serious spiritual traditions from which it originated.

The three Eastern religious traditions of Taoism, Hinduism and Buddhism made in-depth studies of the potential of sexuality as a spiritual vehicle to shorten the time needed to attain authentic enlightenment. All three of these old spiritual traditions recognized that sexual pleasure can be used within spiritual practice, although pleasure by itself was not the main spiritual point and it was a relatively small part of the overall practice. They did agree about the value of deriving maximum sexual satisfaction, bliss, and psychological well-being from better lovemaking, but the totality of the paths they walked was quite different. For example, in the Hindu, Buddhist and Taoist traditions, daily nonsexual, sitting meditation or yoga-like practices comprise the bulk of the practices. Sex was icing on the cake. Within Taoism, sexual meditation was considered only one of five basic modalities of following a spiritual path toward enlightenment.

EXPERIENTIAL KNOWLEDGE: THE CORNERSTONE OF LEARNING

It is important to understand how the Taoists came upon their knowledge, because it is different from the method used by science. Scientists value objectivity and empirical knowledge that can be obtained and validated through observation, measurement and experiment. The scientific method relies on establishing protocols and replicable methodologies, such as double-blind studies, to establish objective credibility for their results. Certainly such methods are important in fields such as medicine, environmental sciences and chemistry.

In the scientific paradigm, experiential or subjective knowledge is orphaned as "anecdotal," sidelined as "unscientific" or dismissed entirely as "spurious."

Genuine inner meditation experiences cannot always be replicated on demand, measured and calculated, or controlled in experimental subgroups as currently we still lack sufficiently sensitive and capable instruments. Scientific methods severely limit the utterly subjective reality of subtle energetic anatomy and invalidate knowledge obtained from directly inside the human psyche. Subjective reality constitutes the core of Taoist and some other inner traditions.

In the literature of all these meditation traditions, we can find similar testimonials to central "mystical" experiences that can create profound inner and outer change. For example, Taoist meditators created the health science of acupuncture by delving into their inner world, locating the specific energy channels and hundreds of points that influence health and well-being, and then objectifying and codifying their findings. This enabled acupuncturists to have predictable, verifiable results.

Discoveries such as these are made possible because every human contains a microcosm of the whole universe within himself or herself. The premise and subjective experience of nearly every mystical tradition is this: if a human mind can penetrate its own consciousness to a sufficient degree, nature will reveal its secrets, both in terms of objective reality and in the natural transactions between matter, energy and spirit.

How do we "know" that something is real in our inner world? How do we discern subtle realities from wishful thinking, self-delusion or hallucination? Validation and confirmation come about when multiple people have the same subjective experience. We genuinely "know" when what is experienced causes a shift or change at some fundamental—and yes, observable—level of our Being.

Taoist meditation is not mere mental contemplation. By entering stillness, insights or capacities are unleashed spontaneously, springing from somewhere other than logic or analytical thought.

Ancient Taoists were able to comprehend complex bodily functions intuitively through direct experiential contact with the subtle internal levels of the body and brain. Their knowledge, obtained by inner awareness, has led to the vast compendium of Taoist practices and written texts. When you decide to follow the Taoist path, then you do practices so that you have direct experience. This is how true soul transformation occurs.

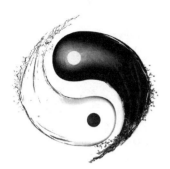

CHAPTER 3

Taoist Energy Anatomy

The Taoists are considered the scientists of the ancient world. *Science and Civilisation in China,* a seven-volume series begun in 1954, edited by British biochemist and sinologist Joseph Needham, gives numerous examples of ancient Taoist contributions to all manner of sciences, including medicine, mathematics, physics, engineering and military technology.[1] Taoists also did in-depth research into what was true in all times, places and energy bodies. They discovered a subtle world governed by qi and then applied this knowledge to how energy flows in healing, martial arts, medicine and spiritual evolution.

In *The Tao of Physics,* Fritjof Capra[2] describes how parallels to modern quantum physics appear in the *I Ching,* and states, "The careful observation of nature, combined with a strong mystical intuition, led the Taoist sages to profound insights which are confirmed by modern scientific theories."

This chapter explores some of the primary energy maps the Taoists created as guides for the human energetic system. These maps and diagrams provide the foundation for learning Taoist sexual qigong and sexual meditation. Many of the ordinary sex, sexual qigong and sexual meditation practices in this book draw on these energetic maps and diagrams.

EIGHT ENERGY BODIES

In the process of mapping qi pathways, Taoists made a remarkable discovery—that human beings encompass eight energy bodies. The eight energy bodies are the entire energetic structural framework within which all of us live. For most people, the awareness of these bodies is completely unconscious. All of the eight energy

1. Needham, Joseph, ed., *Science and Civilisation in China* (Cambridge: Cambridge University Press, 1954, 2008), 7 volumes comprising 27 books to date.

2. Capra, Fritjof, *The Tao of Physics* (Boston: Shambhala, 1999), 114.

bodies are contained within each energy channel of the body. However it easier to initially access some energy bodies in specific energy channels than in others. Through Taoist practices, this energy matrix can be made quite conscious.

Taoists made a remarkable discovery—that human beings encompass eight energy bodies. Through Taoist practices, this energy matrix can be made quite conscious.

According to the Taoists, the eight energy bodies form not only the underlying energetic matrix of all humans but also that of all beings in all universes. This matrix determines how consciously or unconsciously all reincarnated beings undergo their existence, and, depending on the beings' level of awareness, how consciously or unconsciously they function.

How these eight energy bodies experientially manifest in a person depends on the environmental specifics of that human being's incarnation. Laozi's Water tradition is based on the process of dissolving blocked energy within the first seven energy bodies in a clear, tiered system—the physical body, qi or etheric body, emotional body, mental body, psychic body, causal or karmic body and body of individuality or essence—before reaching the eighth body of Tao.

Both sexual qigong and sexual meditation are systems for clearing any blockages in the eight energy bodies and for overcoming the limitations of them in terms of how humans connect or do not connect to them. Sexual qigong is concerned primarily with clearing energy blockages no further than the first four bodies at best. Sexual meditation is used to clear energy blockages in all bodies, but often the focus is on the demanding spiritual work in the psychic and karmic bodies. Once this necessary preparatory work is complete, a practitioner then has a foundation from which to approach his or her seventh energetic body, known as the body of individuality or essence.

The following summaries briefly describe the challenges and benefits of sexual practices as they relate to each of your energy bodies. These summaries are equally relevant to those engaged in solo meditation practices.

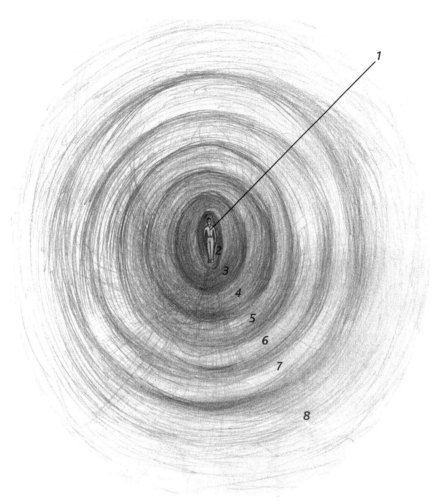

1—*Physical body*
2—*Etheric (qi) body or aura*
3—*Emotional body*
4—*Mental body*
5—*Psychic body*
6—*Karmic (causal) body*
7—*Essence or body of individuality*
8—*Body of the Tao (extends to infinity)*

Figure 3-1: The Eight Energy Bodies

PHYSICAL ENERGY BODY

The first challenge for many practitioners is to get out of their head and into their physical body. The next challenge is to fully inhabit the body and to feel comfortable and relaxed, even in challenging circumstances, sexual or otherwise. This is why traditional Taoist training always begins with body-centered systems such as qigong, tai chi, Taoist yoga and, later, tai chi push hands. If you went to a Taoist monastery, the first practice they might prescribe for you would be tai chi or qigong. These complete mind-body energy arts enable you to drop your consciousness into your body, feel your body and become fully present to what is going on inside you. These energetic practices also allow you to learn to isolate any part of your body and work with specific techniques within that area.

All of the sexual practices in this book help you get your consciousness into your body. Once you know what is going on in your physical body, then you can make choices on what to do with the new awareness. An advanced practitioner can actually feel and move his or her awareness into a lover's body and identify the location of specific blockages in the muscles, organs and bodily tissues. He or she can feel where the body and mind are not relaxed, where tension is gripping them. The goal is to help you and your partner fully resolve the causes of minor or major physical pain and discomfort; this brings you both closer to the deep intimacy and freedom that sexual qigong and meditation can provide.

QI (ETHERIC) ENERGY BODY OR AURA

Sex upgrades the qi that runs the physical body and opens up energy channels that govern physicality and the lower emotions such as fear, anger, possessiveness or jealousy. These emotions are derived from your internal organs and animal ancestors.

The energy channels that regulate your physicality intersect, overlap, go parallel to, extend beyond and exist simultaneously within those that govern your emotions, thoughts, psychic capacities, karma and essence aspects of being.

Although every channel can run all the energetic frequencies with equal strength, some channels run the qi of some energy bodies more easily than others. Without practice, the qi of the higher energy bodies and higher emotions, for most people, simply remains weak or dormant. This is why people can get lost in the physical sensations that accompany the lower emotions.

Many have insufficient strength in the channels to move easily from the lower emotions to the higher emotions such as love, generosity and kindness, or to link to the mental, psychic, karmic or essence aspects of self. As you strengthen the energy in your channels, you will find it less difficult to make the jump from lower negative emotions to the higher positive emotions. You will also be able to stabilize higher emotional states as a natural way of being.

To develop the second energy body, Taoists saw the need to consciously develop and upgrade the central nervous system by enhancing both its sensitivity and strength. They developed and worked comprehensively with the body's energy channels and centers using methods like qigong, tai chi and Taoist yoga.

EMOTIONAL ENERGY BODY

The most basic benefit of sexual qigong and sexual meditation is greater emotional satisfaction. The process of releasing emotional blockages within yourself and your partner can reduce, eliminate and dissolve whatever prevents the two of you from truly connecting. Any one of a thousand sub-shades of emotions can be ameliorated, whether dealing with perpetual emotional wounds or dysfunctional emotions such as anger, greed, insensitivity, sadness or hysteria.

Taking into account the whole range of human energies, emotional energy is still a relatively gross phenomenon. It is essential on the spiritual path that a person first becomes stable, open, balanced, and mature in the energy of his or her physical body, qi, and emotions before embarking on work at the higher levels. Although many people would like to rush the process, Taoists found it can often take as much as five to ten years for people to become stable at the level of body and qi. This is why, in the classical tradition, qigong was practiced before Taoist meditation, and why sexual qigong was learned before sexual meditation. It is also the reason that some traditions would only accept people as initiates after a certain age, where the probability was higher that the person had accumulated enough real world experience and emotional maturity to handle spiritual work.

Once you have done your preparatory qi practices it is critical to consciously open up and fully clear your overt and subliminal emotions. This enables you to experientially feel and develop more emotional intelligence, rather than merely possess a disassociated mental construct of your emotions. Clearing the emotions must be done before you move on to work with the higher energy bodies, such as the psychic body. Stabilizing your emotional body is essential so that real problems do not surface and sabotage your efforts downstream.

MENTAL ENERGY BODY

Sexual practices can help you release and resolve the energy that causes your mind to excessively churn, endlessly repeating the same themes with related words and internal images. There are many techniques that can help you calm down and relax your mental energy. Mental churning explains why many people remain dissatisfied even when they are incredibly successful. The reason behind this dissatisfaction has little to do with what occurs in the outer world and everything to do with mental constructs people use to interpret situations. Mental energy, including the meaning you infer from the facts, is what can make you unhappy and never at peace. This is especially true because your thoughts are directly linked with your emotions, so that negative or confused thoughts feed negative emotions.

On the positive side, when you can consciously and directly contact your unconscious mind, you can trigger the higher possibilities of sex. These include: unimaginable pleasure, expanded joy, ecstasy, and various forms of increased happiness and satisfaction that penetrate right to your core. The mind is what can help you relax, focus and develop your consciousness.

PSYCHIC ENERGY BODY

As sexual pleasure moves into the psychic, karmic and essence energy bodies, the level of potential ecstasy goes beyond what can make you happy from a human perspective. These higher energy bodies can take you into new states that would make a God happy. Clearing out and releasing what is suppressed in the deepest levels of your subconscious or unconscious mind allows you to successfully navigate these unknown waters.

Most are not aware of how they are subliminally affected by psychic energy. We mistake intuition, which is a simple form of psychic energy, with the massive energies of the psychic realm. Like everything, psychic capacities exist in varying degrees along a continuum. Teachers and psychotherapists often use it in their work, often conscious of only a small part of what they are tapping into, while others—professional psychics, medical intuitives, astrologers and meditation masters, for example—consciously recognize and utilize psychic energy for all kinds of specific purposes.

Although in common usage the word "psychic" has become nearly synonymous with "clairvoyant," that is not the only meaning of the word here. The psychic level (the fifth energy body) is vast and far reaching, beyond the limits of time and space in ordinary experience. "Psychic," in this sense, also means being able to see the invisible—what's inside a human being that you cannot see with your ordinary senses, but only with the highly refined internal senses that are inactive for most people. It also means being able to read and potentially flow with a person's energy at the psychic level.

Sexual meditation not only develops recognition and varying degrees of psychic capacity, it also dissolves and releases the negative qualities that remain bound inside the psychic body. These negative energies can manifest in a myriad of ways, making your life anywhere from disjointed to flat-out spooky or miserable. This is also why first stabilizing and clearing the four lower energy bodies is essential before working with the fifth and higher energy bodies, as you can run into real trouble without a solid foundation.

Without a real emotional component at the psychic level, people's empathic pathways remain barricaded. They relate to the suffering of others as if they were mere ideas or ants in the fashion of the gods of ancient Greece, who played with mortals in cruel and capricious ways, giving their egos full play. To become truly energetically sensitive, a person must wake up to the psychic realm.

KARMIC (CAUSAL) ENERGY BODY

After gaining psychic sensitivity, you can *start* the process of directly perceiving and then comprehending how karma gets blocked in people, including yourself. At this level it becomes possible, in varying degrees, to directly perceive karmic blockages as they manifest in the body and its energy channels, as well as how karmic energy plays out in worldly events.

By the time you are able to work with the karmic body, you should already be able to feel and work with qi. If this is not the case, you just get inference rather than the direct experience or evidence. There is a natural progression and unfolding of awareness when you work with the eight energy bodies. Each higher body requires more refinement.

Working with the karmic body enables people to understand the long-term effects they have on others and what long-term effects other people have on them. At the more advanced levels you can consciously and directly consider karmic obligations and possibly resolve them. In fact, working through and resolving karma is a primary reason why souls incarnate in a human body.

Through sexual meditation practices, because both lovers each have access to four times more energy than if they are practicing alone, it becomes infinitely more possible to bring up and recognize qualities of psychic and karmic awareness. The energies must become known quantities in order to be effectively released and resolved. This is the door that must be opened if you want to deal with and ultimately free up whatever blocks the karmic body.

When you come into contact with the events of karma, you learn to recognize the different energies encoded within and how they interact when they come together. You directly feel the energy of karma. Feeling the energy itself is not the same thing as making mental references about something. When you make mental references you may be recognizing its discernible effects and watching how it has gelled within manifestation, but there is a danger that you might get stuck mentally on cataloging manifestations rather than understanding the actual energy itself. It is useful to be aware of this subtle trap.

The first four Taoist energy bodies (physical, qi, emotional and mental bodies) are observances of manifestations in form. Most of the world operates only from these levels. Working within these first four energy bodies allows people to create in our world. This is what science is all about. However, working only with these four energy bodies will not allow you become a free individual at the level of the essence or soul. Many more important issues may be bound in the higher energy bodies.

If you want to be free and enlightened, sooner or later you will have to do the deeper work that includes working with the psychic body, then going through and clearing all your karma. This requires a higher level of presence and awareness developed through disciplined practice.

Reincarnation

It has been said that all spiritual paths lead to the same place, that there are as many paths as there are people on the road. Although true in the absolute sense, in the relative sense, some paths are more direct or have different twists in the road. If you accept the premise of reincarnation, the question becomes, "If you are seeking to fully awaken spiritually, are you going to pursue a path that will take one, ten or ten thousand lifetimes?"

The Taoists generally don't discuss reincarnation in the early stages of a spiritual path, as one might find in Hindu and Buddhist circles. Taoists have always had very scientific minds. They understand that approaching the subject of reincarnation in any authentic way first requires a certain degree of internal stability and sensibility within a spiritual seeker. Without that stability, even talking about reincarnation can degenerate into a blind belief, which Taoists simply won't support. Taoists would say that until you know about your past lives or can start to access them directly, in general, talking about reincarnation has very little value.

Any blind belief a person adopts sets them up to deal with more thoughts making them more deeply conditioned. This is the opposite of progress. On the other hand, if a person arrives at a belief because they have soberly experienced it, they generally don't get conditioned—they have become clearer, because they have had a direct experience. A knowing has been created rather than a belief.

The beginning of any spiritual process may not be what it becomes later on. On the early rungs of the spiritual ladder, the work is about getting real in the here and now. In the here and now, it is absolutely true that everything is reincarnating moment to moment. Your energy, your perception of what you are, and, in fact, everything you are in contact with and perceive as happening is actually generated by you in every moment. To the Taoists, this continuous reincarnation process is part of the constant flux of yin and yang.

Rather than live in the present moment, many unconsciously form attachments to a range of identities about who they are, what they are supposed to do, and how the world is supposed to be. Many get lost in the daily experience of their mind, constantly generating thought form after thought form. This limits perception and crowds out the freshness of each new moment.

Humans have all sorts of experiences, of course. However, it's when we cling to our experience and make it a solid, concrete reality, with thoughts of I am this or that… I can or can't do that… I had this experience and that means this… that we reduce ourselves to an identity and a conditioned way of being. In the Taoist view, 99.9% of everyday experience is intrinsically meaningless, or wu so hui. When you cease building an identity around each new experience, you begin to fully reincarnate at every moment and start to taste real freedom.

BODY OF INDIVIDUALITY (ESSENCE)

Beyond the challenging task of sorting out your physical, emotional and mental blockages, there is an immense amount of psychic and karmic content that must be resolved before it becomes possible to approach blockages in your seventh energetic body, which is called the body of individuality or essence. You may intermittently see glimpses of this seventh energy body, and your life may even be driven by the essence inside you, but it will still be fuzzy and unclear, until you have done enough clearing on your previous energy bodies.

At the level of the seventh body, you become aware of that which enables the actual birth of the full spiritual being, commonly referred to as your essence. In many Taoist Fire alchemical traditions this is called the "Immortal Fetus." The energetic qualities of essence are even subtler and more difficult to transcend than that which has come before, as they are beyond anything related to personal history or personality in any form. The primary spiritual purpose for the beginning and intermediate stage of Taoist meditation involves gathering all the energies of an individual into one integrated, whole energy or consciousness. The unified energy creates a *ling*, which can be translated into English as "soul."

When you and your lover release all the blockages within yourselves and each other, you can arrive at and live from your natural state. Within Taoism the body of individuality is sometimes compared to the human body. The human body has trillions of cells and, likewise, it has trillions of potentially different kinds of essences. At the level of stem cells in the body, the cells are all the same, but their nature is they can differentiate into specific types of cells, such as a liver cell or a brain cell. At the base level, the cell is still a cell, but it now it has a specific purpose for the body. Like this, a person's underlying essence (the body of individuality) can vibrate with a particular quality to fulfill some need within the universe beyond any personal agenda that he or she might have.

The body of individuality is about finding out at the level of consciousness what cell you are in the universe—your soul, or what is known in Chinese as your *ling* —so the nature of your cell can manifest. When you reach this point, you have found your essence—something that is not invented, but just is. This is a major accomplishment on the ladder of enlightenment.

Once you have found your *ling*, you can then start the process of what Taoists call internal alchemy practices on the cell (your nature or body of individuality) and consciously change it. This process could be compared metaphorically to changing, for example, the liver cell mentioned earlier into a brain cell. This is how your energy then manifests through the universe.

All Taoist internal alchemy from the seventh to eighth body is about learning how a cell can *transfigure* into different types of cells that can manifest. These are the different ways your energy can arise in the universe. *Transforming* is parallel to changing milk into yogurt or cheese. *Transfiguring* is parallel to changing milk into sand, lead into gold or a rabbit into a mountain.

Just as all the deities in Tibetan Buddhism are different aspects (or essences) of what is essentially the same deity, this metaphor of a cell transfiguring in different ways represents the different ways Universal Consciousness can manifest in all times and places. After arriving at the body of individuality, you practice internal alchemy on your essence as many times as is appropriate, until by intimately experiencing and not being separate with everything out there, you can cross over into the eighth energy body—that of the Tao.

Taoists do not have the prevailing view of reincarnation that is common in the Western world. They believe that the vast majority of human beings do not have the capacity to reincarnate intact. They believe that when a soul dies, it often breaks up, like an egg hitting the ground, shattering into many parts. If lucky, it breaks just into a few parts, and if not, who knows how many. These pieces then recombine with separated fragments of other souls, which then combine and fuse into a new reincarnating composite soul—another *ling*.

If this new *ling* contains a composite of too many fragmented pieces, it may result in a soul that can never become fully comfortable living on this earth. This is why some people, even from infancy, seem so strongly torn in different directions. The more pieces they come in with, the more difficult it will be to unify their energy through dissolving practices. If this is the case, it will be harder to reach the body of individuality, where it is possible to develop a soul that can reincarnate intact and continue to progress toward its ultimate spiritual destination.

Since many Taoists believe that most people will not come back as a unified being because they have not created a *ling*, they postpone talking about reincarnation until someone has walked the path toward the Tao for a while. At that point Taoists do discuss karma, which is often called the Law of Return. This law states that whatever energy you put out eventually comes back to you in some form or another.

A major purpose behind Taoist meditation is to work toward achieving the body of individuality. Taoists perceive that only a unified being can reincarnate sufficiently to attain the body of the Tao, which is the ultimate purpose of spirituality in Taoism.

Achieving the body of individuality accomplishes self-realization and personal enlightenment; this is not, however, universal enlightenment.

BODY OF THE TAO

The final destination in Taoism is known as the body of the Tao, where the body is like the entire universe in all its aspects. While each individual has the body of individuality in varying degrees, or an original essence beyond his or her personality, experiences and karma, the body of the Tao—the eighth energy body—goes beyond and includes all and everything in all universes, places and times. This is the Taoist parallel to what is called "God," although not in the sense of a supernatural being. It is the totality of everything that is, was and will ever exist.

According to Taoist teachings, the ultimate goal of sexual meditation is to clear all the blockages to the eighth energy body, so that a person can reach his or her fullest potential within the universe as is explained in Chapter 18. The Water tradition of internal alchemy contains the methods to go from the seventh to the eighth body. The eighth body is where a Taoist Spiritual Immortal, or Buddha, arrives.

ENERGY CHANNELS OF THE BODY

Within sexual qigong and sexual meditation three primary channels[3] are the main conduits of qi for all energetic practices. There is also possibility for another energetic channel to be created between the central channels of two lovers, the neo-central channel, through advanced Taoist meditation practices.

The *Tao Te Ching* says, "The One created the Two, the Two created the Three and the Three created the myriad of things." This saying has multiple layers of meaning. One interpretation is that, at the moment of conception and shortly thereafter, the

---

3. The left, right and central channels are the main energy pathways, but Taoists have found a total of four to five thousand channels (depending on the method of classification), all with specific functions.

"One" is the central channel through which one's current essence is embodied. Although the intrinsic energy of the central channel is not polarized into yin and yang, within it is the ability to create them. In Taoist cosmology this is called *tai chi*. The "One" (central channel) then creates the "Two." The "One" and "Two" in combination then create the "Three." In human energetics, the "Two" and "Three" are other names for the left and right energy channels of the body. Depending on circumstances, sometimes the right channel will be the "Two" and the left will be the "Three", and sometimes it will be the other way round.

CENTRAL CHANNEL

In the physical body, the central channel is located both in the torso and the limbs. In the arms and legs, it is within the bone marrow in the center of each bone, including the two bones of the forearm and lower leg. It lies along a very thin line in the exact center of the torso—equidistant from the front, sides and spine of the body. It begins from the center of the perineum, extending through the center of the torso, neck and head to the crown (called *bai hui* in Chinese) and finishes above the head at the boundary of your etheric body, where the eighth and ninth chakras of Indian yoga are also located.

The bai hui point is at the exact center of the crown of the head and is known in Traditional Chinese Medicine as the "meeting of a hundred energy points." Likewise, all the chakras of Indian and Tibetan yoga and the three tantiens of Taoism (see Figure 3-4) are also located along the central channel. In the legs, if you are standing, the central channel ends at the boundary of the etheric body, below the feet, where it connects with the energy of the earth.

The central channel has two major functions: to absorb and to project. By absorbing within it any other energy in the body, it can balance it and also release any bound energy or combinations of energies in any of your energy bodies into emptiness and thereby free them. The central channel can also project energy to energize all your other energy channels and all eight energy bodies. Furthermore, it can enable the consciousness within your human body to contact, communicate, influence and be influenced by all and everything throughout time and space.

In sexual qigong, the central channel is primarily used to balance and energize the yin and yang energies flowing through the body. Sexual meditation includes and goes beyond this, emphasizing the central channel's ability to:

• Dissolve spiritual blockages into emptiness

• Attain the body of individuality

• Resolve the fact that your blockages have hampered your ability to connect with all and everything.

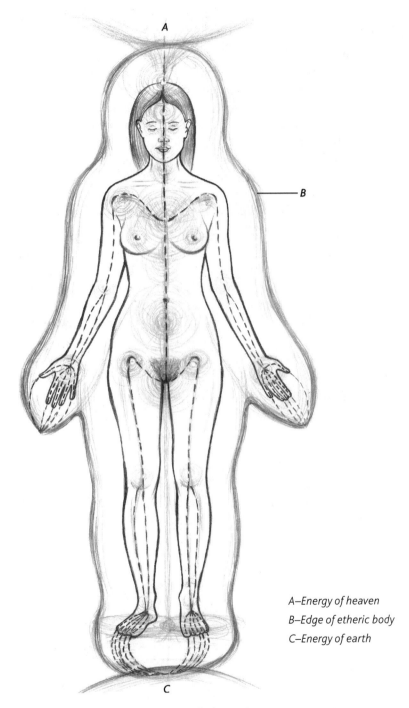

A—Energy of heaven
B—Edge of etheric body
C—Energy of earth

Figure 3-2: The Central Channel

RIGHT AND LEFT CHANNELS

In the physical body, the left and right channels are located both in the torso and the limbs. From the top of the etheric body to the bai hui point at the crown of the head, the left and right channels continue down the center of the brain. At the upper tantien (third eye), the distance between the left and right channels widens, and they continue down to the center of each eye, to the nostrils, down each side of the mouth, down the throat, to the level of the collarbone. At this point on the body, the left and right channels branch off on a line, to the left and right. First they go to the point on the front of each shoulder called the shoulder's nest,[4] then to the armpits and onward within the hard part of each bone (cortex) inside the arms all the way to the fingertips and to the boundary of the etheric body.

Next from both shoulder's nests, the left and right channels descend within the torso to each kwa. The kwa is the Chinese word for the area on each side of the body extending from the inguinal ligaments through the inside of the pelvis to the top of the hip bones. After this, the channels go from each kwa down the legs and feet within the hard part (cortex) of the bones of each leg. This is in contrast to the central channel, which goes through the bone marrow in the center of the bones. Then the right and left channels go to the boundary of the etheric body below the feet, where they join the central channel.

The right and left channels govern the manner in which you experience all essential yang and yin differentiations of energy. At the higher levels of sexual qigong, qi is continuously circulated through these channels to facilitate the unblocking of stuck energies. This enables the practitioner to recognize yin and yang manifestations. Sexual meditation employs the energetic power circulating between left and right channels to bring forth the deeper and more pervasive higher-level blockages within you, so they can ultimately be resolved in the central channel. Often you have to work extensively with the right and left channels before fully moving into the central channel work.

---

4. For more on the shoulder's nest, see Frantzis, Bruce, *Opening the Energy Gates of Your Body: Qigong for Lifelong Health,* rev. ed. (Berkeley, CA: North Atlantic Books, 2006), 133–34.

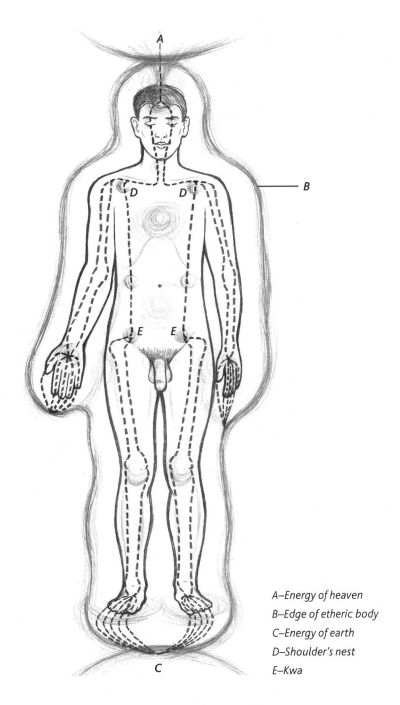

A—Energy of heaven
B—Edge of etheric body
C—Energy of earth
D—Shoulder's nest
E—Kwa

Figure 3-3: The Right and Left Channels

NEO-CENTRAL CHANNEL

Practices in the final chapters of this book work with the neo-central channel. In advanced sexual meditation practices, a neo-central channel is birthed when the two central channels of a man and a woman link and then merge into one to create a new third channel that exists non-physically between the two lovers.

THE THREE TANTIENS

Tantiens are specific energy centers in the body, sometimes called "elixir fields," where qi collects, like a storage or water tank, and from which it is dispersed and circulated throughout the human body, mind and Spirit. There are three tantiens—the lower, middle and upper.

From the Taoist perspective, a woman is usually more active in her middle tantien, while a man is more active in his lower tantien. Directly connected to each of the three tantiens is the *lao gong* point located in the center of each palm. This is the place in the body that can most easily and directly transmit energy into another person.

Sometimes referred to as the lower, middle and upper palaces, the tantiens contain the three treasures—*jing* (sperm/ovary generative energy), *qi* (vital energy, including thoughts, emotions and psychic energy), and *shen* (Spirit or karmic and essence energy).

LOWER TANTIEN

The lower tantien is located below the navel, about one-third of the distance to the genitals, just slightly above the pubic hair. It is in the center of the abdomen, midway between the surface of the belly and the spine. Resting directly on the central channel, it is the energetic center in the body that controls and regulates all energies that affect physical health and bodily functions. The more robust and active this center, the more physically strong, masculine and inherently sexual a man will be.

During sex, a man's lower tantien naturally becomes more activated and alive. The lower tantien governs and enables his physicality; the emotional context and content of sex tends to be less important and less evident to him. In the afterglow of lovemaking, a woman is often full of emotion; she feels bonded and in love, craving pillow talk and cuddling. The man, on the other hand, will often be satisfied by the physical act alone. Much to his ladylove's disappointment, he may even immediately roll over and fall asleep.

Understanding the energetic centers in the body from the perspective of basic priorities of the yin and yang energy of the sexes can relieve some of the stress associated with these differences. If a woman takes a man's lack of emotional response personally and reacts with hurt and anger or becomes demanding, she may end up pushing him away.

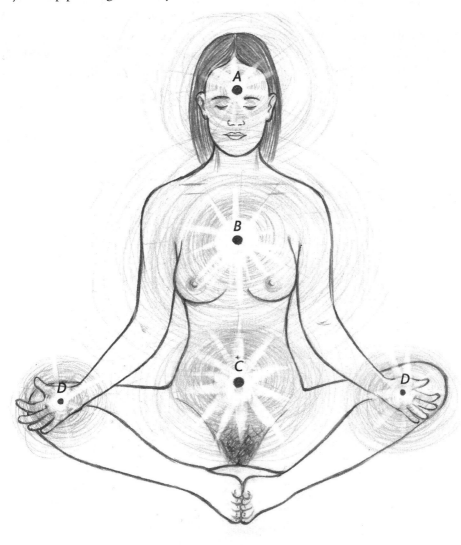

A—Upper tantien
B—Middle tantien
C—Lower tantien
D—Lao gong points

Figure 3-4: The Three Tantiens —Sitting

MIDDLE TANTIEN

The middle tantien is located near the heart on the central channel. It governs all relationships, including how you connect to your essence and the Tao. As both the center and ruler of the emotions, the aliveness in a woman's middle tantien will naturally flow outward toward her lover during sexual intercourse. This activation in her heart is what gives her the feeling of "falling in love." The more robust and active this center, the more nurturing and feminine the woman will be and, likewise, the more emotionally sensitive a man can become.

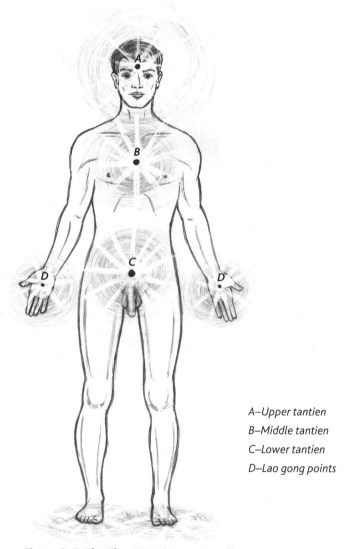

A–Upper tantien
B–Middle tantien
C–Lower tantien
D–Lao gong points

Figure 3-5: The Three Tantiens—Standing

UPPER TANTIEN

In the advanced stages of both solo meditation and sexual meditation, the upper tantien in a person is fully activated. The Taoists identified thirty distinct energetic centers in the brain, which all together are called the upper tantien. The two best-known energetic centers in the head are the "third eye," in the center of the forehead slightly above the eyebrows, and the pineal gland, just below the crown of the head, which often are termed the sixth and seventh chakras within Buddhist and Hindu yoga traditions.

ENERGETIC ANATOMY OF THE GENITALS

Anyone who has seen a reflexology chart will be familiar with the idea that specific zones on the feet correspond to various internal organs. A similar correspondence exists between our internal organs and genitalia. The Taoists have mapped these linkages in the subtle energetic anatomy as well, revealing the intricate connection between the genitals and the tantiens, energy channels and the eight energy bodies. In Taoist sex practices you learn to activate different areas of the body by stimulating different parts of the genitals.

MEN'S ENERGETIC ANATOMY

First let's look at the physical anatomy of the man's erection.

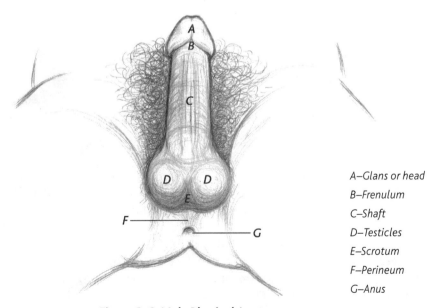

A—Glans or head
B—Frenulum
C—Shaft
D—Testicles
E—Scrotum
F—Perineum
G—Anus

Figure 3-6: Male Physical Anatomy

Both the distance from the base of the penis to the head, and the depth from the outer surface of his skin to the center of the penis, correspond to specific internal organs, energy channels, and centers in the body. A firm grip at the base of the shaft will activate a man's lower tantien; stroking the middle of the shaft will activate his middle tantien; stimulation of the frenulum and head of his penis will feed his upper tantien. The frenulum and nearby tissue is the most sensitive part of the penis, stimulation of which tends to lead to ejaculation.

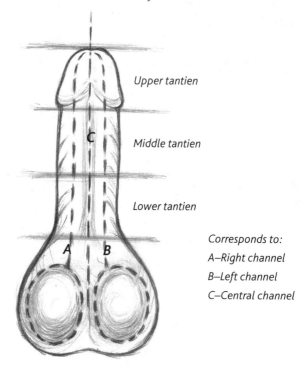

Upper tantien

Middle tantien

Lower tantien

Corresponds to:
A—Right channel
B—Left channel
C—Central channel

Figure 3–7: How the Penis Connects to the Energy Channels and Tantiens

A similar correspondence can be found between the various layers of the penis from the epidermis to the innermost tissue at the center of the shaft. Stimulation of the surface skin activates the physical energy body, whereas the very center of the shaft activates the central channel, and also corresponds to the body of individuality and the Tao (see Figures 3-7 and 3-8). The in-between layers, concentrically deeper and deeper much like the rings of a tree, activate the other energy bodies, layer by layer. Beginning with the outermost ring just a little bit in from the skin, you can stimulate the etheric body. Go one level deeper to activate the emotional body, deeper still to the mental body and deeper still to the psychic, karmic and essence bodies. The harder the penis is handled, obviously within reasonable limits, the more it will activate the higher energy bodies.

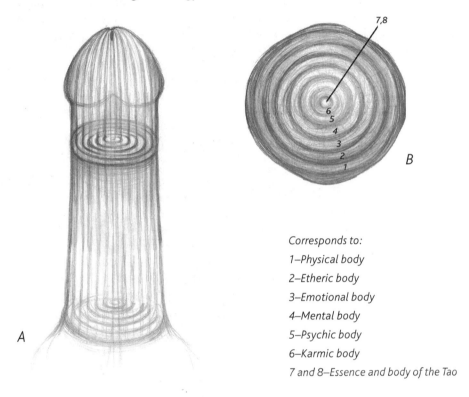

Corresponds to:

1–Physical body

2–Etheric body

3–Emotional body

4–Mental body

5–Psychic body

6–Karmic body

7 and 8–Essence and body of the Tao

A) Longitudinal View.   B) Cross Section.

Figure 3-8: How the Penis Connects to the Eight Energy Bodies

Similarly, any touching along the left and right sides of a man's penis or testicles will activate his left and right channels. The head of the penis activates all the man's yang meridians and his upper body, and the bottom of the penis activates all his yin meridians and his lower body. The middle of the penis activates the internal organs. If a woman wishes to awaken the more subtle parts of her man, she can try to activate all the parts of his penis during foreplay and intercourse. The middle shaft and base of the penis can stimulate a man's internal organs more strongly than the foreskin and head area, ultimately leading to a more powerful overall sexual response than can be achieved by focusing on the more excitable head alone.

WOMEN'S ENERGETIC ANATOMY

Understanding the physical anatomy of a man's penis is fairly straightforward as it hangs outside the body. However, the anatomy of a woman's genitalia tends to be unfamiliar, especially to men, as much of it is hidden inside the body. It is quite useful for both women and men to learn more about the anatomy of a vagina, as it is important in all types of sexual practices.

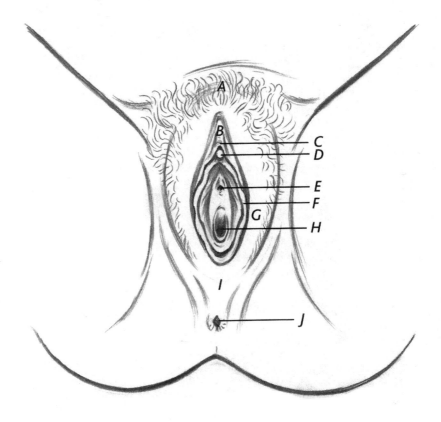

A–Mons pubis (pubic mound)   F–Labia minora

B–Hidden shaft of clitoris   G–Labia majora

C–Clitoral hood   H–Vaginal opening

D–Glans of clitoris   I–Perineum

E–Urethra   J–Anus

Figure 3-9: Female Anatomy

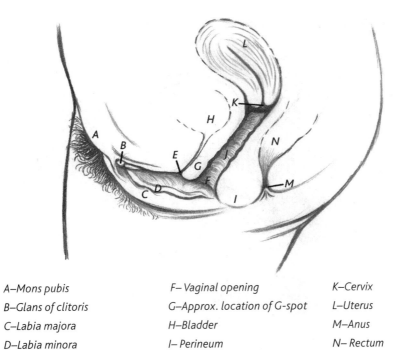

A—Mons pubis

B—Glans of clitoris

C—Labia majora

D—Labia minora

E—Urethra

F— Vaginal opening

G—Approx. location of G-spot

H—Bladder

I— Perineum

J— Vagina

K—Cervix

L—Uterus

M—Anus

N— Rectum

Figure 3-10 A: Female Anatomy in Cross Section

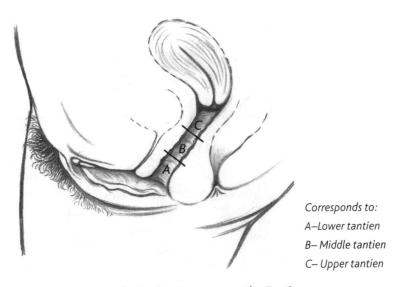

Corresponds to:

A—Lower tantien

B— Middle tantien

C— Upper tantien

Figure 3-10 B: How the Vagina Connects to the Tantiens

A woman's vagina also corresponds to different organs and the three tantiens at each level of penetration along the vaginal canal. When a man who is trained in Taoist sexual techniques plays with a woman's vagina, he can feel subtle concentric rings radiating from the center of the cervix to the vaginal walls. These directly tap into the energies of her body, mind and spirit.

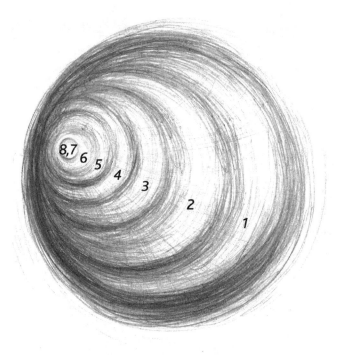

Corresponds to:

1–Physical body

2–Etheric body

3–Emotional body

4–Mental body

5–Psychic body

6–Karmic body

7 and 8–Essence and body of the Tao

Figure 3–11: How the Vagina Connects to the Energy Bodies

The vaginal complex is in the shape of a dome, with the cervix at the top. The cervix corresponds to the central channel and connects to the body of individuality and the body of the Tao. The walls of the dome that slope down toward the entrance of the vagina correspond progressively to her karmic, psychic, mental, emotional, and qi bodies, with the layer nearest the opening of her vagina corresponding to her physical body.

The left and right sides of her vagina correspond to her left and right channels. From the first layer of the vaginal walls (including the famous G-spot) and moving toward the sides of her body, you can touch progressively deeper and deeper inside, stimulating, activating, and energizing each of her progressively higher energy bodies.

THE FLUX OF YIN AND YANG

> The ceaseless intermingling of Heaven and Earth gives form to all things.
> The sexual union of male and female gives life to all things.— *I Ching*

Through Taoist practices, as you begin to directly experience your eight energy bodies, three primary energy channels and three tantiens, you simultaneously will begin to feel the different ways energy flows through your energetic anatomy. At the most basic level, in all Taoist practices you work with the interplay of two primordial energies, yin and yang.

According to classical Taoist philosophy, all men and women are composed of yin and yang energies that flow through each of the energy bodies. Yin is commonly associated with women and yang with men. Although one of these energies will dominate, men and women contain both energies within themselves in varying degrees, and these change and morph, depending on circumstances and how partners interact with each other. Yin and yang cannot exist without containing the other. They are interdependent and weave together in a continuously unfolding cosmic dance. In effect, yin and yang make up the binary code that creates all manifestation.

In effect, yin and yang make up the binary code that creates all manifestation.

MASCULINE AND FEMININE ESSENCES

In exploring various types of personal and sexual interactions, Taoists asked the question, "How can you feel what energetic qualities of the opposite sex are inside you, as well as energetically experience what is going on in your partner?"

In order to experience a partner's energy, the woman must first find the masculine essence, or entire range of yang energies, within herself, and a man must find the feminine essence, or entire range of yin energies, within himself. This is especially true within the emotional, mental, psychic, karmic and essence energy bodies. The ways and experiences of yin or yang energies in each energy body can be quite different, both in quality and as motivating forces.

The symbol for the constant morphing and integration of yin and yang energies is the familiar yin-yang circle (Figure 3-12). The perfect symmetry of this symbol speaks volumes. Half light, half dark, ascending and descending, each contains a drop of the other energy as the balance point within itself. United within a single circle, these two primordial forces give way to one another, each rising as the other falls in perpetual motion.

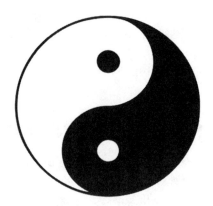

Figure 3-12: Yin-Yang Symbol

According to classical Taoist cosmology, there is an undifferentiated, limitless void called *wu chi* (also spelled *wu ji*), a place that holds all universal possibilities within itself, but is beyond the need to take form. It is also called the Tao. *Wu chi* is the most common interpretation of the "One" in the saying from the *Tao Te Ching*, "The One created the Two, the Two created the Three and the Three created the myriad of things." In order for any specific manifestation within creation to come into existence, there needs to be a creative force, which the Taoists call *tai chi*, the primordial power that brings all phenomena—seen and unseen, large and small—into being. This is the "Two."

This concept is eloquently expressed in Taoist poetry from the twelfth century C.E., written by Taoist Immortal and priestess Sun Bu'er:

> Before our body existed,
> One energy was already there.
> Like jade, more lustrous as it's polished,
> Like gold, brighter as it's refined.[5]

Inside this undifferentiated birthing room, *tai chi* then separates, differentiates and combines into *liang yi*—yin and yang energies, such as night-day, man-woman, matter-spirit, fire-water, this-that, and the left and right channels. These energies are not purely opposites, but ones that weave in and out of each other in a seamless, complementary flow. Yin and yang together—the "Three"—create "the myriad of things."

One meaning of the Taoist saying, "The wise person sits in his room and knows the worlds," is that he or she knows what yin and yang energy are universally beyond the limited confines of how we experience them in this world and in the forms of

---

5. As translated by Thomas Cleary in *The Taoist Classics: Volume Three* (Boston: Shambhala, 1991), 402.

men and women. He or she who knows the universe—who knows the way it works and is aware of it all—has realized *wu chi.*

PRIMARY QUALITIES OF YIN AND YANG

Although the strengths of yin and yang are quite equal, they have primary qualities that are quite distinct. Pure yang energy wants to go outward, like fire or a beam of light. It penetrates and moves through anything in its way. Its strong force can equally create, destroy or damage whatever is in its path. On the positive side, yang energy is what drives people to do, create and accomplish in life. In its pure state however, it is irrelevant to the yang force whether or not something grows from it, so long as it initiates the creative spark. Whether or not it sticks to anything and whether or not it has an ongoing relationship to it is mostly irrelevant to yang energy.

The opposite is true of yin energy, which, like water, naturally wants to absorb, receive and attach itself to and enter into relationship with whatever moves toward it. Yin exists to let in yang, and to allow whatever comes out of that merging to grow by nourishing the manifestation of their combined energies. Yin energy abhors destruction. Enamored of growth in all forms, the primary yin energy of many women has a natural biological propensity to merge with another and make a nest. A woman's yin predisposes her to pair bonding as well as to motherhood; producing and preserving offspring is the quintessential human and animal expression of yin. Without yin, yang can never take manifested form through birth.

Conversely, the quintessential expression of yang energy has a very different agenda, one that is evidenced in the predominance of war among members of our species. All warring ways are an expression of yang. Watch the behavior of alpha male chimpanzees and you will see pure, unabashed biological yang energy. Pure yang will happily create offspring, and will just as happily kill it,[6] often regardless of whether it sprang from its own seed or that of another. Most societies mimic this behavior in the relentless drive toward excessive competition and war.

Nesting and nourishing are not on yang's primary agenda. This places yang at the far opposite pole of yin, which naturally abhors and will do anything to avoid the death of a child, whether its own or that of another, or even that of another species altogether. The tender, protective feelings we experience in the presence of a child— or when we see a playful puppy or kitten for that matter—are tangible expressions of yin.

The proportions of yin and yang in any given individual can vary over time and according to circumstance. For example, a man might spend his late teens and early twenties pursuing goals that amp up his yang energy. He will often channel

---

6. See Wrangham, Richard, and Peterson, Dale, *Demonic Males* (Boston: Houghton Mifflin, 1996), for an in-depth analysis of male and female chimpanzee behavior and its implications as regards human society.

his yang energy into sports, business and other pursuits. His yang energy will increase with each accomplishment. He might become quite the ladies' man, or quite the "dog," depending on his personal style and level of sophistication. He may go from woman to woman, breaking hearts and burning bridges without a thought. He may also get married and create offspring. He is yang energy personified.

Years later, we might meet this same man and be surprised to discover a very different person. He may have burned out this yang energy through excessive competition, injuries, heartbreaks and broken relationships. He will have had to become more receptive to heal. This man will find himself expressing much more of his yin energy, or at least be more balanced.

Likewise a woman may choose in the early part of her life to start a family and raise children, expressing more of her yin nature. Later in life, we might see she comes more into her yang power. She may then turn toward pursuing goals, often by including networks of relationships, expressing yang energy in her own yin way.

Everyone's personal history has ebbs and flows—a man or woman can start life primarily yin and finish yang or the opposite. Look at your own life and see if there haven't been times when you were incredibly productive and creative in the world (yang), while at others you were introspective, preoccupied with caring for your needs and the needs of others (yin). Everyone carries these possibilities within.

FEELING YIN AND YANG

Understanding how to be aware of and how to move comfortably between female and male energetic qualities is an important and achievable goal in Taoism. The practice of all energy arts—health arts such as qigong and Taoist yoga, martial arts such as bagua and tai chi, and Taoist meditation—develop your sensitivity to directly perceive and engage yin and yang energies within yourself and during interactions.

These are not mental, visualization, theoretical or symbolic practices, but pragmatic ones whose goal is to help you feel qi as a living, tangible energetic experience within your body, mind and spirit. These energetic practices make it possible to directly experience universal energies from the gross phenomena of our visible physical world, including sexual interactions, to the most refined spiritual energies of unseen realms that connect to our world. The energetic anatomy presented in this chapter gives you a basic blueprint for how yin and yang energies flow in your body in all Taoist practices.

Feeling the qualities of your energy and that of the other person can be used to resolve blockages within each other's energetic bodies. Ultimately, the goal is to become one unified being. This resolution can only occur after a woman first fully activates her female yin essence energy and a man fully activates his male yang essence energy. Only then is it possible for men and women to completely appreciate and embody the opposite energy within their own body and being. The intent is to unite the fractured opposites within each partner and thereby resolve the tendency to feel separate, a feeling that causes people to always want something more and always feel fundamentally unfulfilled.

BALANCING YIN AND YANG IN THE ENERGY BODIES

The Taoists have a very old phrase, "Let men be men and women be women." When a man's yang energy is balanced and he is comfortable with his masculinity, his sheer presence will feed a woman's yin. In the same way, when a woman is comfortable with her femininity, she will naturally feed his yang.

It's important to understand that all of us have both yin and yang energy in varying proportions at all eight energetic levels. For a man's development to be balanced, he must have some yin in every part of his system. Likewise, a woman needs some yang at every level of her being for her development to evolve in the smoothest fashion.

This yin-yang balance is expressed in the eight energy bodies, which flip their natural predominance from yin to yang between them in the first six energy bodies. A man's physical body will tend to be more yang; his qi body, yin; his emotional body, yang; his mental body, yin; his psychic body, yang; his karmic body, yin. In a woman, it's the opposite: her physical body tends to be more yin, her qi body, yang; her emotional body, yin; her mental body, yang; her psychic body, yin; her karmic body, yang. The essence body mostly goes beyond yin and yang, as does the body of Tao. From a Taoist point of view, recognizing imbalance in any of the energy bodies is the first step toward making a positive change.

According to the Taoists, becoming aware of the female or male essence within each of the first seven energy bodies is crucial; this is so because it is only after a woman fully activates her yin and a man fully activates his yang that either sex can truly appreciate and embody the opposite energy. The goal is for the full range of yin and yang within the individual to be harmonious rather than incomplete, unbalanced or disturbed.

You might ask, "What does balance do for me?" Achieving this unique, even radical integration gives inner stability, allowing you to feel more complete and better able to take action (yang) or connect (yin) as situations arise. When you feel balanced, you can move through blockages quickly and change with circumstances instead of getting fixated and bogged down. Balance helps you develop the higher stage of emptiness and the prized Taoist qualities of real compassion, love, joy and generosity of spirit.

The I Ching: Book of Changes

The *I Ching*, with an oral tradition going back five thousand years, is considered to be the bible of Taoism. It is concerned with the underlying energetic nature and function of all change.

Historically, people in China and the West have used this ancient scripture as a tool to explore the nature of the universe and the relationships and events of their own personal lives. The three most common uses of the *I Ching* are as follows:

1. An oracle for foretelling the future

2. A book of wisdom

3. A mathematical tool.

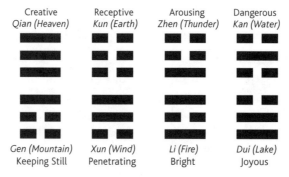

Figure 3-13: The Eight Trigrams of the I Ching

Uncommon uses are the practice methods through which Taoists deconstruct the incredibly complex world of yin and yang as it relates to how qi manifests on all levels.

Taoist adepts who developed the essential sections of the *I Ching* used techniques of observation and meditation to explore and experience the entire interplay of yin and yang energies within relationships.

Within the *I Ching*, possible energetic or qi interactions of yin and yang in human beings are represented by sixty-four hexagrams and accompanying text. Each hexagram represents combinations of unbroken lines (yang) or broken lines (yin). For example, the first hexagram, the "Creative," which consists of six yang lines, represents the active, strong and primordial power of yang. The second, the "Receptive," contains only yin lines, and represents the yielding, receptive primordial power of yin. Other hexagrams show how yin and yang energies can combine, morph, interact and change, depending on circumstances.

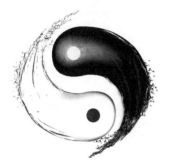

CHAPTER 4

Taoist Morality—
Mind of Man,
Mind of Tao

Every spiritual, religious and philosophical system, including Taoism, has positions on morality. Taoist morality is unique in that it is based on the flows of energy, rather than a set of intellectual beliefs and rules of what is right or wrong. Taoist morality looks at what is constant in the universe in terms of the eight energy bodies, the five elements (see Chapter 6) and the flows of yin and yang rather than purely mental ideas or rigid belief systems.

Laozi in the *Tao Te Ching* said, "If the Great Way perishes, there will be morality and duty." What is the Great Way that Laozi is referring to? It is the Tao that can't be defined with conventional words. Taoism seeks to give people the tools and training so they can reach a place where they follow the universal energy in any situation to choose the best course of action. This is the Great Way rather than the Lesser Way, which is based on dogma.

Through all kinds of physical, energetic and meditative practices, Taoists helped people reach a clearer understanding of the external world and more importantly become more conscious of their own internal content and programming. The Taoists found that after people had evolved enough spiritually, they would naturally act in accordance with what would be the most beneficial in any situation, without creating discord or karma.

The dominant spiritual influence for many Westerners is Christianity. Taoists would agree with the position that it would be wonderful if anyone with genuine awareness could simply and genuinely follow the Golden Rule of Christianity, which is also found in many other religions, "Do to others as you would have them do to you," with its variation, "Love your neighbor as yourself." If this could be so, virtually all word-based morality and ethics would become redundant. There would already be a clear path to the most ethical resolution possible.

Taoist practices progressively teach you how to energetically free the mind and body so that the morality of the Golden Rule can become internally stabilized and balanced within. Rather than adhere to external constraints on behavior, you learn to directly experience the actual energy that manifests in any situation and align yourself with the Taoist principles of naturalness and balance. When you are in full possession of what Taoists call virtue, you will no longer need rules.

> **When you are in full possession of what Taoists call virtue, you will no longer need rules.**

By learning Taoist practices, you can shape how you think and behave with conscious agreement to align your choices with a more universal view of morality—one that aims to use awareness, love and compassion to bring about the greatest possible benefit to all that are affected by those choices.

It may be that the Taoist alternative to morality presented in this chapter is not for you—each must make his or her own choices. However, you may find the Taoist ideas on morality contain a timeless wisdom that makes sense and, if so, then you can incorporate it into your life.

ANCIENT SOURCES OF TAOIST MORALITY

Laozi's famous book, the *Tao Te Ching*, is one of the main texts of the Water tradition of Taoism. Laozi was the keeper of the imperial archives and as such he had direct access to most literary works of the time. The common story that has been passed down is that Laozi was on his way to become a hermit when one of his students, a border guard, refused him passage, asking that he leave behind some principles in writing before going into seclusion. Thus the *Tao Te Ching* was born. If not for this slim but profound piece of literature, most outside China would not even know that Taoism exists.

The *Tao Te Ching* is often translated as "The Way and Its Power" or "The Way and Its Virtue." *Tao* means

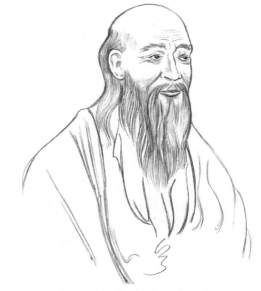

Figure 4-1: Taoist Sage Laozi

"way," "road" or "path"; *Te* means "power," "virtue" or "morality" and *Ching* means "a classic text." Looking at the meaning of these individual words gives us a deeper insight into the Taoist Water tradition's views on morality. In English we are used to a word having just one meaning, but in Chinese each character has multiple layers of interpretation.

The word *Tao* has many meanings. First, there is the *Tao* of doing anything that refers to the ideal way of doing something. You must travel on a particular path in order to wind up where that leads. Going a little deeper, the word *Tao*

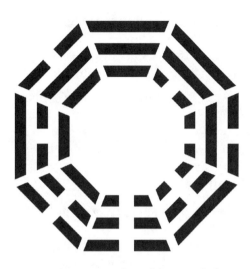

Figure 4-2: The I Ching *Symbol*

considers the question, what connects all and everything and yet has no specific quality of its own? This is the emptiness that lies at the center of the *I Ching* surrounded by the eight trigrams. It has no quality and yet everything is connected to it, comes out of it and flows through it.

The words *Tao* and *qi* are inexorably linked. To do anything in the world a person also needs energy or qi, which is often defined as the power to do some type of work. Qi is a necessary prerequisite for something to accomplish its purpose or to walk the path. Each of the eight energy bodies requires the power of qi to manifest its natural sphere of activities or influence.

Te as "power" sums up the way and the context for how all gross and subtle manifestations happen. Inherent in the word *te* is the concept of virtue. It includes the doctrine known within Hindu and Buddhist traditions as "karma" or "cause and effect," which in Taoism is sometimes called the "Law of Return." When virtue, qi and *te* as "power" emanate at any level of the eight energy bodies, they control and flavor the manner in which the effects of karma or resulting future manifestations will occur. Generally, the words *Tao* and *te* combined in Chinese represent the ordinary morality of how people should behave and think. At this most basic level, *Tao te* (morals) provides a sensible path to effectively and ethically deal with the many trials and tribulations of human interactions, including those that are within a sexual context.

Within the inner Taoist tradition, *Tao te* has deeper implications. It means the morality of the Tao, which also takes into account the ways karma and reincarnation function. Karma is directly tied to the utterly impersonal qi or power mechanics of how *te* works rather than to conceptual ideals of how a human being "should" think or act. In this sense the universal qi or power of virtue inherent in *te* is directly connected to anything that could imply subtle or overt morality.

In essence, this means that Taoist morality is based on the ongoing spiritual evolution of beings rather than perceived moral appropriateness based on any current moment in time or space. As such, Taoists may or may not agree with any specific piece of conventional morality as defined by any particular culture.

THE DILEMMA OF RIGID RULES

Taoists view rigid moral rules as a lesser form of ethics—an accommodation for the unaware masses. Based on fear and maintaining security, such rules provide a means of curbing the nastier tendencies of the human talking ape. In other words, as Laozi said, "The more legal matters are made prominent, the more thieves and robbers there will be."[1]

Taoists observe that when words and rules predominate in a culture or historical age, what often follows, sadly, is incredible hypocrisy, disenchantment, self-righteousness and corruption. Similarly, the more sexual repression that exists within a culture, the higher the prevalence of violence, rape and exploitation because sexual energy, which should be a natural part of life, easily gets deranged and emerges in unhealthy ways.

More often than not, what passes for rules of morality puts an invisible chain around people's necks. For all practical purposes, these chains prevent us from becoming balanced and rarely encourage us to be spiritually free. The Taoist Outer and Inner Dissolving methods give you a pragmatic method to help you find a moral compass based on inner guidance, not on outward rules.

GUILT IN THE WEST, SHAME IN THE EAST

In today's society, there is often confusion about what is and what is not sexually appropriate. In most industrialized nations, sexual repression, which is very common, exists side by side with a consensual hedonism that is without regard to deeper human values. There is very little understanding of what is natural and in balance as regards to sex.

The East and the West are influenced by very different drivers of morality. The primary emphasis in the West is on *individual freedom of choice* and its consequences. In the classic biblical story, Eve plucked the forbidden fruit from the tree of knowledge; Adam chose to eat it and therefore Adam and Eve were banished from the Garden of Eden. Thus guilt became the moral compass.

---

1. Lao-Tzu, *Tao Te Ching,* trans. Robert G. Henricks (New York: Ballantine Books, 1989).

Guilt pervades Western culture. Its origins revolve around making God happy. The primary religious cultural matrix of the West is loaded with terms like *should, must,* and *ought to,* all underwritten with a basic supposition that asserts: if a person doesn't believe this belief and behave this way then there'll be hell to pay.

The truth is that, for thousands of years, guilt has been used as a powerful weapon by those who want control populations. Belief systems, including sexual ones, are embedded at a young age before a person has developed the ability of critical thinking. A well-known quote commonly attributed to the Jesuits is "Give me a child until the age of seven and he is mine for life." Of course, religion is not the only agent that conditions us: government, media, economic institutions businesses and social organizations all have their agendas which usually go unquestioned. There tends to be little discussion about what the entire context of appropriate sexual education should consist of.

Historically Eastern cultures have been much more collectivistic and interdependent rather than individualistic. In contrast with personal freedom in the West, the primary emphasis in the East is *group harmony*. Blind duty to one's family trumps personal choice; the individual is steeped in tradition and hierarchy. Honor and duty form the moral compass. People aren't controlled by guilt so much as fear of being shamed or "losing face" within their society and peer groups.

Traditionally in China, people faced an even longer, more exhaustive list of rules. If you think Western morality is a burden, consider the weight of Confucianism. Confucianism had more than 3,300 rules of propriety and etiquette! Every aspect of life was governed by these rules. When so much of life is regulated, few will bother to ask, "Does this or that rule make sense?" They just follow along blindly.

In an advanced spiritual society, the enlightened mind would simply, even elegantly, know what to do. In a society dominated by the ordinary mind and its conditionings, however, people tend to bow to an outer authority unconsciously. Through Taoist meditation practices, you can begin to find out what is true. You can find your essence and connect with the Tao, which are beyond the morality of any one system. Using Taoist meditation techniques you can learn to become permanently free from both guilt and shame, which releases a tremendous amount of energy and leads you into natural states of compassion, joy, peace, intelligence and happiness.

TAOIST SAGES AND UNIVERSAL MORALITY

Sages viewed morality, or the *te* of *Tao te,* as that which would further everything sooner or later and, in the best-case scenario, in the here and now. For them, morality was a powerful factor for helping humans or any other beings to become enlightened, no matter where or when.

From the Taoist perspective, the morality most known in the West primarily focuses on the first four energy bodies combined with God. This includes all the physical, energetic, emotional and mental ideas and rules of our culture. This is what most can see and feel in the material world. When you move into Taoist morality, not only do you look at what is true in terms of the first four energy bodies but also the last four—psychic, karmic, essence and Tao.

This takes the focus of morality to a higher level that incorporates any place where you can reincarnate in future lives. Your morality is no longer just about the specifics of the earth. After this life a person may not even reincarnate on earth, but on other planets, in other universes and so on. These other reincarnation zones can be so radically different that the moral principles in place on earth may not be useful.

The Taoist mystic sages saw morality as a bigger, more universal event than merely what happened on earth. They looked at developing a higher form of morality, one that was true regardless of where you ended up in the universe beyond your current life. Relatively speaking, they considered the morality of the Tao, in all times and places, as significantly more important than human morality that constantly changes across religions, countries and cultures. To attain universal, rather than worldly knowledge, requires a Being to actually know the universe rather than speculate about it. Through cultivating and fully opening their inner awareness, both the Buddha and Taoist Immortal mystics are said to be capable, in real time, of knowing all and everything, or what is commonly known as omniscience. They gained this knowledge experientially through meditation by directly and internally perceiving the immense workings of the universe across all time and space.

Moment by moment, this enables such mystics to consciously and directly experience what goes on simultaneously in every location, dimension and time that is, has been or will exist throughout all time and in all universes. All places include more corporeal and noncorporeal beings than the human mind can ever hope to accommodate, no matter how fertile the imagination. In all the dimensions of all the possible situations, the interconnecting flows have countless variables within which the flow of karmic qi or *te* can manifest.

Two often-quoted equivalent phrases in the East mention this. The Taoist version says, "The Sage sits alone in his room and thereby knows the worlds," and the Buddhist phrase is, "The Buddha knows as many worlds as there are grains of sand along the Ganges River." Both of these quotes refer to the higher spiritual state of omniscience. The *Tao Te Ching*, when properly understood, provides us with a guide to this universal morality.

LIMITATIONS OF BEING HUMAN-CENTRIC

To understand Taoist morality, a practitioner has to go beyond a human-centric view. When a culture is human-centric, just like being egocentric, it means that at a deep level, people think they are the center of the universe. With a few rare exceptions, most human beings have no direct experience of what happens after death, and thus form their beliefs based on their current reincarnation. Even for those who believe in the afterlife, at the end of the day, for most, there is still no direct experience of other worlds.

A human-centric view often fails to consider the myriad of other life forms on our planet and to see that the earth itself is a living being. Without this perspective it becomes easy to treat the other forms of life and our planet as a resource to be used, dominated and controlled, rather than treated with a morality that is based on reverence, cooperation and respect.

The human-centric view also imposes severe limitations on the ability to experience what scenarios a soul may undergo through the totality of time. Many humans have difficulty seeing past the present moment. They can be extremely tribal in the broadest sense. They have different tribes based on infinite sets of criteria such as location (nationality); belief systems; identifications both intellectual and emotional; political, economic, and social habits, and needs and desires. Many common moral ideas, although easy to grasp and emotionally satisfying, may be misleading and partial because they don't take the whole picture or context into account.

Simply recognizing that there is more out there than you can possibly know is a starting point to developing a wider sense of morality. By realizing your mind is limited, you can become more conscious of when its conditioning is not serving you or those around you.

ONLY ACQUIRE WHAT YOU WILL USE

Another aspect of Taoist morality considers greed and acquisition. In the modern era, some people are driven by an insatiable appetite to own and consume, the energy of which is sometimes brought into sex. Taoists, in general, are not attached to having or acquiring "stuff." They have a simple philosophy: it's fine to acquire or keep anything, as long as you actually use it. This includes obtaining supplies or reserves as a buffer against hard times.

Conversely, it is unwise to possess what you know you won't use. To do so is to put a "black karmic mark" on your soul—a debt that sooner or later will come due. However, if you only have what you use, you don't particularly create that kind of karma, so everything is very clean and smooth.

MIND OF MAN VERSUS MIND OF TAO

Taoism's main moral perspective is universal in scope, which is why Taoists constantly contrast the Mind of Man and Mind of Tao, two concepts identified in the *I Ching*.

MIND OF TAO

Taoist morality is based on the ongoing spiritual evolution of Beings, or the Mind of Tao, rather than perceived moral appropriateness, or on any current moment in time or space. The Mind of Tao leads to a natural, open state of mind that is guided and moves from an inner source of love and pure awareness. This Mind needs no rules imposed from outside—it trusts the moment and allows life to unfold. It is the Great Way that enables virtue to unfold naturally within a human being.

In Taoist thought, the circle of life includes both the external world and the internal realm of soul and Spirit. Every great religion and spiritual system expresses this universal truth in some way. No matter how beautiful the poetry used to describe the external world, it only hints at the vastness that becomes available once we turn within. This draws us toward essence and carries us over the threshold to the infinite perfection and wordless wonder of the Tao.

In the absence of at least some hint of this, the attraction to externals is all-consuming and covers us with spiritual malaise. We're addicted to the hollow promises of the rules of man and the safety of not having to deal with our afflictions. This, however, leads people into a spiritual dead end.

MIND OF MAN

The *I Ching* has a term for external fixations: the Mind of Man. This external mind is constantly processing all the rules about right and wrong, and good and bad that we have learned. The mind generates a nonstop stream of unfocused thought that dwells in the past and projects its fears and everything else into the future. It avoids the now. It is a mind that constantly ruminates, believing itself to be all-important and solid, when actually the opposite is true.

The Mind of Man is driven by short-term satisfactions and worldly pleasures that don't touch the hunger of the soul. Our innermost being craves something far more lasting and real. A key passage in the New Testament points to this dilemma by asking the question, "For what does it profit a man to gain the whole world, and forfeit his soul?"[2]

---

2. Mark 8:36

The Mind of Man squeezes people into little corners or boxes and makes life miserable through all the conditioning and rules imposed by religion, morality systems, legal rules, parents, culture and so on. Not all these rules are negative, but they are often dictated by the family, society and culture a person was born into. Many beliefs and assumptions are taken as true with no conscious reflection or choice.

Unfortunately, few make it through childhood with an intact awareness of who they truly are beyond conditioning. We all begin as naturally joyous, potentially cooperative beings and then get socialized into long-suffering but nonetheless "civilized" adults. No surviving large society consistently ushers children into adulthood without leaving them with psychological issues and problems.[3] We stray far from our essence as natural, spiritual beings.

Settling the Red Dust

Absorbed in the details of daily life, in the wants and desires of the moment, many are lulled into directing their attention outward to focus primarily on the external world. Our energy swirls around, this way and that, attempting to understand and control what is outside us. Taoists call this the "red dust." On this point, Taoists and Buddhists agree—everything changes, and nothing is as solid as it seems.

This important lesson was brought home to me in my studies with Liu Hung Chieh. First he mixed some reddish dirt in a glass of clear water. "This dirt," he said, "is like all the bound energies inside all the levels of your eight bodies." He shook the dirt up, and as we watched it swirl, then settle, he told me, "The settling of the dust is just the beginning of clearing out your energies in the first four energy bodies." He shook the dirt up again. Meditation is a process of shaking up the dust inside you and clearing it out of all of the first seven energy bodies until nothing remains but pure water, the essence of your natural self. Then even the water disappears when you join with the Tao.

The need to manage our circumstances and the drama of people, places and things constantly draws us to the churning of the red dust. People are easily fooled into believing the physical, external reality is all there is. They forget that we are all spiritual beings inhabiting a body.

SEXUAL CONDITIONING AND BURDENS

Although our sexual nature isn't inherently a burden, many of us carry a tremendous amount of baggage in the form of fear, anxiety, repression, confusion, guilt and

---

3. Some of these issues are discussed in Liedloff, Jean, *The Continuum Concept* (Cambridge: Perseus, 1975).

dissatisfaction as regards sex. The sexual attitudes of our parents seep into our consciousness from a very young age, as do the prevalent attitudes of the culture and language in which we're raised. Ideas about what is morally good and right, bad and evil or hip and cool among our peer group overlay what we feel drawn to experience and explore. The current Western culture, which promotes sex as a commodity or uses it to sell products, creates another barrier to moral clarity about sexual issues.

This heavy sexual baggage results in a very shaky foundation to develop a sense of natural ease and balance toward sex. Instead, many are pushed out of shape about this essential aspect of our nature and what is natural. Many develop skewed, unhealthy perspectives on sexuality—or at least stop exploring and shut off this essential aspect of humanity. These perspectives, in turn, create reactive internal pressures that affect moral behavior.

The result is that many lose their inner guidance system, which has been usurped and swamped by the burdens of conditioning. Buried beneath all sorts of overt and implied assumptions, beliefs, demands and expectations, it no wonder that people cannot perceive from a relaxed and open state of being. Rather they adopt ideas like "this is right, that is wrong," that have been drilled into them from an early age, unconsciously shaping how they think and behave.

Here are common internal burdens:

- Scars of abuse, rape and incest
- Thinking that sex is only for procreation
- Religious attitudes that invoke guilt about pleasure
- Legal or illegal addictions
- Needs for approval/disapproval
- Expectations about how people should act, feel or think
- Issues with perceived authority figures
- Destructive emotions
- Negative self-esteem

These burdens, especially when not consciously worked out, can put people out of touch with themselves and warp their moral thinking. In sexual relationships this can be as obvious as a partner who is afraid of sex, refuses sex consistently, can't get erections or is nonorgasmic. It can also be as obscure as a partner who complains of tiredness, headaches and low energy. These burdens can also cause people to have attitudes about sex that are actively destructive.

Once put into the unconscious mind, any conditioned attitude takes root. Just like the roots of a plant, these beliefs draw their nourishment from below the surface of awareness (consciousness itself) and feed what is visible above ground (our personality and behaviors). In this way, any moral attitude or belief becomes part of a person's neurology, which recreates that belief at every turn.

Most lose track of the extent to which they are controlled by these unconscious forces and mistake them for who they are. Such is the nature of conditioning. What's most unfortunate is that most people don't even recognize that they have been conditioned. As with the previous examples, they remain enslaved to subliminal forces, oblivious and unaware of behavior patterns that run internal emotions and dialogue. Their moral compass easily becomes skewed.

It is common for people to return again and again to the external world for answers. They falsely belief if they can master the outer world beyond their physical body then all will be well. Meanwhile, much of what is inside goes unnoticed. They fail to get to the root of the problem.

Modern Media, Sex and Youth

Throughout their early years, boys and girls of impressionable ages are fed a constant diet of unhealthy, unattainable sexual images in the media that often have nothing to do with reality or how to relate to the opposite sex in a human fashion. Repetitive and graphic, these powerful images program youth on how they should feel about themselves and the opposite sex. This conditioning is often done at a young age, when they do not have the discernment to distinguish truth from falsehood.

This constant barrage of images and programming comes from a full spectrum of media, including magazines, film, television, mobile applications, billboards and the Internet, including porn sites. Both sexes suffer from negative influences that become implanted and internalized within the developing psyche and personality.

Much of what both sexes are conditioned into believing about sex is simply not true. Although boys and girls don't need to buy into these ideas, they often end up basing their lives on them, rarely questioning these initial influences. Why does this happen? Often it is because of greed, exploitation and consumerism.

As Erich Fromm noted in *The Art of Loving*,[4] "(Western) culture is based on the appetite for buying, on the idea of a mutually favorable exchange…two persons thus fall in love when they feel they have found the best object available on the market, considering the limitations of their own exchange values."

---

4. Fromm, Erich, *The Art of Loving* (New York: Perennial Classics, 1956, 2000), 3.

Girls will be led to believe that they shouldn't feel good about themselves unless they have the perfect boyfriend, the "really something" body without imperfections, the right weight or attitude or else the boys won't like them. Then there are the fantasy images of whom a girl should reflexively be attracted to as potentially desirable or repulsed by as a useless lover. Arising in the wake of such conditioning are anxiety, depression, loneliness, isolation and extreme behaviors like anorexia, bulimia, and so on.

Boys are conditioned with parallel stereotypes. Those having the "nerd syndrome," or who are less conventionally handsome believe they should fear not being worthy of girls. Even for the "good looking," this social conditioning often results in reflexive posing, bravado or a nasty disdain for girls who "don't measure up." Many shy boys and nerds even at a later age will still find it quite difficult simply to talk to the opposite sex for fear of rejection or ridicule. The media also reinforces the message that only weak men show very human emotional vulnerability. Thus boys learn not to trust that girls can be open to feeling what they do. Yet, in reality most of these media-induced images of manhood are untrue.

The young usually don't have role models with serious sexual experience who can give them the straight story regarding what commonly happens between the sheets. Instead, for sexual education they turn to the distorted and unrealistic images shown in magazines, books or films. Thus they are woefully unprepared for the point when a relationship leads to real sex.

THE PERMISSION TO HAVE SEX

When someone asks, "What about Taoist ethics and morality?" nine times out of ten, the person really wants to know about sexual ethics. They often want to get permission for having regular, satisfying sex that may be denied to them in the particular moral system to which they adhere, or they want to obtain justification to condemn what isn't in accord with their current sexual moral beliefs. This really misses the point of the Taoist way. Rarely do people realize that, in Taoism and many other religions, the moral answers do not primarily lie in the external realm, but rather within.

Sex to Taoists is generally *wu so hui,* or it's okay if you do or don't. As such, Taoists believe that as long as there is no forceful external coercion, consenting adults need no special permission to either have or not have sex with each other. The primary caveat is that both individuals take care to keep the karma genuinely clean.

SEXUAL FREEDOM AND THE MIND OF MAN

There are countless games that get played out in the sexual arena. Lovers come and go. Women and men have umpteen agendas and expectations that they confuse with natural desires and needs. Even those who appear to be wild and free have hang-ups. Sex is a loaded topic on the singles circuit, regardless of age.

A Taoist would ask, "Why is this basic and natural human need riddled with so much confusion and discontent? Why have people shut off this essential aspect of their nature and humanity? What gets in the way of developing a real sense of ease and balance about sex?"

The answer would be that the Mind of Man makes people constantly preoccupied with a whole array of mental, emotional and physical blocks in their energetic bodies that keep them out of touch with direct experience. The limited perspective of the Mind of Man—with all its attitudes, stories and excuses—keeps people's dissatisfaction in place and their minds constantly churning.

Taoists would pragmatically look at issues of the Mind of Man and suggest the following:

1. Apply your full awareness to any individual situation.

2. Do your best to understand the entire context of the situation and its range of implications.

3. Attempt to act ethically by moving forward with as much balance and compassion as possible.

Taoists would also prescribe meditation as a way to see the patterns of the Mind of Man and become aware of the Mind of Tao within. At the beginning stages this would be a solo meditation practice, often done sitting. This is the easiest place to start to see how the deeper levels of the mind work. Later, meditation advances to interactive practices, such as sexual meditation with a partner.

Taoist sexual qigong and sexual meditation are renowned for giving people practices that free them from dead-end journeys. By focusing on internal energies and progressively building awareness, many of life's dissatisfactions dissipate. Taoist practices help to develop a new view of morality based not on conditioning but on recognizing what is universally right or at least sensible in the light of karma. Until a person becomes aware of his or her conditioning and the attitudes that bind them, they are not in a position to be free of that conditioning. As the ancient Greek philosopher Socrates said, "The unexamined life is not worth living."[5]

Another ancient Greek proverb offers perhaps some of the wisest, most succinct spiritual advice ever given: "Know thyself." One of the single most effective ways to

---

5. Plato, *Apology* 38a.

do this is through meditation, including Taoist sexual meditation, combined with such preparatory practices as qigong, sexual qigong, tai chi, Indian or Taoist yoga, or tai chi push hands. These practices can lead to freedom from conditioning and the various belief systems that enslave people. Taoist meditation does not force you to do anything against your will, quite the contrary. It enables you to make the best choices according to your own inward nature, depending on the ever-changing conditions that surround events and your relationships with other souls.

Genuine meditation is not about thinking and intellectual analysis. Beyond ordinary perception, it involves becoming aware of awareness itself. This eventually allows you to relax your mind so that it can open and eliminate boundaries, big or small, either in this or any other world. Meditation provides a direct method for accessing all that is inside you and revealing and eventually clearing your blockages.

> *Genuine meditation is not about thinking and intellectual analysis. Beyond ordinary perception, it involves becoming aware of awareness itself.*

AWARENESS AND YOUR MORAL COMPASS

Taoists believe that for people to have a chance at becoming spiritually free and reaching moral bedrock, they must at some point choose whether to play solely by the moral rules provided in their culture or religion or to move beyond in the direction of greater and greater awareness.

Understanding and living by Taoist morality is arrived at through inner cultivation and ongoing practice. There are two major stages to arrive at this morality:

Stage One: Here you deeply investigate all your moral values, ethics and cultural conditioning. For many, this can involve an extended inner struggle, often quite unique to each individual. Over time, with humility, you penetrate to your core. At this point you can decide if any of your moral positions make sense, and if so, to what degree, given a range of variable circumstances. This enables you live with a personal internal sense of morality generated from the underlying spirit of the Golden Rule, to do to others as you would have them do to you. Then you attempt to act within the moral framework that makes sense to you and minimizes internal conflict and strain. At the end of this stage you find a stable, moral common sense, something quite rare in our current times.

Stage Two: Next you deal practically with and work to go beyond the polarization of opposites within yourself so that you can be solid in the beginning stages of your meditation practice. The goal here is to stably enter emptiness, and from there, eventually arrive at nonduality. These two concepts form the bedrock of both Taoist and Buddhist thought. They can simply be described as "what is both beyond and includes all opposites simultaneously." This stage is required to arrive at a morality based on pure awareness. If someone can't get past the conditioning and the polarization that opposites create, it's very difficult, if not impossible, for that person to look at any situation morally from the lens of pure awareness.

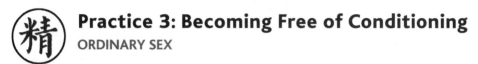

Practice 3: Becoming Free of Conditioning
ORDINARY SEX

To begin unraveling the Mind of Man and your internal conditioning, look at any cultural assumption you hold and then really take it apart. Ask yourself, "If I could start fresh and remake my life, is this something I would agree to?" If you start your investigation with that question, you might come up with some startling insights, because it is rare to direct your attention to the existing beliefs and assumptions you hold and inherited unconsciously. You might become aware of how unaware you really are.

Here are some questions you might ask yourself:

1. How did the views of my parents influence my views on sex, how to be in a relationship with a partner, and how to bring up children?

2. What are the views about sex in the religion in which I was brought up?

3. How have my views about morality been influenced by role models I respect or by my peer group?

Begin to see that you may be lost in thought loops and patterns for most of the day, every day. This is the first step toward freedom. Becoming aware that you are unaware instantly gives you access to the next level of higher awareness. More importantly, you might become more open to using the Taoist methods of meditation that can free you from your conditioning. ●

SPECTRUM OF TAOIST PRACTITIONERS

In terms of sexual politics, Taoism has groups within it that have opinions that range from very conservative and celibate, to moderate, liberal and even libertine in the extreme. The following is a summary of the most typical groups or camps, none considered greater or lesser than the other, but all making up the composite of Taoist practitioners.

CONSERVATIVES, MODERATES AND LIBERALS

Taoist conservatives tend to conform to what they perceive as the old reliable ways and cultural patterns of the society in which they live. They like to live extremely disciplined, moderate and regulated lives with clear, repetitive rhythms in their daily affairs, such as when they go to sleep, wake up, practice, work, interact with people and so on. Generally it is difficult to obtain Taoist teachings from them and they are very formal in their approach towards students. Conservatives usually shy away from sexual meditation. Instead they are more likely to prefer solo meditation and, if not celibate, ordinary sex.

The moderate Taoists in the middle hold the position that the ideal and often the only practical environment in which to practice sexual work is within a committed marriage or partnership, or at the very least, a regular relationship. Both partners within the context of their sexual situations must know the techniques, deal with all the pressures of worldly life and work on their spiritual evolution together.

Moderate Taoists often live "normal" lives within society. They go to school, work, run businesses, engage in professions, marry, produce and raise children, and so on. Their daily lives are filled with human activities that would be quite familiar to you in a multitude of aspects.

For two moderate Taoists who choose to practice sexual meditation, the best scenario involves setting up a regular practice schedule. Consistency is important not only because it allows the relationship to develop but also because, over time, that very regularity dramatically increases the speed at which blockages can be resolved.

The most liberal (or left wing) Taoists believe it is not necessarily ideal for two people to be bonded together to learn and benefit from sexual dissolving practices— unless both partners have had sufficient experience and practice to engage at all energetic levels. Members of ordinary, conservative society are not particularly fond of these liberal men and women because of their highly sexual natures. As people, they are dramatically more socially loose and, in addition, they are extremely open and free with their sexuality. In general, the liberal Taoists view any drama or dysfunctional behavior that arises between sexual consorts as a golden opportunity to become more spiritually awake by resolving such behavior at its roots.

However, both moderate and liberal Taoists agree that the greatest benefits from either sexual qigong or meditation liaisons are to be had with another fully-trained practitioner. Being the pragmatics that they are, they recognize that this is not always possible and that we live in less than ideal circumstances. Although you may be a practitioner of Taoist sexual techniques, your partner may not be or even want to be. In addition, either partner may belong to and deeply believe in a different non-Taoist religion or philosophy.

CRAZY WISDOM

Within the tradition of Taoism are the ultra-leftist crazy wisdom practitioners and teachers. One of the most well-known was Zhuangzi (Chuang Tse), who wrote a book under that name. He was a follower of Laozi. Conventional norms don't apply to crazy wisdom teachers. They literally live "out of the box," operating above and beyond the natural adherence to values, including sexual mores, which are held dear by conservatives. In Chinese, the Taoist Water tradition is sometimes called Lao-Zhuang, combining the philosophies of conservative Laozi and ultra-liberal Zhuangzi.

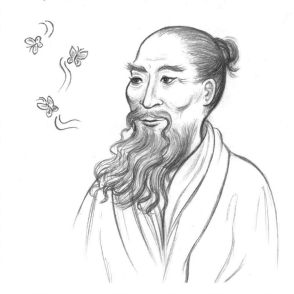

Crazy wisdom teachers[6] aim to enable those they interact with to advance spiritually at the greatest possible speed. They achieve this with what may appear to others as unexpected, radical behavior. They often intentionally seek out and engage (or, at minimum, will not avoid) heated situations that expose and explode hidden karma, so it can be resolved in the fastest manner possible. To crazy wisdom types, bringing the hidden karma to the surface provides an ideal opportunity to most rapidly work through, dissolve and finish it.

A well-known quote attributed to Zhuangzi is "I dreamed I was a butterfly, but now I wonder, am I a man dreaming of being a butterfly, or am I a butterfly dreaming of being a man?"

Figure 4-3: Taoist Crazy Wisdom Teacher Zhuangzi

The actions of crazy wisdom teachers are more often than not incomprehensible to those who do not have access to karmic vision. Someone who can truly "see" in the karmic dimension has an ability to grasp and understand the forces influencing a person's life from a frame of reference that extends far beyond what most can deal with, much less comprehend. This is why these teachers rarely explain what they are doing. Their purposeful secrecy is not so much covert as compassionate. Disclosing what the crazy wisdom teacher sees at the karmic level and his or her methods of intervention, including what potential effects they may have over time, would enable recipients to derail the process. To their detriment, they would find some way to unintentionally compromise or nullify the potential benefits of the crazy wisdom that's being sent their way.

---

6. The author belonged to this tradition during his training to become a Taoist priest.

Crazy wisdom is not a game for spiritual children. Crazy wisdom practitioners and teachers do not exploit others. A genuine teacher of this tradition would not condone those who might put on a charade of crazy wisdom simply because they philosophically like the idea, feel it suits their personality or desire to create a cult. Most crazy wisdom teachers are highly advanced practitioners, not beginners. Their path demands that they first acquire immense experience, emotional stability and personal evolution before moving toward spiritual realization, otherwise they could self-destruct. They have developed great integrity, wisdom and compassion.

Within Taoism, the role of crazy wisdom teachers is to be catalysts for spiritual awakening and, as such, to be comfortable with extremes in people and situations. They will let the winds blow regardless of how strongly they challenge an individual's ego. To them, nothing within a person—or a society—is more important than serving the greater karmic good.

A Radical Approach to Depolarization

In the absence of balance and integration of yin and yang in a person, what often results is the painful polarizations that feed the battle between the sexes. Because this problem is so deeply entrenched and severe in the human condition, some Taoists took up a radical sexual practice designed to depolarize the man-woman dynamic. According to their reasoning, an extreme method had to be used and had a far greater chance of succeeding than the other classic Eastern approach of solo meditation and solitary retreat.

As part of the training for the Taoist priesthood in some groups, male initiates were instructed to sleep with a thousand different women. Female initiates were required to sleep with a minimum of one hundred different men.[7] The goal was to completely balance yin and yang through full engagement with these energies. This radical approach would be considered outright sinful in God-fearing religions. The Taoists of this group saw this approach as the shortest and most direct route to transcendence. Rather than sex addiction or selfish, promiscuous behavior, this was an intentional method to encounter and fully balance inner male and female energies.

Why was there such a difference in the number of lovers required? Because yin energy naturally wants to bond with yang—it is, in fact, yin's most powerful urge. Due to her natural inclination, and the fact that yin gives birth to yang, a woman will find it relatively easy to access the male energy of her partner. Her intrinsic nature and life conditions accelerate the process, whereas a man's intrinsic nature

---

7. Similarly, there was a "mystery school" tradition in Ancient Egypt where female priestesses would have sex with large numbers of men for religious and spiritual purposes.

is to constantly put on the brakes. Staying with this metaphor, it could even be said that a man's natural tendency is to throw it in reverse! For a woman to reach a point at which sex transcends the inclination to attachment and becomes pure yang is relatively easy compared to what is required of a man to transcend to pure yin. His natural yang aversion to bonding makes it infinitely harder for a man to directly comprehend the bonding essence of yin's nature.

SEXUAL NONINTERFERENCE PRINCIPLE

The principle of noninterference is an important feature for practitioners in Laozi's Water tradition. Sometimes sexual partners are open to Taoist practices and sometimes they are not. One partner may have an idea of what he or she considers normal, not wanting to do anything he or she considers "weird." That partner may decide that the idea of qi running through energy bodies is not in line with their religious beliefs. The person could vehemently object to knowing that something subtle, much less psychic, is occurring during sex. This person may deeply love the other partner and be quite satisfied with the sexual and personal relationship. They may just ask not to participate in some or all of the Taoist sex practices.

What do you do if you want to engage in sexual practices but your partner currently says, "Sexual practices are your thing, but not mine" and chooses not to want to know or be involved in them?

The pragmatic Taoists hold the position of noninterference, which encompasses the no coercion, no deception principle. In the Taoist view, you and your partner each have a right to your own sexual beliefs and ways of living. The principle implies that neither do you have the right to interfere in someone's life by either constantly pressuring them to join you in whatever it is you choose to do, nor can you expect or demand that they at least condone what you are doing. It is important not to, in any way, impose and force your sexual ways on the other. You are not to physically or psychologically coerce your partner into participating in your ideas about sexuality.

Likewise, others don't have the right to interfere with your meditating, as long as you are completely present with them and doing your best to make the sexual and personal relationship work. You can simply practice your sexual meditation techniques in silence without any obligation to discuss them.

Although your partner may not gain the maximum amount possible, most likely he or she will benefit sexually from your increased sensitivity and energy, and the smoothing out of subliminal emotional messages that can otherwise become barriers to intimate human communications.

If a practitioner really likes and wishes to teach a partner the Taoist sexual meditation methods, the Taoist noninterference doctrine requires full disclosure. If a partner chooses to engage with you about Taoist sexual techniques, he or she must willingly agree and freely engage in your lifestyle or personal interests—or not. The choice must be freely made, either way.

After broaching the subject and giving your partner a thorough sense of what he or she is getting into and presuming agreement, you must broach that subject again at least three times on different occasions to ensure that your partner is truly willing. Partners must be given every opportunity to change their minds and say no. You must not try to trick them into saying, "Yes, I want to do this." Every opportunity that you can think of must be given to get them off the hook, so that if they engage, it's because they chose to do so of their own free will. Partners must not be manipulated in any fashion, shape or form. This is the Taoist way of being equally pragmatic and moral.

THE KARMA OF SEX

Clearly, sex is an agent of human bonding. Sexual attraction, whether consummated or not, provides a bridge through which two people can connect, when they might not otherwise have come together. Regardless of whether they choose to act on the attraction or whether the sexual liaison is long or short lived, that initial draw can lead two people to form a very strong, intimate bond. Many lifelong friendships are formed as a result of an early sexual attraction that grows into mutual respect and appreciation after the urge is acted on (or not) and the two find their way into a suitable relationship that is right for them.

Taoists would advise against sleeping with someone just to satisfy a sexual urge if the energy, the qi, is not right. To do so will produce rather than resolve negative karma. This principle is folded within a phrase from the *Tao Te Ching:* "The wise man has no enemies." In other words, everyone in the world is your friend. Feeling this truly, from the bottom of your heart, is ever more crucial when it comes to deciding whether to have casual lovers.

Monogamous or not, married or not, Taoists have a basic principle: only have sex with your friends. At minimum, you should care about the humanity of the person you are having sex with. To have sex with someone you really don't like will damage your consciousness, diminish your heart and have negative karmic repercussions.

Taoists observe a more esoteric version of the Golden Rule: "Whatever you do to someone, you have just also done to the depths of your unconscious mind and spiritual consciousness." Karma does exist, and what you put out will come back to bless or haunt you—so be good to yourself and each other.

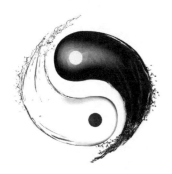

CHAPTER 5

The Path of Taoist Sexual Practice

Let's face it: people make a big deal about sex, especially in a milieu that represses or attempts to curb our sexual expression in a myriad of ways. From the Taoist point of view, sex is a function of life and is neither special nor shameful. As such, the Taoists approach sex as a practical concern to be explored with intelligence.

Taoists take a clear stand: as you explore, make sure you can actually learn something of value from each experience. Recognizing where you are and what's going on within can take you to the next place. This is true both for sex and for spirituality in general.

Once you start the path, you'll go deeper and deeper with each practice. Expect to face various obstacles, issues and fears on the journey ever more inward. It's like going through a series of locks or gates—as you progress, you must resolve and unlock each one before moving forward. Some will be difficult and some easy. Consistent practice over time affords you the time to dissolve blockage after blockage, even the most difficult ones, to reveal what is true. Often as you proceed, you'll find that what once was important to you becomes less so as your awareness grows and your consciousness shifts. Each resolution brings you closer to the essence of who you are.

As you proceed on the journey inward, you'll find that what once was important to you becomes less so as your awareness grows and your consciousness shifts. Each resolution brings you closer to the essence of who you are.

GUIDELINES ON THE TAOIST SEXUAL PATH

Here are some useful guidelines for those who choose to explore and start Taoist sexual practices.

FOCUS ON FEELING, NOT THINKING

A great problem for many people is the tendency to think about what they feel and intellectualize emotions. When a person is not open to the *felt* reality of his or her emotions they are unable to know what is happening within because the energy rises to their head. Moreover, when deeper emotional garbage rises to the surface, it often gets expressed in destructive ways. As a result, seemingly normal people may shift into negative states that could hurt themselves and others. A common example in Western culture is road rage, a kind of knee-jerk response arising from anger, impatience or fear bubbling up from under the surface.

Rather than relate to others on a human level, overly mind-dominated people override their shared humanity and lose access to higher positive emotions. An overarching intellectual stance, such as "all is well with the world," "it's all good" or "might makes right," can allow a person's deep, unconscious neuroses to fester, leading him or her to become increasingly disturbed without even realizing this is the case.

Not feeling hidden emotions has many real consequences above and beyond reducing sexual pleasure. Even though many people have deep emotional issues, *the ability to feel that pain and discomfort and to feel remorse for their actions* is the saving grace that stops them from doing really sick and crazy stuff. Our ability to feel both pain and pleasure is a critical component of true humility and compassion.

Taoist practices are first and foremost about accessing your ability to feel, not just think about your feelings. Many Taoist techniques develop higher levels of internal awareness, connecting your feelings directly to your heart, and your heart to your mind.

GO INWARD TO FACE WHAT IS THERE

Directly confronting the burdens of conditioning takes courage, because it requires that you turn inward, begin to feel your body and notice how it responds when you get uptight, disturbed and fearful. This is very different from the standard approach of going into denial.

Once you can become fully present to your inner world, although you may find things that make you uncomfortable, you can then make choices to begin to heal yourself of any emotional and mental scars. The Taoist practices, especially meditation, can help you to live in the world with joy, balance and compassion, regardless of whatever chaos may be occurring around you.

Taoist sexual practices make achieving this goal a little easier, because you have a partner to help you navigate what can be some pretty tricky inner shoals. The practices are about healing yourself and helping your partner heal from his or her scars. The practices utilize the qi naturally generated during the sexual act to dissolve inner blockages.

There are many common patterns of avoidance. Some may wait to enter into relationships until they meet what they consider the perfect partner or until they find someone who doesn't reject them. Others may fantasize about withdrawing from life in the manner of a monk who, rather than deal with or transcend sexual needs or lust, must never allow his eyes to meet a woman's.

Rather than avoiding our humanness with its many temptations and vulnerabilities, a liberal Taoist would advise going right to the heart of the matter and, once there, dissolving all of whatever arises. In this way you can become free of what otherwise would continue to keep you in invisible chains. With deliberate practice, you can learn to remain truly open when real pressure hits and your wants and desires are thwarted.

The Taoists have an interesting saying on this fear of looking inside yourself and encountering the demons you might find: "The only thing you will find when you meditate and go inside yourself is what's there, regardless of whether it is good, bad, beautiful or ugly."

> *The only thing you will find when you meditate and go inside yourself is what's there, regardless of whether it is good, bad, beautiful or ugly.*

If you can maintain the courage to stay on the path, you can move out of the Mind of Man and into the Mind of Tao. On the way, you're likely to find out who you are, as the beauty, goodness, strength and truth within you comes forward and your true nature as consciousness is gradually revealed. What makes Taoist practices so potent is that they bring you to a place where you can accept what exists inside you. This leads you away from harsh judgments of good or bad. As the Tao teaches, everything changes, and as the *I Ching* says, "Everything futhers."

From the narrow perspective of any given moment in time, or the Mind of Man, it is difficult, even impossible, to know the ultimate result of getting or not getting what you want. Meditation helps you realize that it is perfectly fine in itself to want what you want, regardless of whether or not you get it, and ultimately, the only lasting value is the space of stillness inside.

DEVELOP EMOTIONAL STABILITY

Before anyone goes beyond the practices of ordinary sex—which can make lovemaking more pleasurable—and into sexual qigong practices, it is critical they become energetically stable, open, balanced and mature in their physical body, qi and emotions. To quote the Bible,[1] "When I was a child, I spoke as a child, I understood as a child, I thought as a child: but when I became a man, I put away childish things." To "put away childish things" is to gain emotional maturity.

Immature emotions are a perpetual problem of the human condition. Any adult who feels a strong emotion and defaults to dysfunction—for example, acting out, denial, blame-shifting, avoidance, over-personalizing, playing the victim or not accepting responsibility for one's actions—can be considered emotionally immature.

In this overly tense, overwrought Western culture, keeping a lid on emotional meltdowns is exceptionally difficult. Emotional immaturity locks people into the everyday motion of the Mind of Man—habits of thought that occupy their attention and perpetuate their negative ego.

Taoist practices help people reach balance and objectivity in their lives and prevent them from becoming overwhelmed by their emotions. The aim is to reach an emotionally stable place beyond personal hopes, fears, wants and dislikes. This is an important point of the entire universal play of yin and yang. The universe is in play, not the way we wish it to be, but the way it is. You want to reach a place where the conscious and unconscious mind are in harmony with one another and feel smooth and balanced.

BE CONSISTENT AND STEADY

Taoist practices progressively build inner awareness; they loosen old knots from the inside out through a process of energetically releasing them. You become more mature and balanced in stages, allowing you to stabilize your inner turbulences. With each new insight and release, you work to ground the new awareness inwardly. Only after this is done should you move on to the next practice.

As you do this, you increasingly move toward being genuinely honest, inwardly as well as with others, taking into account the unique circumstances surrounding each relationship as it evolves. Each Taoist practice helps you increase your powers of intuitive understanding. These qualities grow gradually over time and cannot be rushed, regardless of whatever goal or timeframe your mind has chosen.

Taoist Water method practices are not associated with the promises of instantaneous success. Expecting instant gratification is a prime reason why people gravitate to

---

1. Corinthians 13:11.

Fire method–oriented workshops, which promise sudden emotional breakthroughs and spectacular orgasmic sex. When you adopt a new view that temporarily allows you to bounce back into an upbeat frame of mind, suddenly you feel incredibly good, even wonderful. But most often these temporary fixes or energy infusions don't last, and very shortly you're right back to where you started.

When you hurtle like a roller coaster between emotional highs and lows, elation and depression, this exacerbates the inability of the nervous system to relax. Instead, it keeps you in a state of constant rev. Even if some of what is taught within these types of Fire methods is positive, it seldom leads to a place of emotional stability. If your underlying imbalances have not been addressed, it usually isn't long until you feel terrible again. If the deep tensions are emotional, they can make you ever more miserable, and if the tensions get strong enough at the psychic level, they can cause some people to break down or even go mad.

In contrast, the Water method practices help you understand morality and energy gradually by direct awareness and perception of your internal processes. These insights help free you from the burdens that conditioning has imposed and help you to develop a sense of natural ease and balance in your life, including in relationships with those around you and with your sexual partners. Your conditioning gets peeled back gradually, layer after layer, in a sensible and sustainable manner that improves your life over time.

A typical response heard from those learning preliminary qigong methods for releasing tension is, "There's so much tension in there. I had no idea how much I was unable to relax." When people realize how disconnected their consciousness is from their body, they can often become discouraged and give up.

A more sensible attitude is to start loosening the internal resistances and tensions knot by knot—a little at a time. This builds confidence and diminishes resistance and fear. Always remember to start with what is easy first and progress from there. Then, once you've seen some success, you will be willing to go further. This strategy works for all Taoist methods, including all the sexual exercises that are done with partners.

This gradual approach is one of the cornerstones of the Water method. Over time, a steady stream of water will open a hole through the rock and widen it until the rock completely disappears. On the Taoist path you first deal with some of the overt physical tension, and then go forward to deal with easier emotional tensions, and so on over time. That way you and your partner build on successes and the ensuing trust that develops will encourage you to go farther.

OVERCOME THE FEAR OF SEXUAL REJECTION

Rejection is unavoidable—it's part of the package of many sexual quests. We all get rejected somewhere along the line, often by those who make us ache with desire. Fear of rejection and the strategic avoidance of that particular pain can put a serious torque in our emotional world. For some of us, the fear of rejection causes significant suffering in the form of anticipatory dread or social withdrawal.

To diminish or fully resolve this common problem, Taoists begin with Outer Dissolving methods and progressively go deeper using Inner Dissolving meditation agendas.[2] If you were working with the question, "How can I get past this fear?" you might initially use Outer Dissolving methods in sitting meditation or the practices of standing dissolving within Opening the Energy Gates of Your Body™ Qigong.[3] However, if you want a full resolution on the question, "How can I resolve the root of this rejection issue?" it might be more effective to use not only sexual qigong but also Inner Dissolving within sexual meditation where you work with both your own energy and that of your partner (see Chapter 15, Practice 32, "Dissolving the Fear of Sexual Rejection").

A common Taoist way to deal with negative emotions such as fear of rejection is to do the opposite of what most people do—steer directly toward them rather than back away. In this way, any drama or dysfunctional behavior that arises between sexual partners is viewed as an opportunity to become more aware, rather than something to be avoided. In those moments, the energy revs up and is more accessible to you and to your partner to be meditated upon and overcome.

Using dissolving methods, any upheaval can be used to uncover and overcome blockages within the lower (first through seventh) energy bodies. In fact, among sexual meditation practitioners, that is overtly stated as the goal: to continuously seek and resolve the essential nature of the primal human emotions such as fear, jealousy, greed, manipulation or anger. Ultimately, the hope is that the fluctuating contents of an individual's consciousness can be recognized, unraveled and dissolved to reveal the transcendent changelessness from which everything arises and to which all things return.

AVOID BECOMING A SEXUAL SAVIOR OR MARTYR

Whatever problem you encounter in your partner, you are faced with a decision: Is it worth the effort required to ignite this person's sexual flame? Although the practices of dissolving in sexual qigong and sexual meditation can help resolve your own and your partner's blockages, a practitioner should avoid wanting to

---

2. See Frantzis, Bruce, *The Great Stillness* (Berkeley, CA: North Atlantic Books, 2001), 138–39.

3. See Frantzis, Bruce, *Opening the Energy Gates of Your Body: Qigong for Lifelong Health,* rev. ed. (Berkeley, CA: North Atlantic Books, 2006), chapters 6 and 7.

become a sexual savior or martyr. These qualities can easily become associated with ego, power or foolish compassion issues. Your level of enjoyment in both the short and long run (as best you can assess) should be the determining factor.

A Taoist friend told a story that illustrates the point. He met a woman he really enjoyed who was incapable of orgasm. Within four months of working together she became orgasmic. His attention and expertise paid off and the two spent a number of satisfying years together. A key indicator in the man's decision to continue the relationship was his own enjoyment.

The same principle applies to female practitioners. A Taoist woman in China trained a man to be a great lover over the course of a year. She was a highly orgasmic woman with a healthy sexual appetite, while the man initially was a total dead fish in the sack. But she really liked the man. She spent a month and a half with him before he would allow her to do fellatio without freaking out or shutting down. Then another three months passed after which he finally began to realize that she was his girlfriend and not his mother. Shortly thereafter, his sexual energy started to come alive. Before long, they hit a sweet spot and stayed together for a long time.

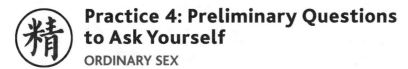

Practice 4: Preliminary Questions to Ask Yourself
ORDINARY SEX

If you and your partner are willing to go further with the Taoist sexual practices, you must face some crucial questions and honestly grapple with the fact that everyone's psyche contains unknowns. If you do not agree to take on this issue, the process will not work between two people.

When you endeavor to resolve your own and your partner's blocked emotional energies at the level of qigong or meditation, success is possible only via the route of moving toward unconditional acceptance. What's inside you sooner or later is bound to come out, just as is whatever might lurk deep in your lover's unconscious.

In the privacy of your own mind and heart, ask yourself these questions:

1. Am I willing to take on and dissolve whatever should arise for my partner, no matter how strong or disconcerting it may be?

2. Can I remain nonjudgmental, regardless of what arises?

3. Can I simply stay present, without assigning meaning to what my partner does?

4. Can I resist the temptation to interpret or read into what my partner says?

5. Can I listen without laying a guilt trip on my partner?

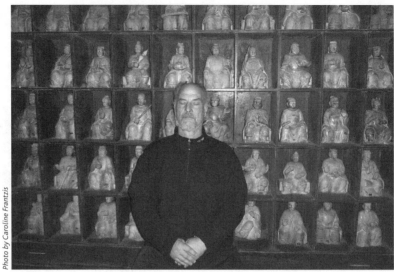

Photo by Caroline Frantzis

The author practices Inner Dissolving meditation
inside the Taoist Reed Flute Cave in Guilin, China.

Taoists invite you to consider these questions deeply, because being fully present with another can be more difficult than it sounds. It is absolutely crucial for you to recognize that resolution comes when the bound-up energy an individual has kept buried inside is expressed and dealt with, rather than denied. Without the needed equanimity, the release of bound energy can ignite a blame game or an attitude of either "You're not worthy to be with me," or "I'm not worthy to be with you." Dynamics like these will not only limit your success, they will poison the psychic and sexual waters between you. This can lead to constant emotional warfare or more subtle forms of disharmony, such as withholding, cold indifference, one partner taking an "I've given up" stance or the age-old "I got my thing, you get your thing" syndrome.

With sexual meditation, a different attitude prevails—one that encompasses a person's whole soul or Being. The sexual experience becomes satisfying at the physical, energetic and emotional level. Beyond that, orgasm expands the Spirit, giving peace and unity to the soul by opening into emptiness and touching the Tao, if only for a moment. ●

HOW TAOIST SEXUAL PRACTICES WERE TRADITIONALLY TAUGHT

In China, sexual qigong and meditation techniques were always taught both intellectually and by hands-on (body-on-body) coaching by masters of sexual meditation. It is of utmost importance to understand that these sexual practices were and are taught in a very specific context—that of meditation and enlightenment.

In some Taoist groups, these techniques were part of the traditional training given to students who wanted to be Taoist priests. Priests, both female and male, were then responsible for sharing the knowledge with the general Taoist community of practitioners. All the practices occurred only between a man and a woman.

These techniques were neither easy, nor perceived as being easy. Sexual practices require great courage and fearlessness. Again and again, the practitioner must bring forth the willingness to directly encounter difficult inner obstacles that prevent the full flowering of awareness that leads to freedom. All of the practices within Taoism's Water school start by using the energy naturally generated during the sexual act to access and release locked up energy. These blockages are personal in nature and unique to you, although they may have archetypal roots and societal origins.

FIVE MODALITIES OF TAOIST PRACTICES

Within Taoism there are five different types or modalities of practices—sitting, standing, moving, lying down and interactive methods, which include sex. All these practices exist along a continuum. It is often easier to learn something within a solo practice first before working with a partner.

Through Outer and Inner Dissolving methods you initially learn techniques while standing or sitting. Next you might put this into a moving practice, such as qigong, tai chi or the interactive practice of tai chi push hands, and only then would you integrate the method into another interactive practice like sexual meditation. In the later stages of development, the qualities and results indicative of true attainment are the same, whether achieved through sitting meditation or sexual meditation.

The major difference between sexual practices and the other four modalities of practice is that, *with the proper training,* a practitioner can get results much faster, because there is more available energy or qi.

TAOIST SEXUAL TRAINING METHODS

Traditionally, membership in Taoist groups that specialized in sexuality was secretive and new initiates were only admitted by invitation from existing members. The techniques were not available to the general public. Potential members were interviewed to ensure they were physically, emotionally and mentally stable before they were given an invitation to join. This invitation was not offered or taken lightly. Once a Taoist initiate was accepted he or she was then required to take various vows upon entry. Most initiates were ordinary members but some were in a more formal program to become Taoist priests. The training of priests within the group would be considerably more intensive than that undergone by ordinary members. The trainee priests were held to a much higher standard, as once ordained, they would be expected to be able to teach all aspects of the curriculum to the lay members of the group.

Regardless of the stage of training in sexual practices, the progression presented below was commonly used in most stages of a student's journey.

First the teacher would discuss the energetic context and provide instructions about how the trainee priests were to practice various sexual methods. After the information was imparted, it was the trainees' responsibility to find a partner and practice as best as they could.

The instruction was to practice with as many partners as needed until trainees "got the practical point of the exercise." It was preferred, but not mandatory, that practice partners be members of the same secret Taoist group, who liked being chosen to participate. If none were available, students were to find willing partners on their own. With a sex partner from outside the group who was interested in sex but not personally doing the sexual practices, students were taught how the practice could benefit that person as much as possible.

Once a trainee had fully absorbed and applied a particular lesson or practice, he or she would move ahead and learn more. Sometimes, the students would return to the teacher and say, "I got it" or "No problem, it worked." Then, when the teacher felt that it was time for a new subject, a new session would be scheduled.

However, sometimes students would return and say, "I'm not exactly sure what you meant, I'm fuzzy on the meaning of the details, I'm having this or that problem," and so on. In this situation, teachers would try to help them resolve the glitches by talking them through it and making suggestions for subsequent practice.

If, however, after sufficient attempts, a student had not fully embodied a lesson, a more direct approach was used. Two trainees would be instructed to make love in the presence of male or female coaches or elders as appropriate. The teacher would analyze what was missing and then coach the lovers.

Coaches might use one or a combination of these techniques:

- They would verbally, in a very gentle and intimate manner, but without physical contact, guide the students accurately through the process.
- They would use non-tactile energetic transmissions until a specific technique could be done with pleasure and awareness.
- Coaches might put their hands on either or both trainees, move body parts, enter orifices; or a male coach would switch places with the male trainee; or a female coach would switch with the female trainee until both trainees got it right.

- A male and a female coach might have sex in front of the students, demonstrating proper application of the techniques involved, while a third coach would be explaining what was going on and answering relevant questions.
- Two students would have sex, and along with talking, the coaches would physically guide them through it. The coaches would touch and direct the movements of all the students' relevant body parts, moving qi through the students' energy channels the way they ultimately wanted the students to be able to do by themselves. All the while the coaches would be transmitting and linking to the students, overcoming their habits of inner resistance and subliminally training the students' awareness. The coaches would tailor their instruction to the needs of the moment, such as when students got stuck or confused.

At the emergence of a student's glitch point, the students would stop having sex and watch the two coaches having sex to be shown how to resolve the glitch. Verbal explanations might originate from either of the coaches, or be given by a third coach on the sidelines who might also be physically moving the two coaches having sex to make it crystal clear what the students should be aiming for in future.

This is some of the more practical, hands-on sexual instruction for effectively and efficiently training students. The methods were not all that different than those used by athletic coaches or music instructors, except that the subject matter was sex.

As students progressed in their training, they were taught how to navigate completely new and uncharted psychic and karmic territories, where any form of conventional sexual morality based on the rules of society or religion would become meaningless. Such externally imposed values would literally disappear as practitioners moved into these realms, then further into various levels of emptiness and ultimately the Tao.

The time it took to learn sexual qigong and meditation would vary considerably. Students, particularly those who were not in the intensive priesthood training, might take five to ten years to become stable at the level of body and qi. This is the reason why, in the classical tradition, qigong would be practiced before Taoist meditation, and sexual qigong would be learned before sexual meditation.

For talented adults, each of the first three energy bodies requires at least one year of work. The physical body is addressed first, and then the qi body. Only then can the work on the emotional body begin—clearing inner ghosts and entering into emotional maturity. The mental body requires two or more years of work, and an open-ended amount of time is needed to clear the psychic body. The amount of time needed to work with the highest three bodies—karmic, essence and Tao—is indeterminate, because in the final stages the focus is on internal alchemy.

Learning Taoist Sexual Practices in the West

Sex is a highly charged subject in Western society. This is the main reason I have rarely taught Taoist sexual qigong or meditation, and the few courses I offered were mostly outside America. Rather than having a sincere interest in the tradition, some participants were just looking for permission to have sex, or they were simply seeking a social group in which they could freely express their sexual nature without an overlay of guilt or shame.

In the United States, effectively teaching Taoist sexual practices in the traditional manner would be difficult, if not impossible. As part of the Taoist priesthood training I underwent, initiates were required to develop considerable sexual experience that was not expected of ordinary members of the group to which I belonged: the recommendations for trainee priests were that men should complete Taoist sexual practices with one thousand women and women with at least one hundred men before having children. Among even the most liberal of Westerners, this amount of sex might seem daunting. Attempting to train students using the methodology of the Taoist priesthood would be severely hampered by the constraints of law, Western morality and social conventions.

The more challenging problem for Westerners wishing to learn Taoist sexual practices is that there are very few masters in the West who know enough to teach these techniques at the level of sexual qigong, and even fewer still who can teach the higher level practices of sexual meditation.

CONNECTING TO THE HEART-MIND

Once a Taoist teacher saw that a prospective student had a reasonable and responsible grasp of his or her first three energetic bodies (physical, qi and emotional), he or she would begin to teach the practices that begin with the fourth—the mental body—and move into what the Taoists call the heart-mind. Heart-mind is the undifferentiated source from which your intent and cognition originates prior to language, and from which thoughts emerge before they filter into your conscious awareness. This source is directly discernible in deep states of meditation.

Here the work is to dissolve and transcend the data-driven process of mundane, everyday consciousness in the interest of stumbling into the open and often silent stillness within. This place of openness, which may or may not be experienced as quietude, is the origin of Consciousness or the Tao.

The formless place of the heart-mind is a very refined space. It is the middle ground between qigong and serious meditation. It is the threshold where you move beyond the limits of qigong and enter into the deep, emotional clearing processes of meditation.

LEARNING CURVES

Different practitioners will have different learning curves and individual rhythms. Much of what may be initially learned in terms of qi and meditation can be quite challenging. Some techniques will be natural to you and easy to pick up. Others will require great struggle. However, at the end of the day, through steadfastness and perseverance, it may be that what was initially seemingly difficult or impossible you can now do in an even more relaxed, skillful and effortless manner than those things that seemed easy at first.

When you can do it, it's easy, and how difficult it may have been before becomes irrelevant. Regardless of whether it happens sooner or later, the main point is to get there. This is the same whether it's the ability to move qi in the body or, through meditation practices, to let go of the biggest stuck points in your soul. The more you can stay within the seventy-percent rule, the faster your practice will go from struggle to ease.

HOW TAOISTS WOULD TEACH ADOLESCENTS ABOUT SEX

The easiest way to cure a disease or a problem is to prevent it from ever occurring. Adolescents usually carry less mental and emotional baggage than adults for two prime reasons. They have not had the time to be exposed to a lot of physical, emotional and other problems that harden in their bodies over decades. Second, their bodily energy naturally flows more strongly.

Within traditional Taoist communities, young people were taught the physical and energetic nature of sexuality, as well as a sense of moral responsibility. This education generally began before puberty, thus smoothing the path into adolescence. A trained Taoist adolescent would have a comprehensive view of sex—in terms of the energy men and women put out, exchange and absorb—above and beyond the the purely physical aspects of sex.

If an adolescent was willing to learn, Taoist parents, or more likely aunts, uncles or elder members of a Taoist community, began to teach more advanced sexual methods a little before the age of fourteen to sixteen (a common age for marriage in ancient times). Each phase of this uniquely energy-based sex education emphasized fully engaging and balancing the eight energy bodies one at a time.

The foundational work of developing a general level of proficiency in controlling qi, either through qigong or meditation practices, would be a prerequisite.

By the age of sixteen the adolescent might have spent at least one or possibly two or even ten years clearing his or her first three energy bodies through qigong and sitting meditation. Many Taoist children began qigong at the age of six. If an adolescent began early, this foundation could be well set before the onset of puberty. Work on the physical, energetic and emotional bodies would then be revisited later, using essentially the same techniques while engaged in sexual activity.

Teaching youngsters so early about sexuality and related matters might well offend current Western sensibilities. However, ancient Taoists would find the unhealthy attitudes towards sex that the modern media instills in young people to be equally disturbing (see Chapter 4, "Modern Media, Sex and Youth").

SEX ACROSS THE LIFESPAN

Taoist teachings address the issues of our cyclic existence with respect for the many peaks and valleys every life takes along its long, winding journey. We are fortunate to have the type of body that is capable of being highly sexual into our eighties, nineties, or even longer. Whether sexually active or not, every person's sexual energy is tied to his or her first seven energy bodies. The precious opportunity we are given to actualize our potential hinges on our ability to utilize the natural resources available to us at each stage of life.

Understanding what underlies the emotional, mental, psychic and even karmic implications of sexuality is extremely valuable. The earlier we take up this investigation, the more progress we can make. Unfortunately, many never deal with this issue at all or only begin to do so after many failed relationships or a failed marriage.

It is important to examine your internal life before failures happen. Even so, the Taoist view is that whatever baseline or age you start from, the practices will nourish you and help you resolve the blockages that have gotten in the way of becoming a happy human being and of having a fulfilling sex life.

It is wise that while you still have sexual desire, you should enjoy and use it, because there's no guarantee it will be lifelong. Later in life, or even early in life, energetic elements within you sometimes shift, or you could find yourself in an internal space where sexual desire is absent.

YOUTH

Young people today have easy access through the Internet to all sorts of information about physical sex that historically was not available. What is often lacking, however, is guidance as to what it takes to interact with another human being on primal energetic levels. Without this type of input, young people go through all sorts of ups and downs trying to define what it means to be in a relationship. The predominant emotional energy that rides on the surface consumes their full attention. Rarely do they investigate what is happening at the depths or recognize the underlying energies that are in play.

Unrealistic self-judgments and expectations full of "should, ought to, must," based on inner images and ideas that no human could ever live up to, just perpetuate the confusion. Psychic interactions that go on subliminally before, during and after sex further exacerbate the situation. Most people are never trained to recognize telltale overt and subtle psychic signals. Add to this the dimension of karma and you can begin to sense the real complexity that exists the minute we engage in sex. No wonder the young can easily get frustrated, crestfallen and confused!

Among the Taoists, young people become interested in sexual meditation to learn how to fully open up their body's energies and maximize this naturally energetic phase of life. Youth is commonly the most sexual period of life. Young people may try many things in an effort to take the edge off the force of their hormones. Mood swings

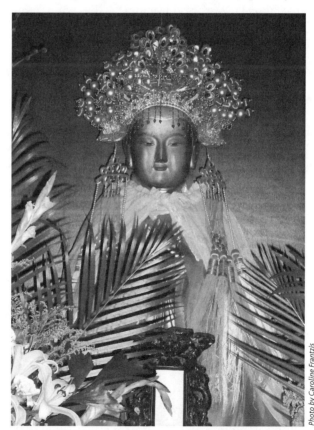

Photo by Caroline Frantzis

The Goddess Bixia Yuanjun in the Yuanjun Deity Hall at the Bai Yun Guan (White Cloud Taoist Temple) in Beijing.This is one of the most important Taoist sites in China.Bixia Yuanjun is said to bring lovers together and bless them with peace and harmony.

and stark emotional peaks and valleys that go from elation to depression at lightning speed drive sensible youths to look for ways to mature faster. When youthful foolishness is accompanied by genuine remorse, young people are in an excellent position to leave immature ways behind.

Young people who take up Taoist practices can leverage strong hormones, a vigorous body and natural youthful energy to open up their ordinary mind and expand their consciousness. Natural youthful energy is offered only once in a life, and it usually brings both happiness and misery. Sexual meditation can help young people resolve and remove inner blockages affecting many common issues that accompany this stage of life, including:

- Reducing sadness and enhancing joy.
- Moving beyond mood swings, malaise and depression.
- Resolving the "I don't know what I want to do with my life" syndrome.
- Turning early relationships into true awakenings and growth experiences rather than emotional roller-coaster rides that leave many young people in tense states of confusion.
- Empowering the individual to take control of his or her energy to build a happy life and stable relationships with partners and friends.

From a Taoist perspective, issues with the physical body are relatively easy to deal with. Far more complex are factors that arise from the third through seventh energy bodies. Educating the young about the energetic functions of sexuality is extremely helpful to enable them to have a smoother ride through this difficult stage of life.

MIDLIFE

Talk to an old Taoist about your midlife crisis and he or she is likely to say, "The clock is ticking and now is the time to truly resolve your karma." Now is the time to protect and build sexual energy because it has such a strong influence over the mechanisms of qi flow within all eight energy bodies. If an individual does not work with and make smooth his or her sexual energy before entering the golden years, then their emotional, mental and psychic energy won't be smooth either.

In this regard, sexual meditation is an accessible gateway to open your heart center and explore all relationships in depth. Having survived the excesses and vicissitudes of youth, midlife is the time to calm your body and mind for the long haul. Emphasis shifts from the body as the primary concern toward energy and spirit. The goal at this stage of life, specifically as regards sexuality, is to become emotionally and psychically clear.

Both Taoism and the Jewish mystical tradition of the Kabbalah place tremendous emphasis on spiritual maturity. Traditionally, the Kabbalah was never taught until the student had reached at least the age of forty. By this point, many people will have raised their children and developed the ability to recognize childishness for what it is, whether expressed by little ones, teenagers, themselves or even their elders. The key is a visceral understanding of the negative consequences that are created by lack of maturity.

By middle age most are less prone to self-righteous, explosive or overly naïve views. Spiritual maturity is mandatory for the person who wishes to awaken in this life.

To this end, midlife is a time for clearing out the psychic and karmic cobwebs. Those who are married or pair bonded often find that while physical sex may have declined, psychic bonding increases to naturally compensate for this loss. Midlife is the natural season for moving beyond a strong identification with the physical body. This makes it progressively easier to be completely comfortable with a partner, whether the two of you are sexually active or not.

Midlife presents an excellent opportunity to develop equanimity with respect to sexual desire, allowing it to exist in a relaxed way without unrelenting physical, emotional and psychic demands for physical contact. This internal freedom is one of the boons of midlife.

SENIORS

In the West and in many places around the globe, a new type of sexual revolution—led by seniors—has begun to emerge. Having moved beyond concern for what people think, seniors experience unprecedented freedom of expression. Pregnancy is generally off the table, as is the guilt associated with sleeping around. Senior sex swap and swinging clubs are not uncommon; nor is sex in senior care facilities.

Relieved of self-consciousness, seniors can enjoy sex with renewed enthusiasm, embracing what may have been unthinkable in their younger years, including threesomes, foursomes and even group sex. As one charming older woman put it, "I had five kids with the same man, but I never had any fun with sex. Then, in my seventies, my God, I found out that I actually enjoy it!"

After people have lived many years, they may well have moved past the limited viewpoints and negative conditioning that inhibits sexual expression. They can just take sex for what it is without all the drama. Usually they no longer bring all sorts of mental and emotional issues into bed. If some baggage persists, sexual qigong is truly valuable as a form of physical and psychological therapy.

A current reality of aging is that women live longer than men. Senior women who outnumber senior men have a number of options to choose from. Many simply become celibate and live out their lives in an asexual state. Some remain pair bonded or bond with someone new. It is possible that changing demographics and the relatively lower numbers of older men may make it become common for several women to share one man without the confusion of ethical and moral stances.

In terms of meditation, seniors have both potential advantages and pitfalls. As death becomes ever more relevant, so does the importance of clearing karma, especially if people are interested in moving on to the next place as awake as possible.

Meditation is the key for transcending any remaining conditioning that still cuts deep. Whatever still binds the soul at mental, emotional, psychic, karmic or essence levels can be dissolved and released. Now is the time to transcend the deep karma of this life. For seniors who are ready to practice sexual meditation, this can be a very exciting time of life.

Meditation is the key for transcending any remaining conditioning that still cuts deep. Whatever still binds the soul at mental, emotional, psychic, karmic or essence levels can be dissolved and released.

ELDERS

Our final years present a unique opportunity to mentor the younger generation and give back to the world. Here it is important to make the distinction between the word "senior," which just means older, and "elder," which denotes a person who has lived life and has accumulated wisdom. From the most basic standpoint, the more outer and inner work a person has cumulatively done in life, the more they could be considered an elder. Real elders have also been fully initiated both by direct experience and by being passed on knowledge from previous generations.

Like many traditional societies, "elder" is a title of respect among the Taoists. The term indicates the acquisition of real knowledge. Furthermore, beyond book knowledge and the wisdom that comes with age, an elder knows the exquisite richness of silence. Among the Taoists, the title is not conferred automatically with age—elders are made.

COMMON QUESTIONS ON THE PATH

Throughout time the following four considerations have arisen for those who decide to engage in Taoist sexual practices.

WHAT IF YOUR PARTNER ISN'T INTERESTED?

Different people have different views on sex and often one partner may be more interested than the other. Often this question of partner interest is accompanied by internal feelings that your partner is rejecting your choices in life or rejecting you personally. You may feel he or she isn't supporting you, and this may leave you with diminished feelings of intimacy or even hopelessness, even if you are very much in love with the person. These are internal issues that can be best resolved with solo dissolving practices.

These issues can also be somewhat resolved during sex with your partner, even if the person has no interest in Taoist sexual practices, if you dissolve them silently. During sex, you can also practice dissolving on your own. In fact, dissolving silently within yourself without your partner's knowledge will benefit him or her sexually, because of the increase in energetic intensity that results from your blocks dissolving and releasing.

If your partner is not willing to engage in sex at all, then you have to make a choice to just do solo exercises or to find another partner. Of course, the best scenario is when both partners are willing to participate in the Taoist sexual practices together and can pull out all the stops.

WHAT IF A WOMAN IS NONORGASMIC?

From the Taoist perspective, most women with enough practice can learn to have orgasms and even become multi-orgasmic. Sometimes there are known reasons why it is difficult for her to have an orgasm. For example, at very deep levels, many women who have shut down or never had an orgasm may have experienced deep rejection by parents or other loved ones or had some form of sexual trauma when they were younger. Unfortunately, sexual trauma is more common than most people think. To address these issues the woman and her partner can use the Outer and Inner Dissolving methods explained later in this book.

If you are a man, you should recognize you are dealing not only with the woman's predicament, but also possibly some internal fear of your own that her lack of orgasm implies that she is rejecting you or that there is something wrong with you. Just recognize that this situation may not have anything to do with you at all. If you are a man, it is important to make sure your partner knows you care about her and are willing to help. Any subtle indication that you feel something is wrong with her or that you don't like to have sex with her may devastate her emotionally. This is especially true of women who are strongly tied to romantic ideals. Women are as susceptible to performance anxiety as are men. Later in this book we will look at various practices to help a woman become more orgasmic and to assist a man to develop the ability to help the woman.

WHAT IF HE CAN'T GET IT UP OR MAINTAIN AN ERECTION?

A condition parallel to the inability of women to experience orgasm exists for many men. Some can't get it up or can't maintain an erection, both for nonmedical reasons and for medical conditions such as diabetes or heart problems. To try to overcome this, men may use illegal drugs or prescription erectile dysfunction drugs. Practices later in this book explore traditional Taoist methods for men to maintain erections.

A related problem is lack of sensitivity. Some men can pump for a long time and ejaculate. However, although these men may go through the motions and ejaculate, they may have virtually no sensation the entire time. Some, even those who are sexually adept, may experience little joy in the experience of sex. Further, some men don't even realize the degree to which the inside of their body is insensitive or dead, or how much their nerves have shut down. If a man recognizes that his nerves are shut down and wants to increase his energetic sensitivity then he will want to engage in some basic foundational energetic training in qigong and tai chi as explained in Chapter 10. He will also want to focus on mastering the Taoist ordinary sex techniques that increase sensitivity.

WHAT ABOUT SEXUALLY TRANSMITTED DISEASES?

When engaging in sexual activity, sexually transmitted diseases (STDs) are, of course, an important consideration that requires both understanding and proper precautions. Exaggeration, fear and ignorance often cloud salient issues, so it's important to get accurate information and take care of your partners as well as yourself.[4] As Dr. Alex Comfort says in *The New Joy of Sex*,[5] "There is no occasion for panic, or for losing out on the joy of sex—simply for informed caution."

---

4. Planned Parenthood's website, www.plannedparenthood.org, is an excellent online resource with a thorough educational guide to STDs.

5. Comfort, Alex, *The New Joy of Sex* (New York: Pocket Books, 1991), 15.

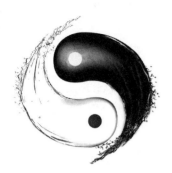

CHAPTER 6

Five Elements, Sex and Relationships

Entering into a relationship with another can bring us into joy or despair. We may be pulled into a relationship because of a deep physical attraction or it may be the unseen force that we call "love." The Taoists looked at all relationships through the lens of the five elements. They found that everyone has a primary element that predisposes them to certain traits and qualities.

Based on the five elements, Taoists developed a comprehensive theory of compatibility for relationships. This theory teaches you to how to recognize the five elements within you and your partner by directly feeling the experience of that energy and linking to the energy itself through sexual qigong and sexual meditation.

The interaction of the five elements is a key factor in determining if two people will be sexually compatible and whether the relationship bond will be short-lived or can be long-lasting. By doing practices with the five elements, you can identify the primary energies that are present at any given moment in time. This can help you to adjust to changing situations, as well as understand sexual proclivities and different ways of being.

Without this understanding, you may ascribe differences to personality or other factors, which may or may not have anything to do with the underlying situation at hand. At the highest levels of spiritual meditation, you learn to go beyond feeling the elements at only a gross level, to tap into and feel these five elements directly within each of the eight energy bodies, including how the elements make themselves known in each energy body. When you are able to do this, you can use the energies of the elements to accelerate your meditation practices.

FIVE ELEMENTS AND SEX

The Taoist perspective looks at the entirety of all and everything—anywhere, any time, any place, any dimension, without exception—and recognizes that only two phenomena ever occur: that which changes and that which is changeless. That which changes sooner or later becomes something else and manifests differently in some shape, manner or form, whatever the conditions or circumstances. However, at the core lies the absolute reality that there is something that truly never changes, once one arrives at a place of genuine emptiness. This is the essential teaching of the *I Ching*—change may be apparent everywhere at the relative level, but underneath it is the nature of changelessness.

Arriving at this place of emptiness is the goal of Taoist spiritual meditation, and once it is achieved a Taoist practitioner has reached what some call "enlightenment." The Taoists found that without a profound understanding of the nature of change, we do not arrive at emptiness.

Five-element theory begins to help you understand the world of change in meaningful ways. According to Taoist tradition, all matter and human dynamics are comprised of some energetic combination of Earth, Water, Wood, Fire and Metal. Just like electricity, which can take millions of forms depending on its use, elements change to match the energy fields in which they're operating. They exist to create matter and are inside everything that is created and within every physical and nonphysical dynamic that manifests.

> *Taoists recognize that only two phenomena ever occur: that which changes and that which is changeless. Within the world of change, all matter and human dynamics are comprised of some energetic combination of Earth, Water, Wood, Fire and Metal.*

Anything that changes is always in a relationship to something else. As the nature of any relationship morphs or stays stable, there is a different kind of change. The five elements underlie how everything relates to everything else. They are the nature of the quantum flux of the universe. As you enter into various human relationships, there is always a mixing and interplay of elements at hand.

The elements take different forms according to which of the eight energy bodies they dominate and how they interact with one another on both intrapersonal and interpersonal levels. Through sexual qigong and meditation, you begin to see how elements flow and continuously morph through each of the energy bodies of you and your partner.

From the perspective of changelessness and genuine emptiness, the five elements are irrelevant. As soon as you enter the world of change and the world of consciousness, understanding the relationships of the five elements becomes *extremely* relevant.

Special Note: The Fire and Water traditions of Taoism specifically refer to the overall methodology and style of how Taoists do all their practices. The terms Fire and Water traditions are not related to the Fire and Water of the five elements. Both Taoist Fire and Water traditions have numerous practices that use all the five elements.

The five elements are interrelated—there are no distinct boundaries. Fire produces Earth; Earth gives birth to Metal; Metal produces Water through condensation; Water grows Wood; Wood feeds Fire. Statements like "Fire means this" and "Metal means that" are tricky, because each element influences, bleeds through and melds into the next one. Although it is difficult for the mind to accept, hard and fast boundaries don't exist. Quite the contrary—the elements only exist within an intricate relational and energetic matrix with one phase yielding to and encompassing the next in a continuous cycle.

Even though you are likely to have one personal element as a foundation, other elements are always at play inside you, depending on ever-changing circumstances and the qi that manifests inside you when you respond to them. A long-term goal is to bring the energetic qualities of the five elements inside you into proper balance.

However, we can look at each of the five elements in terms of their unique characteristics. Later in the chapter is an exercise to help you make a rudimentary assessment of your own or another's personal elemental power. Having an understanding of which elements are active provides a new level of experiential, empirical knowledge to use when considering if someone is right for you now, and if so, for how long.

The important question you will need to ask is not "What element am I?" but rather "How do I use this information?" In the Taoist world, firm distinctions are not useful, because of the inherent flux of everything. Understanding the element in you and your partner may also give you important insights into nature of your sexuality and that of your partner.

While making love, there is also the Taoist art of how you recognize, move and flow in coordination with the infinite ways of how the energy of the five elements can manifest in real time through every moment that you are having sex, including when it's over. Each element goes through cycles that can last from thirty seconds to many minutes before shifting to the next element. The subtleties of how this plays out as regards to the ever-shifting sexual and emotional energy arising is yet another aspect of traditional Taoist sexual qigong and meditation practices.

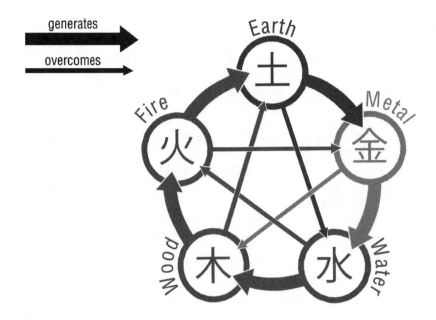

Figure 6-1: Five-Element Creative Cycle

This chapter looks at the five elements from the flow of the creative cycle. It starts with the Earth element rather than following the classic order, which begins with Metal and ends with Earth. The author feels this will make the concepts involved more understandable in the sexual context than would the more traditional sequence that is commonly used for Traditional Chinese Medicine. The creative cycle emphasizes the circular, interconnected nature of the five elements.

EARTH ELEMENT

Earth people have two important qualities. The first is they have a power that allows them to integrate all experiences. The second is Earth people have a sense of stability, an ability to filter out distracting environmental influences. While these strengths keep Earth types grounded and balanced, it can also cause them to get stuck or be stodgy.

The Earth holds Fire, Water, Metal and Wood. Earth integrates all the elements while maintaining inner stability and a delicate gravitational balance. This is its essential nature, which is expressed by those dominated by the Earth element.

According to the Taoists, anyone who does not feel intrinsically stable inside his or her own body, who cannot integrate experiences well or who has trouble feeling comfortable with what happens on this planet probably has minimal Earth qualities in his or her makeup. The lack of integration keeps them anxious, stressed and mentally unfocused.

The Earth element is linked to the spleen. The function of the spleen, energetically speaking, is to integrate and provide stability. People with a healthy predominance of the Earth element have a proclivity for good, grounded thought. Emotionally, they are also quite stable. This element is characterized by fewer emotional swings. They can hear all points of view, integrate them and not be thrown off balance. They intrinsically recognize how to pull everything together. Earth people naturally have the stability, stamina and follow-through to bring all kinds of long-term projects and relationships to a successful conclusion. They do not have to exert a lot of effort to do this—it happens as a matter of course.

However, one of their limitations, which they share with Water people, is that they may have difficulty discerning what is necessary and important in the short term. Everything registers as having the same priority. Often their view is that "everything will be okay," even in the midst of upheaval, but they may be oblivious to what is tactically needed in the moment.

Earth people tend to be less verbal and more strong and silent, with some exceptions. They are also less likely to be inherently active as a matter of habit. In terms of spiritual evolution, "it's all good" is often the general disposition. In terms of dealing with most earthly phenomena, this attitude can potentially undermine timely, effective problem solving. Earth people must cultivate the ability to discriminate between what matters in the ultimate sense and what is less or more important in the timely sense.

Earth People and Sex

Earth types are inherently sexual. Sex naturally puts Earth people completely into the body, which makes them wildly happy and satisfied, amplifying their internal stability. Making love helps them feel utterly comfortable with living. Although capable of monogamy, Earth types are able to simultaneously have a lot of sexual friends and remain loyal to all of them in different yet very real ways.

Many are drawn to Earth people because, at the bodily level, Earth types ground all the other elements. This makes sex with them particularly attractive. During and after sex, Earth types make their partners feel more integrated and more able to feel content on this planet. These powerful feelings emanate effortlessly from the Earth element.

Earth and Wood tend to be very loyal as well as the most unforgiving of disloyalty.

WATER ELEMENT

People whose personality is dominated by the Water element have the quality of vitality, which has in its foundation the ability to stay active. They have an incredible ability to stay connected to an internal sense of joy.

A Water person typically has a highly developed ability to feel. Water people feel things without knowing how or why. They don't ask why water is wet. They simply know. Water types flow and move quite easily from one emotion to the other, without holding back. Often described as mercurial, the feeling state of a Water personality changes rapidly, although not in quite as fast and furious a manner as Fire personalities.

Emotional swings that would drive an Earth person to distraction are no big deal for the Water person, and Water types are often confused when people have a negative response to their emotional flux. Water people are unpredictable—they can be as quiet and still as a calm lake, or as forceful and fast moving as a tidal wave.

Like Earth, Water is integrative by nature. Unlike Earth, Water is active. Water types do not just sit back and integrate information, rather they fully go with the flow and are inherently flexible. They're like streams that move easily around obstacles. They do not find it particularly difficult to adjust to different situations or changing circumstances. Like the ocean, which is not disturbed by what drops in it or how it moves with the currents, Water types have minimal preferences. They can accept and go along with almost anything.

Because Water tends to flow, a predominance of this element can make a person very verbal. Generally, Water people talk more than people with other predominant elements. A Water person feels no difference between words and silence. The idea of only being able to be peaceful by being completely still is irrelevant to a Water person. Water can be internally very still even in its externally turbulent modes, such as during a storm or in a tidal wave. In each circumstance the character of the Water is still the same. Water is still Water. Even though its form changes, it will have a characteristic underlying energy.

The Water element is linked to the kidneys, which bring about a sense of life and flow of energy in your internal organs. Strong kidneys are associated with positive emotions and a strong life force. Weak kidneys are associated with negative emotions of fear and listlessness and a weak life force.

A person who relates to the physical body through the Water element will readily notice the flows within the body. Water people tend to feel their fluids without thinking or trying, whereas other people might be mystified when a Water person might say, for example, that his lymph or blood flow is a bit sluggish that day.

If Water types get too sluggish, they have a tendency toward depression. Think of a river that is blocked from flowing. The water will become brackish and diseased if it cannot move. By releasing the blockage that is preventing the water from flowing, the river is restored to its strong healthy flow. For Water people, it's all about the flow.

Water People and Sex

Sex moves fluids and energy strongly through the human body. Because Water types can feel that flow, they are incredibly sensation-oriented, particularly when they are having sex. Sex is natural to them; they have an internal ability to smoothly go with the flow.

Having sex with a Water person will give the other elemental types a stronger sense of flow, virtually by osmosis. Water people have the internal ability to flow more easily with their partners, as the currents between them change and morph.

Water people just naturally love sex. They have no inherent need to bond and can go from one lover to another with ease. Of all the elemental types, Water people are the least likely to be monogamous. Unlike Fire, which tends to burn bridges when a relationship is done, Water people tend to remain friends with former partners.

Difficulty can arise when a Water person is with a partner whose body lacks fluidity and movement. This deficit can present quite a challenge on more than just the physical level, by acting like a dam that blocks the Water type's ability to relate to the other person.

If a Water person has a proclivity toward psychic energy, sex can feed it, whereas a lack of sex will starve it. An active and strong Water element also makes it the easiest of all the elements to drop into the psychic dimension of sex.

WOOD ELEMENT

Wood's nature is one of stamina and slow, steady and continuous growth. The inherent nature of Wood is that it simultaneously grows high into the air with its trunk and branches, and deep into the ground through its roots. Woods strength comes from its ability to penetrate, join and meld with whatever it encounters. A tree can even push its way through a piece of concrete and continue to grow.

The important challenge for Wood types is to not attempt to grow too quickly at one time. Just as a tree, which can stay stable and grow tall only if its roots go down into the ground, Wood people must maintain their natural boundaries and follow a steady path of growth in everything, including relationships.

As a general proposition, Wood personalities naturally feel. Like trees well rooted in the earth, Wood types have tremendous internal stability. They tend to be emotionally steady. In terms of activity, Wood people get to the root of things and commonly become highly skilled in their area of expertise.

The counterpoint to this strength is that Wood has a hard time letting go. If a person near to a Wood type breaks a bond or betrays him or her, the betrayer can become a potential lifelong enemy. Dissolving practices can help with this.

Wood personalities tend to be strong and silent types. They grow into situations but do not have a massive need to talk about it. Wood people hear the silences and actually speak in silences. If your partner has a predominance of Wood, you must learn to communicate through the silences rather than relying only on words.

The Wood element is connected to the liver, which is responsible for the strength and flexibility of the muscles, tendons and ligaments. A strong liver is associated with positive emotions of perseverance and confidence; and can strengthen your ability to overcome obstacles. A weak liver, however, is associated with negative emotions, such as anger, irritability and failure, accompanied by high blood pressure.

Emotions in Wood people are always trying to grow, take over and be taken over by the other person. Wood types in relationships actually try to penetrate one another. Usually, one dramatically tries to influence the other. In the best scenarios, they penetrate each other in a balanced manner.

Wood People and Sex

Sex helps Wood people grow into themselves. Just like a plant, they need to bond and graft with something. Wood people are monogamous by nature. A Wood person's ideal would be to meet one person and stay with that person forever. If you look at people who have an easy time in their long-term relationship, something in the energy of the couple's bodies allows the Wood elements in them to connect. Over time, they will grow into each other and the relationship will become even stronger.

In sex, Wood types get off and are excited when they feel their blood is about to burst, because they can feel their blood pressure. They tend to build sexual energy slowly and deeply. They like being kissed and to have their muscles and deep tissues dug into with significant pressure. Some like to be bitten and scratched, although not to the point of drawing blood.

FIRE ELEMENT

People whose personalities are dominated by the Fire element have the outward qualities of excitability and the internal positive qualities of clarity, happiness and joy.

The Fire element is linked to the heart. As a result, Fire personalities commonly have strong emotions that emanate from the heart. They may feel their heart, not as an experience of pumping, but as one of incessant moving and jumping around, even if only for a tenth of a second. Unlike Water people, who feel flow, Fire people feel the intrinsic and intermittent agitation of the heart, like the way fire behaves when it burns through a forest.

The highly active heart of Fire people can create extreme joy and love, especially when they have peace in their lives. If peace is lacking, the heart can cause extreme anxiety, anger and sadness.

Fire types are known for being sharp orators and making short, choppy remarks that can scorch their opponents like a flame. They like to one-up other people. Fire personalities are commonly combative and usually start most or many of the fights in relationships. They are always seeking the next fuel source.

Just like a physical fire, which will die unless it constantly jumps around and consumes everything in its path, people who have an extreme amount of the Fire element in their bodies must keep doing something new or they will feel deprived and get uncomfortable and upset.

Fighting and pleasuring are different fuel sources; the Fire element both consumes and produces them with equal ease. Fire people have a natural tendency in their bodies to go through endless cycles of attraction and repulsion. They also tend to flip out a lot and are easily drawn toward the dark sides of their personalities. The most stressed-out people tend to be Fire types.

Emotions in Fire people are always jumping around, moving here, moving there, and always seeking the next new thing. These highly active types have the ability to produce, although they can also be the ones who just talk a lot and shoot energy everywhere but never actually make anything happen. If they didn't jump around in some kind of constant agitation, they would be bored to death.

A bit of Earth in their constitution can help them be more grounded. They feel too much of everything and constantly bounce around. Intrinsically ungrounded, Fire people can easily disturb or, in a worst-case scenario, rip apart those who are sensitive in nature.

Fire is light and Fire types are naturally drawn to finding the light within. They are most easily attracted to following a spiritual path that emphasizes light, which can be found in both the Fire and Water meditation traditions.

Fire People and Sex

Fire people love sex. Generally speaking, they are not naturally monogamous and need to have sex with a number of different people. Unfortunately, they often don't get all that satisfied from jumping around from one lover to the next—they are fueled by compulsion more than the enjoyment of the act itself.

However, if a Fire person meets someone who activates his or her intrinsic sense of physicality, and this fulfills his or her need to feel alive by constantly creating new sexual experiences, the Fire type might be able to settle down with that one person and may even be comfortable having sex only once in a while.

Fire people are often the ones who love to have an argument followed by great "make-up" sex. People who have Fire qi running through their systems could be perfectly happy having a "War of the Roses" against others right up to the day they die.

Conversely, if a Water person were in such a situation, the flow would be interrupted. Put a Wood personality in such a situation and it would destroy him or her. That kind of lifestyle would ravage that person like a fire does a forest. On the other hand, Earth can accommodate Fire—even if uncomfortably scorched, it can't be damaged that much. Metal is indeterminate, as it depends how strong the Metal and how hot the fire. Because they can keep inciting the flames within, two Fire people either generally work well together or quite the opposite. It depends on whether the directions of their interactions tends toward the positive or negative because Fire is equally drawn to and feeds on both love and conflict.

METAL ELEMENT

Metal people have a lot of strength, which comes from their mental energy. They have tremendously active thoughts and are incessantly planning and strategizing. They have great enthusiasm for ideas.

In relationships, Metal personalities rely on mental exchanges with their partners, families and coworkers and tend to treat emotions as ideas. They love to classify and categorize everything. They either analyze situations to death or are oblivious. They tend to be judgmental in their relationships: "You shouldn't be this way; you should be that way." They continuously try to use their minds to change, reconfigure or manipulate what they see, and they can become very fixated on their points of view.

The dark side of Metal personalities can be their nearly complete lack of feeling. They are often disconnected from the planet and especially from the world of emotions. Metal types often relate to the body and to emotions as ideas. Rather than feeling an emotion or experiencing the body as living and vibrant, Metal personalities observe it as a congealed thought. In extreme cases, Metal people may try to understand what someone is doing by looking at that person and analyzing the situation, but may not be able to feel any empathy.

Metal types have a tendency to be auditory, particularly within their own heads. Many must talk something through in order for it to make sense. These people are great conversationalists, as long as the conversation is not emotional in nature.

The body parts associated with the Metal element are the lungs and spine. The lungs can make them prone to sadness and melancholy on one end of the spectrum, and on the other, highly enthusiastic about mental ideas. Metal people have an intrinsic ability to connect with the spine, brain, and the rest of the central nervous system.

Too much Metal can be a problem in relationships. The mental rigidity of Metal people means that when something hits deep down, they shut down. They often cannot relate to the fact that their partner is a living, changing being rather than a known quantity in an equation. Metal types can only move forward with someone so long as their idea of that person remains stable and sound.

Metal People and Sex

People for whom the Metal element predominates are the natural-born celibates of the universe. Sex is often nothing more than a notion for Metal types. Many of them would be happier reading a book than making love.

When Metal personalities do engage in sex, they first recognize the sexual energy inside of their body as an *idea*. Only over time can they actually start to *feel* sexual energy. During sex, they can go anywhere in their minds. They love visualizations, which are mental pictures. In terms of sexual qigong or meditation, the challenge for Metal types is to actually experience what is happening rather than just think about it.

Sex between two Metal people can be just fine. The conversation may begin with what is happening during sex, and then move on to history, computers, or the like. This could work well for two Metal types, as it could give them another access point to Taoist meditation processes.

People who are looking for back-and-forth emotional sharing may find that a person who has Metal dominating their personality is incapable of this kind of communication.

Sex for the Nonsexual

My main teacher, Liu Hung Chieh, was a natural-born celibate as regards sex. He told me that when he was younger and a Confucian, he had sex only as many times as was required for him to have children in order to fulfill his ancestral obligation for descendants. After he had fathered two children, he never had sex with his wife, or with anybody else for that matter.

I asked him if he had ever enjoyed having sex, and he told me he could get through it, but that for him sex was a nonevent. He found practicing martial art punches or reading a book to be more complete experiences and significantly more enjoyable than having sex. He then told me that asexual people can use sex as a valuable tool to clear out their spiritual blockages.

Liu said in terms of Taoist spirituality, being a natural-born celibate or not is neither an advantage nor disadvantage. If people are naturally asexual, they may still have a mildly sexual lifestyle if they deeply care for someone who requires some small amount of sexuality to feel bonded. What is important is that they have sex only when their mind and body naturally turns toward it. Otherwise their mind can become distracted during sex and will naturally flow away from being present into various mental meandering such as chess, math or other visualizations that have nothing to do with their partner.

People of combined Metal and Wood personalities are particularly capable of this kind of uninvolved sex. Even if their partner is the true love of their life, the person who can turn them on beyond all others, an asexual must be turned on by the idea of making love in each specific instance. If not, the act of making love can become extremely boring and deadening.

During either sexual qigong or meditation, partners of asexual people must be able to wake up their partner's nerves, because very commonly their nerves, particularly the psychic nerves that that govern the sexual body, will be relatively weak. If you live with or intermittently have sex with such a person, at times he or she may have a certain higher range of sexual response, but most of the time will revert to a much lower response level. In this situation, it is very healthy if you can bring that person's response level more toward the upper range, because this can help flush his or her stagnant bodily qi.

However, a potentially likely and untoward consequence of taking asexuals too far past their natural sexual limitations on an ongoing basis is that the overall sexual response level of asexual people will simply drop, and they may, to their partner's sorrow, easily revert to celibacy. Therefore it behooves the partner of an asexual lover to encourage the maximum level of their sexual capacity when possible, without putting pressure on that person to go beyond what they naturally cannot. The point is more but not too much. Applying the seventy-percent rule is the best course of action.

One of the great differences between people on the higher and lower ends of the sexual desire scale is that those on the higher end have naturally stronger sexual nerves than those on the lower end. People on the higher end of the scale (who tend to have a preponderance of Earth, Water and Fire elements) are more capable of feeling and enjoying sensual experience than can an average person or an asexual. It's a question of how much pleasure your sexual nerves can tolerate before losing the capacity to enjoy the feeling. It is useful to recognize and accept your natural situation rather than attempt to make it what your mind thinks it should be. This means finding out what your and your lover's natural sexual level is, accepting it, nourishing it and working with it within your sexual relationship.

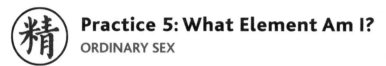

Practice 5: What Element Am I?
ORDINARY SEX

Once you are past your twenties, you have most likely had enough life experience to perceive which elements are active and which are not in your body. Generally speaking, every person is born with an essential underlying energetic frequency that predominates. Although the other elements are always present, for the vast majority of people, this underlying frequency is characterized by a single predominant element throughout their lifespan, and in a relative minority, two. The predominant element forms the basis from which any of the other minor elements can rise and take over. For example, someone who is predominantly Earth or Water might come upon a circumstance that suddenly raises the Fire element within so that it temporarily dominates.

A person's dominant element tends to remain stable throughout his or her life. Exceptions to this are the rare individual who has two elements that are equally dominant, or the man or woman for whom one element is extremely powerful until the age of thirty or forty, and then, at midlife, another element ascends and becomes dominant.

Since the following exercise is based only on self-reflection, first sit down and breathe until your breath is relaxed and smooth and your thoughts and emotions are somewhat quiet. This could take a few minutes.

To figure out which one or two elements are predominant within you, go back and review your entire life. Notice patterns in relationships that worked or didn't. What relationships were you usually drawn into? What do you commonly accept or reject? Notice hints and trends and the types of internal resistance that block you from recognizing what's going on or what makes it easy for you to figure this out. Do not think you need to be anything different from what is in you. Once you understand what your element is, simply focus on making peace with your interactions and what is inside you. ●

SEXUAL COMPATIBILITY IN RELATIONSHIPS

If you want to sustain a relationship, you must find an element in your partner to which you strongly connect and that is comfortable and stabilizing for you. Your partner should not make you feel destabilized. After you see what is going on elementally in the relationship, you can then decide whether you want to continue to be in it or not.

When you examine energetic reactions, learn to recognize the flows of qi. Does the energy between you continue, stop or freeze? If the fluidity stops on a regular basis, negative qualities can worsen. If the negativity is not released and dissolved, most likely the relationship will continue to get worse, going through a hundred different variations that keep both of you stuck.

Once you recognize the reality of the energies involved, stop focusing your thoughts around what the relationship and dynamic "should be." Instead consider the five elements and ask, "What can be done to make it work for you, rather than against you?" If you do not deal with reality, you can expect things to fall apart. It is only a matter of time before illusions crumble.

Compatibility is as simple as the energy that comprises our bodies—the result can be negative, neutral or positive. Thus, it is not about any myopic idea of "good" or "bad." The Taoist approach is that everything that has a specific form has a natural duration—a beginning, middle and end.

Relating comes down, quite simply, to whether you can connect and be useful and satisfying to one another. If you make choices that are not useful and not functional, things fall apart. Of course, if you don't mind things falling apart, go ahead! But if you like things succeed, realize that your inner world has ways that it works *for* you or *against* you, just like in the external world.

If you understand these basic concepts and begin to make yourself aware of which element is at play, when you experience blockages internally or with people, you will cultivate the ability to understand what you are getting into, what is happening when you are in it and what you should do about it when situations continue or change. One of the tricks is to have all of the elements within you active and balanced so that you do not go off into deep extremes in one direction or the other. You may find when your primary element is strongly active, you naturally and unconsciously incite or trigger some of the people around you through your interactions, for good or for bad. Eventually, you can actually learn how to tune your elements. If both you and your partner can tune in to the same element with Taoist sexual qigong and meditation practices, you can more rapidly release the other person's blockages while uncovering the ones you have in the same area.

ATTRACTION VERSUS SEXUAL COMPATIBILITY

From the moment you begin to explore your sexuality, you will simultaneously be exploring sexual attraction. How much of initial attraction is little more than sexual curiosity? Or looks? How can you predict more accurately when attraction is likely to lead to a solid relationship beyond just sex? Is the attraction truly sexual, or does it only appear so initially? Are you attracted because of some past karma with this person?

From the Taoist point of view, it is totally natural for human beings to be sexually curious about each other and to be attracted to different people. It's no different than getting a mouth-watering whiff from the kitchen and wondering what the food will taste like. The initial response from your salivary glands is reflexive; it doesn't necessarily mean that you're about to eat, and certainly doesn't mean that you'll want that dish on the menu for the rest of your life. Our desire for food, sex, knowledge, beauty, affection and human warmth are natural human appetites.

What's behind attraction, above and beyond a natural sexual appetite, is a valuable inquiry. The Taoists found that attraction was very different from sexual compatibility. Of all the potential sex partners to whom you might initially feel attracted, only ten to fifteen percent of them will result in relationships that will be enjoyable for both of you. Those aren't great odds. Of course, most will need to confirm this with their own experience before the urge to act on initial attractions is tempered and their tastes and choices become more refined. The Taoists also explored how long-term compatibility was directly linked to the five elements and how those elements were part of the energetic matrix of different people.

NATURAL AND CONDITIONED RESPONSES

The ways individual men or women manifest the same five element disposition can appear be either quite similar or different. Professor Higgins in the musical, *My*

Fair Lady sang, "Why can't a woman be more like a man?" This sentiment is equally echoed by women who ask, "Why can't men be more like us?" The fact is that yin and yang are different, although exactly how is very much a gray zone.

The yin and yang of men and women in their thinking and behavior are strongly influenced by all kinds of conditioning. This determines how either partner will psychologically filter the energetic yin and yang qualities of each element in human interaction. Such factors as family background, education, economic class or peer group pressure can affect the external behavior through which the energies of the five elements will express themselves. For example, this will influence whether you stick up for yourself or not and the way you display such qualities as vulnerability or strength.

From a Taoist perspective, there are some important points to consider when trying to comprehend the many ways that yin and yang in terms of the five elements can manifest. Don't confuse masculine and feminine styles with energetic substance. Get beyond gender politics and its ever-changing red dust definitions of gender roles and appropriate behavior. Seek the direct experience of the elemental energy itself. Observe and recognize how qualities of the five elements emerge in you and those with whom you have relationships. This may bring you some valuable insights. Developing a natural rather than a conditioned response to the five elements is one of the aims of Taoist meditation.

Looking at Someone: Appearance and Reality

While training for Taoist priesthood, I was taught to recognize the element or elements active in a person first by looking. Going beyond the surface to recognize the elements present made me start examining what actually underlies all attraction between people.

Through this inquiry, I learned it was not only about looking, it was also about listening. Then it became not just about listening, but about being able to put out my hand or my mind and telepathically find out which elements were most active in a person. I learned that the appearance of things and the reality of things are often not the same.

LETTING GO OF CONDITIONED MIND IMAGES

Anyone with conditioned brain reflexes could sexually be just as easily attracted as repulsed by the standard markers of attraction, that is by a potential partner's looks, way of speaking and personality. However, this initial attraction or repulsion alone often doesn't give an accurate hint of what will happen between the sheets.

Judging a specific person sexually by his or her physical or mental appearance, although convenient, may be a big mistake.

What initially looks great and fits the image of your ideal partner may at the end of the day be a great disappointment. When this is the case, as your bodies touch, or when you kiss, nuzzle, suck, have manual sex or when the vagina engulfs the erection, there is simply no energy, nothing, zip, nada—just a total nonevent devoid of anything resembling energy and life.

It is not uncommon for people to finally connect with someone who they think should be the ideal Mr. or Miss right, a composite of all their internal favorable images, only to find out that the sex is terrible. This reality can be shocking and quite demoralizing for either sex. It is especially disappointing after a long streak of dead lovers, extended courting rituals or for a person who waits until after marriage to have sex only to discover there is no spark.

Conversely, there is also the possibility that you may find a partner who goes against much of the mental conditioning you have, but who in bed and in the totality of the relationship is nothing less than amazing. This is why quite often you see the "most beautiful" man or woman hand in hand with someone who society might unfairly judge as physically ugly or who in other ways doesn't fit the idealized profile. Given that media-induced images of conditioned expectations may or may not be what lies beneath the surface, it is wise to relax and be open to all possibilities. Rather than judge, learn to have discernment by following what energy flows between you and another.

COMPLEMENTARY ELEMENTS IN RELATIONSHIPS

Being able to look at yourself and your partner from some understanding of what elements are active inside can help you decide about potential compatibility. It is useful to experientially understand which elements complement and support each other moment by moment, and which are intrinsically at war. It is possible to learn to recognize if the elements inside you are compatible with those working inside someone else, or if the combination will continuously drive you mad. Generally, people with the same predominance of elements have the easiest time getting along. Sometimes, however, opposites attract. For example the Fire and Water elements have the potential to damage each other or create steam, which is sexually and spiritually elevating to both.

It may be that your partner's elements complement yours. While anyone can recognize basic states of emotion, few can recognize the elemental energy that's at play and learn how to flow between the rhythms of each element as they emerge. You can achieve this when you cultivate inner awareness, especially through Outer and Inner Dissolving.

Some people lack a certain elemental quality within and somehow, at a subliminal level, know that another person has that desired element. In such a case, they may feel a strong attraction to that person. Taoists generally say that, although this is a common scenario, it's equivalent to a hamster spinning in a wheel. No matter how much the hamsters run, they never get anywhere. If you need something inside yourself, don't bet on reliably getting it from somebody else. A better approach is to find what you need internally and strengthen it, and by doing this, you will have a better chance of successfully sustaining the relationship. Moreover, although you cannot reasonably expect to change others, you do have the power to change yourself.

Each of the eight energy bodies and the five elements has a yin or yang way of manifesting energetically. The more alive the sexual compatibility between partners, the more connected, active and responsive will be energetic qualities between both partner's eight energy bodies, five elements and the yin-yang ways their qualities interact and naturally influence each other. These determine energetic compatibility and, ultimately, the satisfaction people can have from a sexual relationship. Moreover, there is no fixed formula, as each case is highly individual. The same man or woman whom someone might find to be a sexual live wire and perfect match, could for another be rather disappointing.

Knowing the qualities of the elements as described, begin to identify the patterns in your life for what they are. In terms of a relationship with another person, when a negative quality of an element manifests, you can lessen it, but you can't override it by going against it. Whether you want to deal with it depends on who you are with and the circumstances of the situation. You need to decide whether you want to have compassion and try to make things better, or you may just want to get out of the way.

YIN AND YANG WITHIN RELATIONSHIPS

Many of the lessons we learn in life are closely related to the interplay between yin and yang. Yet the underlying energy dynamics remain largely unconscious for many people. The following examples give a sense of how yin and yang express within the individual.

A man with too much yin may tend to be sexually weak. He will approach sex in a timid manner, waiting for his partner to initiate rather than taking charge. His mind rejects all forms of aggression. If he does make a move, he won't do it with confidence and can't sustain his initiative for very long. The Yiddish word for this type of man is *nebish,* which may also mean neurotic and whining. Because he's uncomfortable with directness and confrontation, he is often passive-aggressive, which will most likely frustrate a woman rather than give her yin the complete yang essence that she needs.

On the other end of the spectrum is the macho man. These are the men who beat their wives without remorse, the mega-control freaks who couldn't care less what a woman is getting out of sex as long as he's having a good time. If a man has only yang and no yin, he can only be a conqueror. It has often been said that men like this ought never to leave the war zone. These men validate aggression at every turn; they are out to win, conquer, rape and pillage. "I want it, I get it, it's mine," is their motto. They avoid anything of a softer nature. Human history has seen plenty of extreme yang displays.

A man who has excess yang may give you all his opinions and ideas, but he will have a difficult time receiving anything emotional. The best he can do is sit there and grunt; often he can't accept what's coming from a woman as having much validity.

Just as a man's emotional energy is naturally more yang, a woman's emotions are naturally more yin. Her natural disposition is to care for and protect others. Women with too much yin are slaves, even slaves to their own emotions. They can be overly emotionally sensitive and prone to excessive crying at minimal provocation.

A totally yang woman, on the other hand, is often called an "Iron Lady." She will relate to her children more like a task to be completed, no different than making a good piece of furniture. She will feed them, house them, and make sure they go to school, always demanding, "do this, do that, I expect you be this or that," with little or no nurturing. In the bedroom, the overly yang woman is like a drill sergeant, which often does little to actualize her man's yang essence.

FIVE ELEMENTS AND THE SPIRITUAL PATH

The purpose of Taoist meditation is to move beyond the binding force of a particular element and to open up smoothly to the whole sphere of elements within your body, mind, emotions, psychic body, karma and so on. Eventually, you may reach a point at which you can feel all five elements simultaneously inside you. This is when the fun begins, because you'll begin to see that you can actually morph your system and shift dominance by allowing and even encouraging the less-active elements to come much more strongly into play.

Even so, it is easier for someone to engage on a spiritual path whose methodology accords with the primary elements of their makeup. Conversely it is more difficult if they don't. Swimming upstream has its challenges. Just as the minor elements, along with the major elements, are always present in your energetic composition, so also are they within the methods of every spiritual tradition.

These are the spiritual practices that accord most naturally with different elements:

- Earth people need something that is not frenetic to benefit most from. Since the the nature of the Earth element is to be grounded, for example, sitting is preferred to a wild dancing devotional path. Earth people need a path that seeks to integrate a common thread through what may seem disparate practices.

- Water needs a path that emphasizes flexibility and flow within all practices.
- Wood needs to grow in an environment in which the nature of the practice embodies steady growth. Thus its methods should have clear beginning, middle and end points with minimal variation.
- Fire people need a path that encourages spiritual passion and enables them to directly connect to light.
- Metal people need a path that enables them, through mental clarity, to directly perceive the spiritual nature of things.

Compatibility: The Nose Knows

Over millennia, Taoists have discovered that the single most reliable determinate of whether a sexual relationship can work comes down to smell. We can thank Western science for verifying this by mapping the direct line between the olfactory center in the nose and the limbic center of the brain, but the Taoists discovered this link long before the scientific method came into vogue. Bottom line: if your most primary sense organ is not pleased by a person's scent, odds are that a sexual relationship between the two of you doesn't have a chance.

Imagine trying to relax and enjoy someone when you dislike the smell of their sweat or genital secretions. To override or ignore such bodily responses sets up resistance and builds the relationship on a foundation of stress. You may be able to put up with each other for a while, and you may even enjoy one another for a limited duration, but the relationship most likely will not last beyond a certain point. The same principle applies regarding the taste of your partner's genital fluids.

At minimum, a prospective partner's scent and taste should be neutral and not offensive. Some odors may be due to hygiene, but sometimes it's just a person's basic smells. If, on a scale of one to ten, you find a partner's odor and taste on the low end of the scale, you can be pretty sure that the composite of your sexual relationship at best will go no higher than five or seven out of ten.

Of course, it's optimal that you enjoy your partner's bodily smells and find their taste pleasant as well. If a partner's scent isn't on the higher end of the scale, hidden resistance may express itself unconsciously in any number of confusing ways—irritability, impatience, avoidance, sarcasm, emotional distance, even physical abuse. Put very simply—if someone's scent really bothers you, consider it a real deal-breaker.

Obviously, the most direct way to find out how you respond to a person's genital smells and tastes, which range from extremely subtle to exceedingly strong, is through oral sex. A certain segment of every population feels revulsion toward oral-genital contact, often due to religious or philosophical influences. The Taoists are clear proponents of oral sex. They do not consider the genitals a place of shame any more than the nose, mouth, tongue or the bottom of a foot.

Ian Kerner describes cunnilingus in detail in his book, *She Comes First*.[1] He writes:

"Every woman smells and tastes different. Some are sweeter than others, some are a bit pungent, still others are more neutral and nondescript. Sometimes the differences are subtle, other times they're stark. Nor will the same woman always consistently smell or taste the same."

Rather than focusing only on smelling your partner's genitals, armpits or sweating skin, you can enjoy the preamble to oral sex and perform an unobtrusive genital examination without stifling or breaking the sexual flow. Besides checking out the compatibility of your lover's sexual smells, you can also look for visible signs of sexual disease such as crabs, herpes, gonorrhea and genital warts. Extremely rank or foul smells can indicate a sexual health problem such as a yeast infection or other issue.

Within a continuing relationship, should the smell of a partner's genitals become foul smelling or bad tasting for a period of time, it's best to discontinue sex, as this can be a strong indication that their body is becoming ill. It's time for that person to consult a physician and get the situation checked out. A Chinese herbalist or Ayurvedic practitioner can also be particularly helpful in this situation, as looking at changes in a patient's smells are part of their traditional diagnostic protocols.

If a man observes and recognizes from his smells, and his overall body and energetic fitness level that he is moving into weakness, regardless of the reason and whether it is unknown or known, this is a sign that it is best to avoid sex and/or find a way not to ejaculate. However, if he is moving into a medium or strong cycle, it is normally not a problem if he has sex or ejaculates.

Generally, whether you are a man or a woman, if you feel that you are moving into a weak cycle, it is important to avoid weakening yourself further by any actions that might cause strain.

---

1. Kerner, Ian, *She Comes First* (New York: Harper, 2004), 69–an appropriate page number!

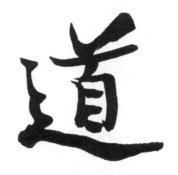

SECTION 2

TAOIST ORDINARY SEX

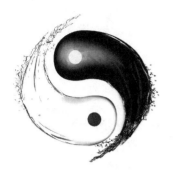

CHAPTER 7

Enhancing Ordinary Sex

The Taoists discovered and tracked hundreds of techniques for increasing pleasure and making sex more enjoyable. They trained people to develop the type of varied, attentive, intelligent touch that can drive a lover wild.

Good, ordinary sex can help couples derive maximum satisfaction and happiness in a relationship; unhappy sex can make them miserable. The goal within ordinary sex is for human beings to learn practices that help them become more satisfied, balanced, loving and compassionate. With a little guidance and the right techniques, both partners can learn various skills to be more sensitive and alive during lovemaking. Learning ordinary sex techniques is an important preliminary step if you want to access higher potentials within sexual qigong and sexual meditation.

Here are four minimum requirements, or areas of skill, that must be achieved to improve ordinary sex and to become a better lover:

1. Develop hand sensitivity for manual sex.

2. Increase sensitivity and stamina of the mouth and tongue for oral sex.

3. For men, delay orgasms while maintaining and prolonging pleasurable erections.

4. For women, learn to have orgasms more easily.

For the average person, improving proficiency in these sexual skills can dramatically increase the pleasure in the bedroom.

SEXUAL SENSITIVITY SKILLS

Traditionally, the starting point in Taoist ordinary sex training is to learn to increase your overall sensitivity to your partner's nerves. You learn to make all parts of your body more sensitive and learn to feel how your touch is received by your partner. Great lovers are able to read their partner's body in real time, adjusting their touch and techniques to what is working and what is not. Each person and body is unique and often the sexual stimulation he or she needs may vary at different times.

Great lovers are able to read their partner's body in real time, adjusting their touch and techniques to what is working and what is not.

NERVE WEAKENING AND OVERSTIMULATION

Both a man's and a woman's genitals need to be handled with care, sensitivity and adroitness, especially if you want the sex act to go on for as long as you desire. Overstimulation of the genitals is a common issue with couples. It overloads the nerves and causes them to shut down. If this happens, both women and men may become numb to more stimulation, more easily sexually exhausted and in some cases may even experience pain. You can overstimulate the genitals with your hands, tongue and mouth or during intercourse.

The problem of overstimulation often surfaces after the first flush of strong attraction. It is well known that a man will often reach orgasm more quickly when he is with a woman for the first time than when he has known her for a while. This is due to the excitement factor, and the way new sensory input affects his nerves. In contrast, a woman typically has orgasms more easily only after she's been with a man a few times—we could call this the familiarity and comfort factor.

After the initial flush of excitement, other issues may surface. A woman may come far later than a man, and either the man or the woman may not want sex to go on long enough for her to reach orgasm. Thus, if the man comes significantly sooner than she, he can potentially leave her unsatisfied.

Even if he drives her to orgasm through manual or oral sex, his yang energy may not sufficiently connect strongly enough to satisfy her deeper yin. Through manual sex alone, she may also fail to fully release her pelvic nerves. Many men don't realize that if a woman's nerves do not fully release, if she does not relax at a deeper level, then her orgasm is far less likely to happen or, if it does, it will be significantly weaker. This may leave her tense and unsatisfied.

Moreover, some women are not aware that a man can have a very strong orgasm without ejaculating fluid, or that he can emit semen during a very weak orgasm that is not particularly pleasurable.

When a man has been making love for a while, the nerves of his penis can become overexcited and thus shut down. This can also occur for a woman's arousal. Her vaginal area can get so tense that she no longer becomes capable of successful lubrication, excitement, genital stimulation or orgasm. This is not due to a sudden lack of interest, appetite or some failing on the man or woman's part. It is simply that the sexually-related nerves are so overloaded they go numb. Often, when the nerves of a man or women go numb it results in the man ceasing to find sex pleasurable and losing his erection and causes the woman to be unable to complete an orgasm. Learning to tune into and monitor your nerves as well as those of your partner through greater sensitivity is a primary skill in all Taoist sexual arts.

OVERALL PRESSURE AND NERVE STRENGTH

The beginning point for greater sexual sensitivity is to become aware of your overall tactile pressure anytime you are touching your partner's body. When having sex you modulate your pressure and methods based on how your partner's body is responding. Take for example the area of a woman's clitoris. While some women require an incredible amount of stimulation in the clitoris area to get the nerves to activate, other women can just as easily become overstimulated and close down with minimal activity and pressure.

The same effect can happen with a man's penis when a woman, either with her hand or mouth, is too rough or conversely, too light. The art is to tune into your lover's body and vary your touch depending on the feedback your lover's body is giving you.

Sexual response is a delicate phenomenon that calls for a person to be sensitive and attentive to what is occurring spontaneously and naturally. A woman's body can bloom and open like a flower if she is handled with tender knowingness and skill, and it can close down quickly if she is not. Men respond to women who know how to turn them on but will equally shut down quickly if her sexual skills are poor.

When sex is hot and the pleasurable sensations particularly strong, you should also be aware that talking can alter the mood. It gets people out of their bodies and back into their heads. The same is true when nerves are becoming overstimulated. It's better to train your nonverbal sense of touch and let it tell you what is going on in your lover's body so that you can then adjust accordingly. However, if your partner has tuned you out—perhaps because he or she is just too turned on to notice or is lost in sensation—you should gently let the person know if you think your nerves are shutting down and guide them to slow down.

You should also take into consideration age in terms of nerve capacity. What was easy for a man and woman to do in their early twenties might not be so easy in their forties, fifties, sixties and beyond. Factors such as tension, disease, lack of sleep or excessive mental work can dramatically weaken human nerves. Nerve strength is linked to the ability of the penis to stay erect and the vagina to engorge. It is also what gives both partners the ability to register sensations.

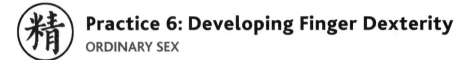

Practice 6: Developing Finger Dexterity
ORDINARY SEX

Working with your hands is one of the easiest ways to learn to improve your sensitivity as regards manual sex and to begin to feel how your touch affects the nerves of your partner. The following hand and finger sensitivity techniques[1] are among the very first practices Taoist initiates in sexual traditions are given to work with. This solo exercise develops tremendous finger dexterity. It also beneficially stimulates and increases the qi of your internal organs, as the acupuncture meridians of these organs end in the fingertips. This exercise also keeps your hands flexible and helps you avoid such problems as arthritis and carpal tunnel syndrome. Musicians report that practicing this technique helps to improve their playing.

Initially, do ten repetitions (five in one direction, five in the other). Then work your way up to one hundred or more over time. You can practice it when you are reading or watching television, for example. Always keep within seventy percent of your range of motion and stamina.

This exercise is done in two phases. Phase 1 has three parts. Do each hand in turn.

Phase 1

Part 1: Finger Rolling Exercise

1. Hold your thumb fixed in space above the middle of your palm.

2. Starting with your little finger and progressing to your index finger (Figures 7-1 A–D), move each fingertip in a rounded, rolling motion so that each touches your steady thumb tip in turn. Do this five times. Concentrate on rolling your fingers slowly and rhythmically.

3. Next, repeat the same action in the opposite direction, starting from your index finger and finishing with your little finger.

4. Progress to having your fingertips touch your thumb more quickly and fluidly, as you stretch the insides of your hands upward from the base of the palms to the fingertips.

---

1. The exercise that follows originally appeared in the author's book *The Great Stillness*.

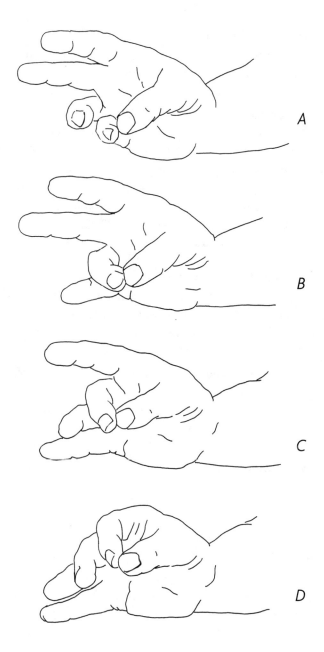

The fingers move to the thumb.

Figure 7-1 A–D: Hand Dexterity Exercise—Part 1

Part 2: Thumb Rolling Exercise

1. Curve your palm so the little finger is well within the borders of your palm and not toward or beyond the fleshy edge of your palm.

2. Move your thumb so that its tip touches the other four fingertips, one by one, beginning with the little finger and moving toward the index finger (Figure 7–2 A–D). The fingertips are held still. First move your thumb slowly and then more quickly and fluidly, stretching your muscles and tendons all the way from your wrist to your fingertips.

3. After your thumb touches your index finger, let it continue as far to the side as possible, stretching the whole hand (Figure 7–2 E) before circling back to again touch your little finger (Figure 7–2 A). After a significant number of repetitions, repeat the exercise in the reverse direction. Touch your index fingers first, little finger last, and as before, continue to move your thumb and spread your hand open (Figure 7–2 E).

Part 3: Combining the Two Moves

After you have separately mastered the finger and thumb motions of Parts 1 and 2, combine these together into one continuous movement, as follows. Begin by touching your little finger first and index finger last. After five times, repeat the same process, only reverse direction and begin touching your index finger first and little finger last.

1. Fingers move: Begin with your little finger and touch each of your four fingertips one by one to your thumb (held fixed in space above your palm). After your index finger has touched your thumb, stretch your hand wide open. Again, sequentially touch your four fingers to your thumb, stretch your hand open, and repeat.

2. Thumb moves: Without stopping or resting your hand, if possible, continue in the other direction as your thumb touches your index finger first and your little finger last, doing all the motions of Part 2.

Phase 2

1. Repeat Phase 1, Part 1, but instead of touching the tip of your thumb, the fingertips now touch the base of the thumb or at least the big muscle below your thumb.

2. Repeat Phase 1, Part 2, but now the thumb tip touches the base of your fingers, rather than their tips. The number of repetitions remains the same. The stretch of your hand muscles, ligaments, and tendons should not only include your palm but also extend all the way down to your forearm. ●

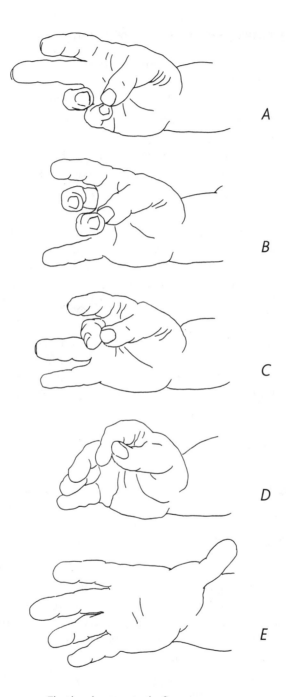

A

B

C

D

E

The thumb moves to the fingers.

Figure 7-2 A–E: Hand Dexterity Exercise—Part 2

SLOW DOWN TO RECOVER FROM OVERSTIMULATION

When couples experience a nerve shutdown during sex, they may start running internal dialogues that blame the other person. Both partners must understand that the problem is nerve shutdown and that they can do something about it.

When you are having sex, at the first sign of overstimulation, one strategy is to leave each other's genitals alone. Shift the focus to another part of the body or simply rest for a few minutes by cuddling and breathing together. It's important to give the nerves a chance to rest, relax and decompress. The nerves need time to process the flood of stimuli. Once the stimuli diminish, the man's erection will usually return and so will the woman's openness.

Unfortunately, many often do the opposite and go for escalating stimulation when an erection starts to fail or the woman doesn't climax. This worsens the situation rather than helping it. Keeping nerve pulsations regular can create stamina and keep pleasure increasing rather than diminishing. You will want to continually tune in and notice when you are overstimulating your partner's nerves or the reverse. Don't hesitate to back off or slow down or ask them to do the same.

If you are having regular issues of nerve overstimulation, the energy practices of qigong and tai chi (explained in Chapter 10) directly help relax the body and strengthen the nerves. Other benefits of these energy practices, such as better circulation of fluids and the toning of internal organs, also make you healthier and more flexible, which in turn will benefit your sex life. This makes it possible for you to eventually go beyond ordinary sex into the higher potentials of sexual qigong and sexual meditation.

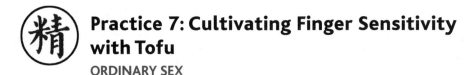 ## Practice 7: Cultivating Finger Sensitivity with Tofu
ORDINARY SEX

One of the most widely used and, to most Westerners, surprising techniques for further developing finger sensitivity involves the use of tofu, the bean-curd cake used in many Chinese and vegetarian recipes. The texture and density of some kinds of tofu closely approximates that of human flesh. Through this exercise you can learn to change the tactile pressure of your fingers to reach different layers with precision. You can use this skill to add more pleasure to your sexual activity.

Tofu training can be done either as an ordinary sex or a sexual qigong practice. These exercises have been used for millennia in Chinese qi-based therapeutic massage, tai chi and internal martial arts to help develop relaxed, flexible yet strong fingers. Qi releases from both fingers and fingertips. The more sensitive your fingers become, the more aware you can be of your own qi and that of others. In sexual qigong, you can project not only physical pressure but also qi from your fingers (gained through tofu training) to turn your partner on and bring him or her to orgasm more pleasurably than with manual sex that is only physical.

Most importantly, these exercises will help you avoid insensitive sexual touching, which can result in rough handling of areas that are exceptionally sensitive or in overstimulating them.

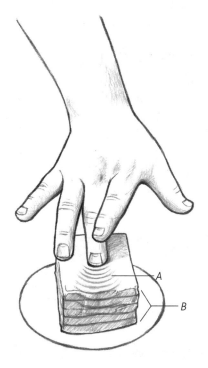

A—Finger pressure waves
    penetrating into tofu

B—Finger pressure can be
    isolated into each of
    the five layers of tofu

Figure 7-3: Finger Exercises with Tofu

Begin by first using your middle or index finger. Eventually progress to where you can use any possible combinations of your fingers, including your thumbs. Keep contact on the same patch of tofu surface without sliding off until you have finished the exercise. Repeat the exercise by moving your finger to a new patch of tofu surface.

1. Touch the top surface of a smooth cake of tofu with either your middle or your index finger as lightly as possible. Adjust your finger pressure and adhesion so you can grip the skin of the tofu without sliding or breaking the bean curd's skin.

2. Vary the degree to which your hand is pressing into the "flesh" to cause the tofu to move, layer-by-layer, deeper toward the bottom. Eventually you will be able to make

the whole cake move with a very light touch on the same patch of skin on the surface.

3. In the beginning, you will probably only be able to get the whole tofu cake to move only as a single unit. With time and copious practice, however, you will be able to identify and isolate exactly which layer of the tofu your finger pressure will move. Stay with it until you can move one specific layer only, leaving the rest of the cake unaffected.

Eventually you want to be able to use all the fingers of your hand equally well, including your thumb. If you practice regularly with tofu, within a year you should be able to use your fingers to stimulate erogenous zones for a prolonged time with skill and without strain. ●

USING HAND SENSITIVITY TECHNIQUES

Apply what you have learned on the tofu to various erogenous zones of your partner, not only the genitals. These techniques will enable you to vary the rhythms of your touch as well as their intensity and help keep you and your partner's nerves smooth while maximizing excitement. The increased sensitivity you've developed will also enable you to feel when you are overstimulating your partner's nerves.

You will find that the sensitivity you have acquired will, with practice, easily transfer to your mouth, tongue and genitals. When you learn to feel in one place, it makes it easier to feel in another.

Some men are often baffled by the mysteries of a woman's body, and women may feel the same way about a man's body, although the mystery can become an adventure if your starting point is one of discovery. First of all, it's important to keep in mind that every woman's and man's body is unique, as are their genital areas. You cannot assume that what your last lover enjoyed will also get your new lover arching and writhing with pleasure.

How a Man Can Help Bring a Woman to Orgasm

Along the length of a woman's vagina, and especially her clitoris, are several small ring-shaped zones that energetically correspond to and activate various areas of her physical and energy anatomy. Each ring can have a differing ability to receive pleasure.

Using various forms of pressure, touch and intensity, explore their effects. Don't fixate solely on her clitoris or any of her unique "hot spots" like her G-spot. Any time you stay on a particular spot too long—no matter how much she moans—you run the risk of "too much of a good thing" and can cause her nerves to become numb and shut down.

The frustration of being so close and yet so far away is no fun for either of you. To remedy this, shift your fingers away from the overstimulated place to where the nerves are fresh. Keep her turned on by shifting your focus and giving her hot spots a rest. Once the nerves have a chance to regenerate and reawaken, they will be open again to pleasurable sensation.

How a Woman Can Help Bring a Man to Orgasm

Although a man's body may be more easily stimulated and aroused than a woman's, hand sensitivity is equally important. All parts of the man's penis and balls have varying levels of sensitivity. Use your new techniques to explore each part. You may find yourself enjoying the varying degrees of hardness and changes in skin texture that occur in a man's penis as he cycles through the different phases of an erection.

Be gentle. A woman who is too rough can cause pain to a man's genitals. A woman needs a light, sensitive touch to gauge if she is stimulating a man's genitals in a way that progressively turns him on or, conversely, is overworking his genital nerves and thereby inhibiting his full sexual response.

What few women realize is that many men won't say anything when a woman is causing him discomfort. His "macho" conditioning simply won't allow him to admit something hurts or is not pleasurable. This means it is doubly important that her hand sensitivity be sufficient to feel his bodily responses, especially if the man is relatively inexperienced and insensitive to his own bodily functions.

As much as the penis likes to take center stage, however, it's important to be sensitive to the pubic mound area around and above the penis as well. Is it becoming overly tense? Is he developing resistance in his body above and beyond his sexual contractions?

Be creative and experiment with the techniques in this chapter to both increase sexual pleasure and avoid the nerve shutdown that can lead to emotional resistance. The more a partner can become sensitive to the other's needs, the better the sex and the relationship becomes.

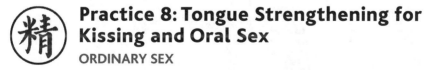

Practice 8: Tongue Strengthening for Kissing and Oral Sex
ORDINARY SEX

The previous practices worked on developing your hand sensitivity. You can use all parts of your body during sex, and one of the most useful is your tongue. However, when using your tongue to please your lover sexually, you may find that the area underneath the root of the tongue becomes fatigued, causing weakness and loss of sensitivity. Here are two useful exercises to remedy this problem:

- Extend your tongue as far beyond your teeth as possible. Move it around, up and down

(Figure 7-4 A and C), side to side (Figure 7-4 B), diagonally (Figure 7-4 D), in circles of varying circumferences (Figure 7-4 A–D and D–A), in figure eights (not shown) or write the alphabet in the air at varying speeds for up to five to ten minutes. This will stretch the ligaments and strengthen the muscles at the root of the tongue, enabling you to stay on the job a lot longer while enjoying it more.

- Curl the tongue outside the teeth, for two or three minutes at a time. Tongue sensitivity, speed and control are equally important for cunnilingus and fellatio. Men usually need more practice than women. One of the problems a woman may have with fellatio, however, is she may not realize when she is attempting to give pleasure that she's actually hurting a man's testicles—she may not have learned how to play the line between sexual excitement, numbness and pressure-inducing pain. In addition, the mouth or tongue pressure on his penis may either be too light or too heavy. ●

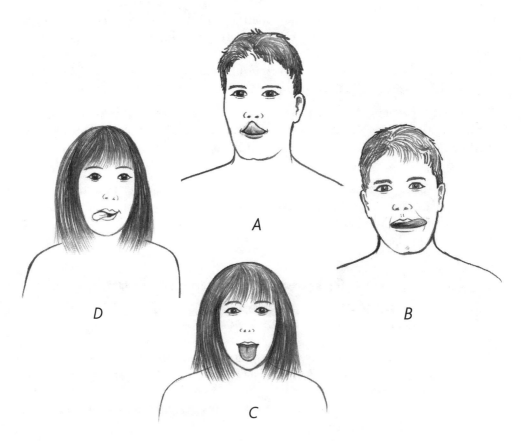

Stretch the tongue to extend its stamina and range of motion.

Figure 7-4 A–D: Tongue Stretching Exercise

Sex and Pregnancy

During pregnancy, it is not uncommon for either or both partners to have strong feelings about intercourse. These feelings can range across a broad spectrum from intense desire to fear and nervousness to feeling completely shut down and unwilling to engage sexually. Some men fear penetration, because they think that in some way it will harm the mother or fetus.

If a woman is feeling down or genuinely does not want to make love during pregnancy, Taoists advise that she does not do so. Rather than risk a potential negative impact on the child, which could take many forms, such as a subliminal resistance to sex later in life, listen to what is arising within. This is an issue of utmost sensitivity that must be carefully weighed, taking into account the differing needs of mother, father and child.

Men are known to get resentful when pregnant wives don't satisfy their sexual needs, especially for intercourse. On the flip side of that issue, many women feel resentful and abandoned when a man fails to meet her emotional needs because she is unwilling to engage in active intercourse. This pregnancy-related resentment has been known to fester after the baby arrives and to lead to marital problems down the road. To remedy the situation before it gets out of hand, couples can use massage, oral sex, mutual masturbation, cuddling or whatever is required to relieve the sexual tension.

When either partner really doesn't want to make love and feels a powerful internal "No!" that message gets communicated energetically to the baby, whether verbalized or not. If the fetus absorbs this energy, it can create subliminal negative conditioning that may have lifelong effects.

Even though Taoists have positive views about sex and encourage sexual expression, they consider the parents' two primary duties far more important than their pleasure. First, parents must do everything possible to ensure the healthy development of their child. Second, they must take great care to avoid negatively conditioning the fetus in any way, to reduce the risk of problems later in the child's life.

MITIGATING NERVE STRAIN WITH PILLOWS

Due to the nature of sexual excitement and other types of physical activity, regular nerve pulsations build stamina while irregular nerve firing rapidly leads to exhaustion. Nerves can also become exhausted if there is strain on the hip and back muscles. Pain in these areas may be an early indicator of weakening sexual nerves.

Depending on who is doing more pelvic thrusting during lovemaking, a man or woman can mitigate nerve strain by using pillows to prop up his or her hips or back. This will allow a lover to use the large muscles of the buttocks to thrust and withdraw rather than the more vulnerable lower back and pelvic muscles, which are comparatively weaker. Pumping by moving the butt muscles rather than the lower back takes much less effort and is less tiring.

AROUSAL THROUGH BITING

Biting can be a highly erotic form of love play. The important issue with biting is degree: depending on how gently or hard you nip, you can either stimulate your partner's nerves in a variety of wonderful ways or shut them down. Play the edge between exciting the nerves and stopping completely to let them release, relax and regenerate. You want to bite harder to get your partner excited and then soften your grip or just hold ever so gently with your teeth until the nerves regroup. Keep your partner in a state of heightened arousal, only rarely pushing it into the one hundred percent excitability zone. This type of play can be quite delightful for both parties.

It is important to note, however, that while some people respond very well to biting and deep scratching, others do not like it at all. From the Taoist perspective, the qualities of the five elements (see Chapter 6) are determining factors. Those with a preponderance of the Fire and Earth elements usually don't respond very well to deep biting or scratching, whereas those with a preponderance of Wood as their elemental type usually do, although not to the point of drawing blood. Metal types tend to be neutral. Bottom line: if you bite or scratch deeply and it gives your partner pleasure and excitement, then it's okay. If biting makes your partner contract or shut down, then don't do it. An inappropriately timed bite has been known to shut down the whole sexual process.

TAOIST VIEWS ON MASTURBATION

Taoists generally view sex through the lens of how it affects your overall qi rather than whether or not it's pleasurable. If a sexual activity makes your qi stronger and your body healthier, it is good. If it brings pleasure but no appreciable benefit to your qi, it is neutral or *wu so hui,* not so important. If the likely outcome is that a sexual activity—regardless of how pleasurable—weakens or damages your qi, then it is not good.

FOR WOMEN

Taoists are neutral regarding female masturbation—so enjoy it if it turns you on. The big benefit of female masturbation from a Taoist view is to learn to use it as a solo practice tool to access and consciously move sexual energy around the body.

Taoists are neutral as regards the use of sex toys, such as vibrators, dildos and so on. They would say these items aren't negative in themselves, but because they can't emit qi into the female body, neither are they preferred.

Taoists approve of anything that promotes physical health without significant downsides. They view sex toys as pragmatic tools for keeping women healthy during sexual dry spells, as they can keep a woman's sexual area in better working order in two ways. First, they can keep her pelvic nerves accustomed to stimulation, so when she is sexually active again, they won't shut down as easily during sex. Second, dildos can help stretch her pelvic chamber, so that it remains more flexible and relaxed. This is particularly helpful if the area has can become overly contracted, for example, as a result of accumulated scar tissue acquired from childbirth or surgery.[2]

FOR MEN

For the most part, Taoists considered male masturbation at best neutral and a pleasurable waste of time. At worst, it is not good or even dangerous. Taoists recommend against it mostly due to its potential to damage a male's qi.

Conservative Taoists insist that a man must never masturbate, due to the risk of losing *jing* (sperm energy), becoming weak and shortening his lifespan.

Of course, the question remains: what can be done with sexual frustration that becomes unhealthy for the mind? If unsatisfied sexual needs cause a disturbance that consumes qi anyway, a man is probably better off masturbating. Here are some additional points:

1. If a man has a very strong physique and doesn't tire afterward, masturbation is probably not too detrimental.

2. If a man is going to masturbate, it's better to do so during the yang period of daytime rather than the yin period of night, as this allows him to reclaim his lost energy more easily.

3. On occasion, masturbation can be valuable as a learning tool for a limited duration. It can teach a man how to:

   • Transfer sexual energy from the genitals to other parts of his body

   • Have weak internal orgasms without ejaculation

   • Sexually generate and direct qi to move through all cells in the body.

---

2. In certain cases, physical therapists who specialize in women's health and rehabilitating the pelvic area can help to alleviate this problem.

FOR ADOLESCENTS

In the case of virgin female adolescents, just as for women in general, masturbation was a neutral event. As regards to boys, however, Taoists were pragmatists—they recognized that most male virgin adolescents were going to masturbate even if told not to, so they would teach them sexual energy control techniques to use during masturbation. Taoists believed it was better for virgin boys approaching the beginning of sexual life to gain energy rather than lose it.

PROSTATE MASSAGE

In Chinese medicine, prostate problems are often resolved with qigong, herbs and mineral therapies. An ordinary sex technique a man can do for himself that is generally beneficial for the prostate is to open and close the kwa (see Chapter 11, Figure 11-8) using medium or strong pressure that will internally massage the prostate area. A woman can address congestion in a man's prostate by making small circles with her fingers massaging his mound area around the pubic hair. It is not advocated by Taoists to use the method of massaging the prostate directly by inserting a finger through the anus that is sometimes advocated in neo-Tantra.

Work very slowly and go quite deep using small circles with the tips of your fingers. Focus especially on the pubic mound area, as this is where the nerve congestion that will reflect to the genitals is likely to be centered. Draw the pressure in his testicles up from the root of the penis all the way out to the tip. Your goal is to get the energy stuck in his testicles to cycle through to completion so the nerves can let go and allow the fluid (blood or lymph) to drain from the body. Releasing nerve congestion in this area can release all the tissue up and into the prostate.

FLUID HIPS FOR BETTER SEX

Your genitals are attached to the inside of your pelvis—to the hips. Many people have hips that are generally stiff in or out of the bedroom. The solo pelvic movement exercises of Practice 9 can help you to increase the fluidity, flexibility, and ease of control of your hips. Being able to move them fully and in multiple angles enables lovers to have greater pleasure. For example, if you can do large hip circles with skill, in time you can do very small ones, which works wonders in bed.

精 Practice 9: Move That Pelvis
ORDINARY SEX

Many people have a fairly limited range of pelvic motion, which can also limit the pleasure a couple can have. Ideally during lovemaking, pelvic movement should be able to make a man's penis or a woman's vagina go any direction—up or down, in and out, side to side and all the connecting angles in between, as well as in shapes such as circles and figure eights. The object of the following exercises is to give you precise pelvic control and to enable you to turn stiff hips into ones that are free-moving like undulating silk.

Pelvic exercises are a very effective and easy way to develop the body for sex. Each exercise can be done first by standing, which is physically the easiest way to do the practice. Later, if you choose, it can be beneficial to practice these pelvic movements in different sexual positions.

For example, you can try the exercises sitting Japanese style with your feet under your buttocks, squatting with one leg higher than or in front of the other, going on all fours and lying down on your back or side. It is important in each of these exercises, no matter what position, to apply your seventy-percent rule. If you are not used to moving your hips or you do not regularly exercise, start with fewer repetitions and gradually build up over time.

To begin, stand with your feet shoulder-width apart and:

1. Move your pelvis on a horizontal plane forward and backward as comfortably as you can go. In the beginning, take it slow and easy so as not to strain your back (Figure 7-5 A–B).

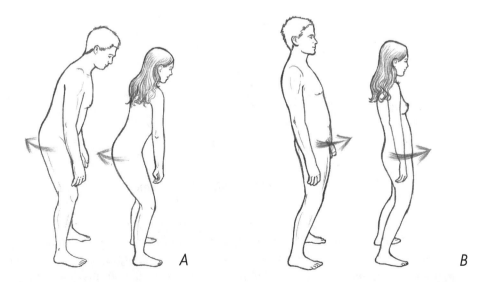

Figure 7-5 A–B: Backward and Forward Hip Movements for Thrusting and Withdrawal

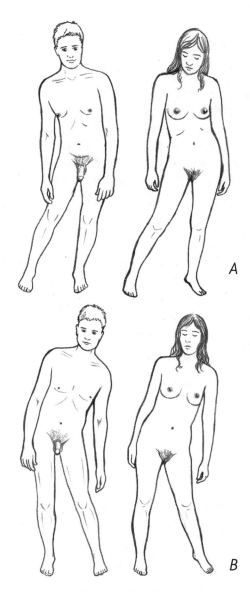

Figure 7-6 A–B: Side-to-Side Hip Movements

2. Continuing to keep your feet planted, move your hips slightly to the left and then right until your hips and associated muscles become warmed up and, as if oiled, move smoothly with minimal or no physical resistance. Gradually extend the sideways motions of your hips until you can go to seventy percent of your maximum range of motion to the left and right sides easily and without strain (Figure 7-6 A–B).

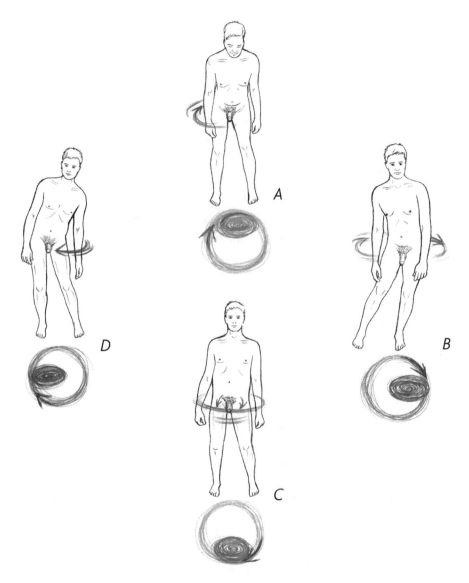

Shaded area of circle represents hip position for each part of the rotation.

Figure 7-7 A–D: Circular Hip Movements

3. Merge the previous two movements (forward, back, left and right) together into a circle. Begin with a small rotation, and as your hips become more relaxed, stretched and "oiled," gradually increase the size of your hip-rotating circle until you have reached seventy percent of your range of motion. Reverse the direction of your rotation every two or three circles (Figure 7-7 A–D).

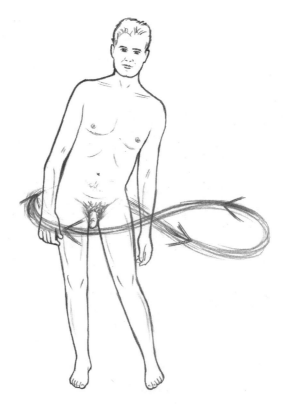

Figure 7-8: Figure Eight Hip Movements

4. Finally turn the circle into a spiral. Gradually make the circle bigger till it reaches its largest circumference, then gradually wind it down to as small a circle as possible, and then enlarge it again, and so on. In a large motion, make figure eights with your pelvis, lowering and raising your pelvis accordingly (Figure 7-8). Without moving large distances either forward, back or sideways, make vertical circles with your hips, so the left side goes down and the right side raises and vice versa. Then make very tight figure eights in every direction, moving your genitals up/down, forward/back, and left/right, both vertically and horizontally. ●

THE VALUE OF HIP EXERCISES FOR THE PHYSICAL BODY

The exercises shown in Practice 9 can be quite physically beneficial. For example, forward and backward hip movements (Figure 7-5 A–B) connect, stretch and lengthen the entire area from the middle of the thighs all the way up to the top of the neck, preventing all the related body parts from tightening. Sex can contract these areas and cause negative results, including back pain. If strained, these areas can also diminish your stamina as regards the hip movements which drive the genitals, causing your hips to tire needlessly early.

In addition, these hip movements can help relax and deepen your breathing during sex. The full stretch, from the feet to the top of your head, usually requires more aerobic capacity than only doing pelvic thrusting either lying down in bed or on all fours. This exercise for developing relaxed hip-thrusting stamina is especially useful, for example, in rear-entry positions (doggie style) or while he stands on the floor and she lies on the bed, and so forth. Loosening the related pelvic muscles and ligaments through this hip exercise will also make it easier to do pelvic forward and backward thrusting.

THE VALUE OF HIP EXERCISES FOR SEXUAL QIGONG

The exercises of Practice 9, done keeping the spine straight while moving the buttocks in all directions, build the necessary foundation in sexual qigong for connecting the energy of the torso, spine, hips, legs and feet. Done standing, these pelvic movements set the physical stage for later in sexual qigong unifying the entire body's energy without it disconnecting at the pelvic or lower back area.

Within sexual qigong, these hip movements are used to consciously activate and direct qi to move in all three primary energy channels as well as in others. For example, one might bring qi from the feet to the crown of the head on forward or upward hip thrusts and then from the crown of the head down the three channels to the feet when the hips go backward or downward. Likewise, smooth, fluid hip movements enable you to move the qi up and down more efficiently at the required speed without breaking the flow.

In sexual qigong, each of these hip movement exercises can be used to work with the three main energy channels of the body (introduced in Chapter 3) in specific ways:

Backward and forward movements (Figure 7-5): Activate energy moving up and down the central channel.

Side-to-side movements (Figure 7-6): Move qi either into the left or right channel.

Circular movements (Figure 7-7): Continuously circulate qi between the left and right channels.

Figure eight movements (Figure 7-8): Circulate energy between the three channels in all possible combinations, such as up one and down the other and vice-versa, from the central to the right only or vice versa, from the central to the left only or vice versa, and combining these configurations in continuous, ever-changing flows as the hips do figure eights.

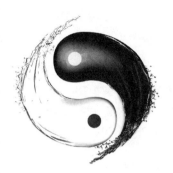

CHAPTER 8

Orgasm—
Hers and His

The essential difference between the sexual nature of a man and that of a woman has a great deal to do with the very unique way each gender experiences—or doesn't experience—satisfaction through an orgasm. The challenges men and women face with orgasms are very distinct. For men, the challenge is obvious: if untrained, most tend to come too soon. Learning to prolong an erection and delay ejaculation is essential for a man to satisfy a woman. Many men also complain of feeling depleted and exhausted after an ejaculation orgasm.

A woman's challenge is quite different: she must learn to turn on and fully ignite her orgasmic nature as well as work with her sexual partner to ensure her needs are met. A large segment of the female population remains nonorgasmic, and those who do experience orgasms often have a fairly limited range of sensations.

Taoists have developed many useful techniques for both men and women to address these practical concerns. As always, the emphasis is on working with internal energies to move toward balance, integration, happiness and, ultimately, spiritual awakening.

ENERGETIC MECHANISM OF A TENSION ORGASM

The Chinese call ordinary genital orgasms "Clouds and Rain." Unless you understand how the Chinese mind works, you'd have no way of knowing that "Clouds and Rain" alludes to the lightning phase in the middle, an apt metaphor for the high-pressure release that accompanies the average man's climax. As a man makes love, his glandular system builds up a highly charged energetic lattice that affects all his internal organs. As he revs up, his insides become tense. The more he revs, the more his body tenses and his nerves tighten.

This buildup is akin to the high-pressure system of clouds that come in before a rainstorm. At the peak of this tension state, he explodes in a dramatic act (the lightning), which is followed by a release (the rain). This "rev, rev, rev...explode" pattern shatters the energetic lattice and disorients his glands and internal organs. The sudden explosion also shocks his qi, and can also be accompanied by adrenaline, which is destructive to a man's health and nerves in the long run.

A tension orgasm hits a man's body like an internal body-slam. Some men feel completely and totally exhausted for hours, even days, after a tension orgasm, whereas women don't. The degree of tiredness is related to the ratio between the internal strength of a man's body and the frequency of sexual contact.

If a man doesn't have a strong constitution, the sudden shock can debilitate him. But a stronger man often doesn't even register the shock to his system; he isn't aware that each tension orgasm is potentially a self-inflicted injury. His situation is analogous to the athlete who, after playing contact sports for years, is considerably weaker and less able-bodied after having sustained cumulative injuries. While he is acquiring these injuries, the athlete may not take them that seriously.

Women also have tension orgasms, although the net effect is quite different. When a tension orgasm shatters the energetic lattice in a woman's body, her yin will naturally reabsorb the energy and draw it back into her system. In the long run, a tension orgasm will not diminish her vitality but instead will energize and invigorate her.

The tension orgasm has an energetic explosive quality, which may or may not accompany a physical explosion. In a man, a tension orgasm and ejaculation can occur even without pleasurable sensation, simply because, at a certain point, the body's nerves go into spontaneous override. This is a cause of nocturnal emissions, or wet dreams, in adolescent boys.

Even in adults, continuous rubbing—whether through vaginal friction or manual stimulation—sooner or later can affect the nerves that go from the penis back to the prostrate, causing automatic reflexes to take over. More often than not, the result is an orgasm or, alternatively, a partial orgasm when the reflexes fire, but ejaculation does not occur.

In the West, neither men nor women commonly know that there are different and better ways to experience orgasms.

FEMALE ORGASM: MAXIMIZE THE YIN

Among the Chinese, where poetic images so often express value, a woman's orgasm is widely known as gao chao, or "High Tide." Her sexual nature is more sensitive as evidenced in simple biological facts: a man's penis has about four thousand nerve endings, whereas eight thousand or so are found in a woman's clitoris.

Unlike the multipurpose penis, which—in addition to housing his primary pleasure circuits—serves as an organ of procreation and elimination, the sole function of the clitoris is ecstasy leading to orgasm. Most women experience orgasm through clitoral stimulation, while far fewer orgasmic women have deeper "vaginal" orgasms with intercourse. In reality, the clitoris is a complex organ that interacts with more than fifteen thousand nerve endings throughout the entire pelvic area. Generally a woman's external orgasmic capacity can far exceed the average man's.

The Taoist approach to the female orgasm is to actualize the maximum amount of yin a woman can absorb through sex. From this perspective, an orgasm that is sourced from direct stimulation of the external portion of the clitoris—the glans or "pearl" that sits at the top of her labia beneath a hood (see Chapter 3, Figure 3-9)—does not activate nearly as much of her yin as an orgasm from deep within.

In addition, when her orgasm issues from the external portion of the clitoris, a woman will generally require a rest period, due to hypersensitivity of the glans. On the other hand, when she experiences a deep orgasm that shudders through the walls of her vagina, this profoundly nourishes her yin. In addition, deeper orgasms tend to build on one another as she comes again and again in wave after pleasurable wave.

A woman is fulfilled in her yin nature when she learns to surrender and fully receive a man's yang energy. He can increase her receptivity by involving as much of her body in the sensation as possible rather than focusing specifically on either the clitoris or the vagina. Both men and women do well to approach her orgasm as an ongoing discovery.

EXPANDING WESTERN VIEWS OF FEMALE ORGASM

It is difficult to say how Westerners viewed the orgasm, much less a woman's orgasmic capacity, before the middle of the twentieth century. We do know that many women were nonorgasmic. Historically, this was not considered a problem, because in the Victorian cultural era (which continues to exert its influence more than we imagine), many women viewed sex as a chore. As long as she "did her duty" and produced offspring, she was believed to have fulfilled her role in life. In previous eras, women with an overt desire for sex were branded as wanton or brazen, suitable for a mistress but not for a respectable wife.

The once popular books of British doctor, William Acton, reflect the repressive and anti-female views on sexuality that were commonplace in Victorian times. Renowned as an expert in gynecology and urology, he states, "I should say that the majority of women (happily for them) are not very much troubled with sexual feeling of any kind."[1]

Indeed, the ludicrous way doctors of that day would deal with female health issues, as Mary Roach describes in *Bonk: The Curious Coupling of Science and Sex,*[2] does not inspire confidence in any conclusions drawn by a Victorian physician regarding women's bodily functions:

"Victorian physicians practiced gynecology and urology on women *without looking.* Even a catheter insertion would typically be done blind, with the doctor's hands under the sheets and his gaze heading off in some polite middle distance."

We know that Sigmund Freud postulated the concept of a vaginal orgasm as distinct from a clitoral orgasm, and that he believed clitoral orgasms to be an adolescent phenomenon that a woman would (and should) outgrow once she reached adulthood. Not until the late 1950s and early 1960s, with the groundbreaking work of Alfred Kinsey, Shere Hite, and the pioneering research team, Masters and Johnson, was the female orgasm liberated from this limited Freudian frame.

In recent years, the female orgasm has become quite the hot topic. Women are now far more likely to want, even demand, a satisfying sex life. Women have come to understand (and even crave) multiple and extended orgasms, gushing orgasms and G-spot orgasms.

BARRIERS TO FEMALE ORGASMS

A woman who wants to activate and awaken her ability to have orgasms must first learn how to get over the physical hurdle to doing so. Many women are minimally orgasmic and have been so throughout their lives. There are a number of possible reasons why some women do not have more orgasms or have difficulty having an orgasm at all:

1. General excessive levels of physical, emotional and mental tension.

2. Frozen sexual pelvic nerves that can't release.

3. Hormonal imbalances—especially during periods of stress—may result in a lowered libido.

4. Inability to surrender fully to a male's yang energy, which may or may not be tied to a need to stay in control.

5. Either physical or psychological trauma.

---

1. Acton, William, *The Functions and Disorders of the Reproductive Organs in Childhood, Youth, Adult Age, and Advanced Life: Considered in Their Physiological, Social, and Moral Relations,* 2nd American from 4th London ed. (Philadelphia: Lindsay and Blakiston, 1867), 144.

2. Roach, Mary, *Bonk: The Curious Coupling of Science and Sex* (New York: W. W. Norton, 2008), 14.

6. Insufficient energy moving from the heart and/or throat to the vagina.

7. Previous sexual karma.

All of these conditions may be due to any number of causes: for example, fear, repression, aggressive or abusive treatment in her past, or lack of positive emotional contact as a child. In these cases, the Taoists' expertise is particularly helpful, because a woman's orgasm derives from the opening of her sexual nerves and the flow of energy throughout her body.

It's important to understand that sexual unresponsiveness is not purely psychological. Once highly sensitive nerves become habitually shut down, the qi also contracts. This contraction normally cannot be reversed all at once, only over time with many major and minor releases. Some take a long time, even years, to become orgasmic, although it can also happen quickly.

One of the easiest ways for a woman to learn to have better orgasms is through masturbation, either with or without a vibrator or other sex toy. Taoists do not generally have specific solo practices beyond this method to help a woman cross the threshold from nonorgasmic to orgasmic. However, Taoist women have found that solo sexual qigong practices helped them go over the edge by increasing their sensitivity and flow of qi. A far more reliable method is to have a man skillfully use his hands, mouth and tongue to guide a woman into her senses and over the finish line. A mechanical vibrator provides a physical orgasm only. An orgasm from sexual activity with a live human being tends to be much more satisfying as it involves an energy transfer and an emotional context.

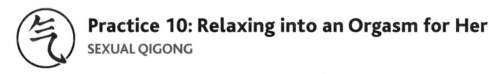

Practice 10: Relaxing into an Orgasm for Her
SEXUAL QIGONG

Guidelines for a woman: You can begin to coax your own orgasm out of hiding by paying attention to sensation and, essentially, getting out of your head and into your body. Begin by noticing how you feel inside your own skin during nonsexual activities of all kinds.

Then, while in the presence of your lover, slow down enough to allow your body to truly respond to his touch. You might do this in the kitchen or anywhere else when he brushes up against you. Simply allow your body to register pleasure and actually respond. When you feel ready, you can ask him to specifically touch you all over with no intention of intercourse.

How a Man Can Help

Here are basic guidelines if a man wants to take on the commitment of enabling a nonorgasmic woman to become orgasmic.

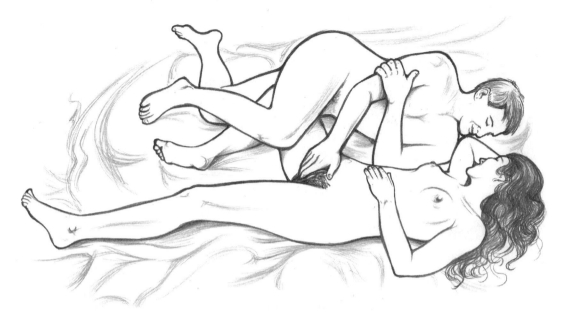

Figure 8-1: Bringing a Woman to Orgasm by Manual Stimulation

1. Understand that her contracted nerves and closed-down energy channels will take time to open. This can involve a lot of nongenital foreplay, including foot and thigh work, as well as manual and tongue stimulation.

2. Do what it takes to establish trust, so she knows you are not going to hurt her in any way.

3. Follow through is key. You must have a genuine and sincere desire to go through this labor of love, otherwise it is just too easy to give up in the middle.

4. On any given night, stoke the fires as far as they can go for a minimum of three rounds. Stimulate her, then let her calm down for a minimum of five minutes before you begin again. This enables her nervous system to stabilize and potentially reach a higher level of nerve input before shutting down the next time. Although three rounds is the minimum, feel free to continue as long as she is willing and indicates that she likes what is happening.

5. Over time, her naturally orgasmic nerve flows will reawaken and start behaving normally. ●

Possible Reactions from Strong Orgasms

Anyone can experience a reaction during or after an orgasm and, while within the range of perfectly normal, certain responses can come as quite a surprise. Ideally, these should be recognized and accepted for what they are—a natural reaction to the intense whole-being release that occurs with an orgasm. Here are a few examples:

- A little bit of urine can become mixed in with copious vaginal secretions. If a woman has this tendency then it is best that she empties her bladder before making love.

- When a woman has a very strong orgasm, besides physical secretions, she may also have a tremendous release of yin qi, which may manifest in tears. A man can benefit greatly by absorbing the yin of her tears if he kisses or licks up his lover's tears.

- The male counterpart to her yin release is a yang release during or after a strong orgasm. He may growl, laugh or have a peculiar, even fierce, look on his face. These are expressions of his yang qi fulfilling itself.

MALE ORGASM: MAXIMIZE THE YANG

Whereas the female belongs to yin and is slow to be aroused, the male belongs to yang and is quickly aroused. His challenge, then, is to pace himself so as not to be viewed as an impatient and insensitive lover.

SEMEN RETENTION: A HALLMARK OF TAOIST SEX TECHNIQUES

There are countless ancient methods that enable a man to slow down or completely stop the emission of semen—some from the inner traditions of Indian Tantra and yoga—for example in classic Hatha Yoga, the advanced *Vajroli Mudra* is a classic technique in which male practitioners are able to suck up and drain water from a glass with their penis to enable them to avoid ejaculating or, if they do, to bring the semen back into their body before it is lost.

There are also numerous techniques from both the Fire and Water traditions of Taoism. Taoist men mastered semen retention thousands of years ago. Their ability to control their orgasms is what gave Taoist men and women the freedom to explore the potential of sex outside reproduction. What's more, the ancient Taoists had no equivalent to Victorian repression. The basic assumption was that both men and women were always interested in maximizing each other's pleasure. Learning to prolong an erection in order to fulfill a woman has always been a primary mandate for Taoist men.

For many people in the Western world, the idea of semen retention is utterly foreign. We're speaking in general here, of course, but in an overarching sense, Westerners have been far less involved in the systematic study of sex, historically speaking, than the Chinese.

Since ancient times in China, both men and women have given a great deal of thought to how to have a lot of satisfying sex without a negative impact on the body. Open discussion was commonplace. Men were concerned for obvious reasons, and women were concerned because unhappy or blaming husbands could make life dismal. Some texts and schools of thought asserted that ejaculation would make a man happy, whereas not ejaculating could make him miserable.

THE CASE FOR SEMEN RETENTION

The idea of holding the sperm inside and not ejaculating is often is credited to Peng Zu (Peng Tzu, Peng Tsu), who purportedly lived for eight hundred years. Among Peng Zu's classic prescriptions for a living a very long life was that a man should have sex three to five times a day (preferably with very young women) and not ejaculate. He was also to sleep with young virgins without having sex (to absorb their yin energy), use herbs and practice qigong.

Peng Zu and others advanced several ideas regarding the negative impact of ejaculation. For example, it was asserted that ejaculation causes:

- Weakness in the body
- Buzzing in the ears
- Soreness in the eyes
- Dryness in the throat
- Degeneration in the bones

According to these theories, not ejaculating or emitting sperm allows a man to avoid these problems with no downside. A man can still be happy and, on top of that, can increase his lifespan, and become more vibrant, healthy and resistant to disease, simply by retaining his semen.

After the Tang Dynasty (618–907 AD), this philosophy formed the basis of the fanatical, often neurotic and even obsessive belief held by neo-Taoists and many Fire-method Taoists that ejaculating semen was a major mistake—one a man should never make.

The belief is predicated on the idea that semen contains the essential nutritional and energetic essence of your body, and that a man cannot readily replenish or replace that essence once it is spent. It was thought that every ejaculation permanently weakens a man's vitality and diminishes his lifespan. Losing a drop of semen was believed to be equivalent to losing the nutritional value of thousands of pounds of food over the next twenty years of a man's life. Among some Taoists and many Chinese generally, the injunction against ejaculation carried the same weight that eternal punishment in Hell from a mortal sin would carry for a good Catholic.

For many men, however, this "just say no" approach is excessive and unworkable. Even the more moderate Fire-method Taoists developed a range of specific formulas for how often one should ejaculate. According to these formulas, for example, a teenager in good health can ejaculate anywhere from two to seven times per week, and progressively fewer times each week as he matures, to fewer and fewer times each month, or none at all after he reaches age sixty or seventy. All these prescriptions are based on the premise than ejaculating semen damages your health.

CLASSIC TAOIST TECHNIQUES FOR PROLONGING SEX

These techniques for extending sex are taken from seven classic Chinese texts on the erotic arts. The methods are presented in order of difficulty, beginning with the easiest to grasp and adopt as part of your sex play. All the techniques that follow have stood the test of time and are either derived from ancient texts, or are commonly practiced in Taoist communities.

Going Slowly

According to *Huang Di Nei Jing Su Wen*,[3] sex should not make men weak and, as such, fewer ejaculations are better than more. Conversely, sexual secretions make women happy and healthy. The book advocates moving slowly and not going too fast when the penis and vagina make contact during sex. If you move overly fast, the ability to feel can be diminished and become less sensitive. Therefore, slower movements are better, as they allow a man to make love longer and lessen his need to ejaculate.

It is wise to apply the seventy-percent rule of moderation and avoid going completely over the moon unless you want to come. This will allow you to maintain a comfort zone that can grow progressively greater each time you make love. Over time, you will find that the automatic ejaculation response begins to recede.

---

3. *Huang Di Nei Jing* (The Yellow Emperor's Inner Canon), believed to have been written between 475–221 BCE and 206 BCE–220 CE, is a seminal work on Chinese medicine. What is known as *Su Wen* (Basic Questions) is the first of the two texts that comprise the book.

Recovery

Another ancient text, *Yang Xing Yan Ming Lu* (Notes on Nurturing One's Nature and Lengthening Life) by Tao Hongjing, recommends moving slowly. If you become tired, rest and recover before you begin again. By practicing patience, you can extend your lovemaking to a very long time, possibly all night.

Try to avoid the Roman candle effect: fast and bright, but short lived. A super-rush of passion can result in the early burnout of a sexual relationship. If you want a sexual relationship to last, alternate periods of revving up and slowing down during lovemaking.

Likewise, allow for a variety of interludes: both of you rev up and calm down together, he gets revved up while she stays calm and vice versa, or both of you

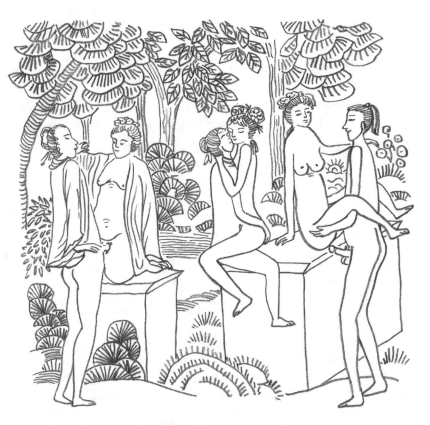

Men and women enjoy sex together at a summer afternoon garden party.
In ancient China, this was the relaxed equivalent of what today is known as "swinging."

Figure 8-2: Swingers of Ancient China

become deeply relaxed. Play around with the ebb and flow—not too excited and yet not overly mellow. Discover and cultivate the middle ground.

Most Important Matters

One of the sections within *Huang Di Nei Jing* is called the *Tian Xia Zhi Dao Tan,* which translates, roughly, as "Talking about Most Important Matters." Here are two suggestions from it:

- The most important issue regarding sex is to make sperm strong and plentiful, that is, more is better. When sperm is abundant, do not hold it back, allow yourself to ejaculate. If not, let it build over time to the maximum extent.
- Before sex, the man and woman should sit or lie together. As they kiss, each will swallow the others saliva. As they do this, let the breath of both partners get very big, breathing either through the nose or mouth in whatever manner that allows the greatest volume of breath to flow.

When swallowing a lover's saliva, most people normally cease to breathe or shorten their breaths considerably. You must move past this common limitation. As you do so, you should feel your body start to build up energy. Only after you feel like your energy is very strong and charged up do you begin sexual intercourse. During sex, continue to take large breaths, especially if either partner feels their energy begin to flag. You want to have the energetic sense of swallowing your own and your partner's saliva down into your lower tantien. This will cause the man's erection to become less sensitive and more enduring. To desensitize a relatively soft erection, penetrate the vagina and once the penis becomes a bit harder, withdraw for a while before continuing.

Long Foreplay

Texts from the Han Dynasty's *Ma Wang Dui* series, *Yu Fang* (Inside the Room), and *Zhi Yao* (Hint of Seduction) both say long foreplay is better. These writings and the related *Ma Wang Dui* text, *He Yin Yang,* give men this advice to improve foreplay and intercourse:

During sexual foreplay, massage and touch the woman's *he gu* (the space at the bottom between the hand's thumb and index finger—see Figure 8-3) and continue up to her elbow on both sides of the arm, up to the armpit, over her ears and head. Massage the back of her neck, then make circles around her neck and her breasts (up to down, but not vice versa), and then make fast movements with your fingers down between her breasts to the pubic bone.

Be light and gentle with your fingernails. Look for beads of sweat on her nose. From there, move to her clitoris and then begin kissing everywhere on her body until your kisses produce copious saliva and her vagina begins to produce copious sexual secretions.

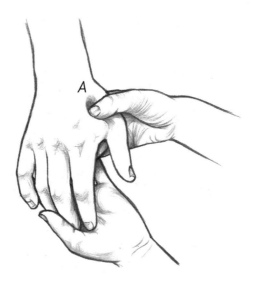

Thumb pressing the he gu point (A).

Figure 8-3: He Gu Acupuncture Point of the Hand

Three-Phase Technique for a Man

The *Yu Fang, Zhi Yao* and the *Huang Di Nei Jing* all advocate a three-phase technique:

1. When you want to ejaculate, use your own or your lover's index and middle finger to press on the perineum. Then, within one breath, immediately inhale and on your exhale, tap your teeth together in a vibrating manner with a "hah" breath sound. Do this several times, and sperm won't be discharged.

2. Next, bring qi from your erection to the *wei lu* (tailbone) up to your head.

3. Hold your breath, raise your head slightly backward, open your eyes wide, look left and right, and pull your sperm from your erection and testicles back into your body. This techniques makes a man's body very strong.

Shallow and Deep Thrusts

The three related texts, *Yu Fang, Zhi Yao* and *He Yin Yang* all propose a series of shallow and deep thrusts to prevent ejaculation and increase sexual excitement.

1. The series of thrusts begin with one deep thrust followed by eight shallow ones, then continues with two deep thrusts followed by seven shallow ones and so on: three deep and six shallow, four deep and five shallow, five deep and four shallow, six deep and three shallow, seven deep and two shallow, eight deep and one shallow.

2. Next use no deep thrusts and nine shallow ones only.

3. The system then reverses itself with eight shallow thrusts followed by one deep thrust, followed by seven shallow and two deep, and so on through to one shallow and eight deep thrusts.

4. Finally, do no shallow thrusts and nine deep ones. Then the system reverses itself again, ad infinitum, or until both decide to stop or the man ejaculates.

Advice for Men: Pause to Increase the Number of Strokes

The *He Yin Yang* and the *Huang Di Nei Jing* both say that more or less after doing ten penetrations and withdrawals (i.e., regular strokes), stop and wait for your body and nerves to settle before you begin again. On the next round, after a few seconds pause, and add another ten strokes to make a total of twenty. Then, after an appropriate regenerative interval, add another ten to reach the new goal of thirty strokes. Continue this process of activity alternating with rest and regeneration before adding more strokes until you reach one hundred strokes.

These texts claim the following benefits:

- If you don't ejaculate during the first twenty strokes, it helps increase the strength of your voice and lungs.
- If you don't ejaculate during the first thirty strokes, it helps your skin become brighter.
- If you don't ejaculate during the first forty strokes, it helps strengthen your spinal vertebrae and ribs.
- If you don't ejaculate during the first fifty strokes, it helps the bones of your hips and spinal vertebrae to become strong.
- If you don't ejaculate during the first sixty strokes, it helps your bladder and urination gain strength.
- If you don't ejaculate during the first seventy strokes, it helps your erection become harder.
- If you don't ejaculate during the first eighty strokes, it helps your skin become more youthful-looking.
- If you don't ejaculate during the first ninety strokes, it helps you become more intelligent.
- If you don't ejaculate during the first one hundred strokes, it helps extend your lifespan.

These ancient texts continue by extolling proposed benefits to be gathered by progressively adding ten new strokes before ejaculating. In certain Taoist priesthood communities, initiates were instructed to start with one hundred strokes, then progress to three hundred, and then to one thousand strokes, after which time semen retention seemed to disappear as an issue. As far as lovemaking in the present day is concerned, the author would say that under normal circumstances there is minimal need to go beyond three hundred strokes. However, if a man can work up to one hundred, this can be very beneficial for him and certainly his lover is likely to appreciate it as well.

Differing Views on Ejaculation

During the 1920s and 1930s when my teacher Liu Hung Chieh was a young man, prostitution was legal in China. It was a period when massive numbers of poor young girls flooded into the cities from the countryside. Such an environment—in which cheap, plentiful sex was readily available—had occurred in Chinese history but rarely to such an extent. According to Liu and others I spoke with who lived at that time, there were a hundred thousand active prostitutes in the center of Shanghai proper, and over a million quite nearby; in Beijing, there were fifty thousand within the city center, and half a million in the greater metropolitan area.

Unlike at other times in China's history, societal and financial obstacles that would prevent the common man from having a lot of sex were minimal during this particular era. Even a moderately prosperous male could have a number of wives and sexual dalliances. Prices for prostitutes were so low that he could easily pay for all the sex he wanted. The only obstacle was a man's endurance. Naturally, the issue of semen retention and ejaculation control—longtime fascinations of the Chinese and an ancient area of study for Taoists—became a major topic of concern. As Liu and others explained it to me, the men of that era tended to express three widely different points of view as regards whether or not a man should ejaculate:

- It's not a problem

- It's advisable to ejaculate only once every X number of days or weeks, depending on your age

- Never ejaculate under any circumstances.

Thus there was not a general consensus that semen retention was always to be considered the best option.

THE CASE AGAINST SEMEN RETENTION

According to the premise of the Taoist Water method, the energetic mechanism of ejaculation is more important than the physical emission of semen. If a man understands and can optimize this energetic mechanism by fully relaxing upon orgasm, it is not necessary to be overly concerned about semen retention. This coincides with Western science, which has found little evidence to confirm the idea that ejaculation is harmful to a man's health or has any major effect on his lifespan.

EJACULATION AND BONDING

From a relationship perspective, a potential problem can arise if a man does not ejaculate; it can prevent or undermine emotional bonding. Culturally, Westerners assume that, for a man, sexual satisfaction hinges on his orgasm and ejaculation. In the absence of a culturally acceptable paradigm that suggests otherwise, the man's *jing* is a crucial ingredient in the bonding process that leads to a long-term relationship.

Western women are likely to complain that they do not feel emotionally complete or have not fulfilled their feminine role if the man does not come. This perceived intrinsic need for a man to ejaculate is also echoed in sexual massage parlors where a man is often asked if he wants to finish the massage with a "happy ending."

REGULARITY IS BEST

Ancient Taoists found that males operate best with regularity for ejaculation. Regularity is also best for sex, as the body adapts to consistent rhythms. Every day at erratic times or only once a year will not give the body what it needs to function optimally. If two to three times a week does not tire you, it is best to keep to a relatively regular schedule. "Bad" or inappropriate scenarios might include:

- Excessive activity followed by an abrupt or long-lasting stop
- Little or no activity (for months or even years) followed by extreme excess (multiple times a day) for a prolonged period.

The male body needs to have internal sense of sexual regularity, so it subliminally knows what to expect. Without that sense of regularity, imbalances can easily arise and result in problems.

DEAD *JING*

Taoists refer to the non-ejaculated sperm left over in a man's body after sexual intercourse as "dead *jing*." The term jing has two implications in Chinese: it can simply refer to the leftover sperm, but it also has a broader meaning that encompasses the overall energetic matrix of the physical body. When a man makes love, certain energy channels inside his body are activated, and the natural outlet for the buildup of sexual energy is completion through the process of ejaculation.

If a man doesn't know how to control the pathways so that the energy naturally moves through his circuitry until it clears out through his entire energetic system, sperm that has not been ejaculated can cause energetic contractions. Such contractions can, over time, become structural. An energetic contraction of this type may then have a negative effect on the functioning of the internal organs and glands. Taoists refer to this larger syndrome as dead *jing*—dead sperm—implying that when sperm do not find a natural outlet, they "die on the vine" and, in a matter of speaking, turn into sour grapes.

Problems can arise from not ejaculating over long periods of time and show up for men when they reach their sixties and seventies. The loss of sexual vitality may start a cascade of minor or serious problems in the body. For a man with a naturally strong body, dead *jing* is rarely a problem, as his system can usually handle the changes that come with age. However, for men who have middling or weak constitutions (these types also tend to be more obsessed with whether they ejaculate or not), this can become a problem as they age.

TOTAL RELAXATION ORGASMS

The habit of over-tensing the body and nervous system to enhance the zing of an ejaculation is ingrained in most males. If the tension is excessive, it can tire and strain a man's body. It's similar to the strain in a man's muscles that occurs from the clutching tension that goes into lifting an excessive weight. The difference is that a strong tension orgasm strains not a man's muscles but his nervous system and internal organs, especially the kidneys and glands.

According to the Taoists, kidney qi is thought to be the prime determinant of a man's overall qi, vitality and sexuality. This means that, energetically, the hit a tension orgasm gives the kidneys is particularly problematic. The effects on the body can be similar to emotional depression and listlessness, which are also indicators of weakened or damaged kidney qi.

Taoists discovered that men could transform the sexual rev and build it into a profoundly relaxing orgasmic response that rejuvenates the body rather than damages it. Instead of riding the tension over the edge, a man can learn to relax his body and genitals just before he ejaculates. This allows the energy in the genitals to release and move in waves that spread throughout the body, eliminating the sudden shock. With practice, a man can learn to have a tension-free orgasm that sends healing waves of qi throughout his entire body, from his genitals to his fingers, toes and head (see Practice 11 later in this chapter). As Margot Anand says in *The Art of Sexual Ecstasy,*[4] "the ordinary orgasm of release is not the only goal to sexual

---

4. Anand, Margot, *The Art of Sexual Ecstasy: The Path of Sacred Sexuality for Western Lovers* (Los Angeles: Jeremy P. Tarcher, 1989), 35.

intimacy. The whole body can be transformed into an erogenous zone, offering many erotic and sensual experiences that become increasingly subtle and ecstatic."

Many women are naturally prone to having orgasms spread through their whole bodies, which leaves them inherently more relaxed and less nerve-shocked. From the Taoist point of view, whole-body orgasms are part of a woman's natural energetic anatomy. However, women can also use the total relaxation orgasm method. For women these total relaxation orgasms can complete or strongly enhance the natural tendency to achieve even greater pleasure and satisfaction from orgasm. For nonorgasmic women who eventually become orgasmic, this practice expands her orgasm into her whole body.

Your first few attempts at a total relaxation orgasm may not be much fun, because you are habituated to the sudden tension release and all the cultural images associated with it. Once you learn to move the energy out of your genitals and into the rest of your body, you will find the relaxation orgasm is at the very least as enjoyable as the tension release. The bonus is that you won't be excessively tired afterward.

It has often been said that Taoist energy practices are gifts that keeps on giving. The more you practice, the more you open yourself internally and directly feel and harness your energy. These are the inherent gifts of all Taoist energy arts, including sexual qigong and meditation.

Students of Taoist energy arts are constantly discovering the importance of the basic principle, "The more you relax, the more energy you have." Along with naturalness and balance, it forms the foundation of every practice. At first, few understand the true implications of the phrase, but as they learn to release strain and tension, this principle's significance becomes tangible.

The more you relax, the more energy you have.

As is true of all the energy arts, the goal of Taoist sexual practices is to enable students to have a direct experience of profound relaxation as a living reality. Ultimately, practitioners learn to sustain that depth of ease in their daily lives. For the non-practitioner, the afterglow of an orgasm offers a fleeting experience of what profound relaxation is like. However, few can sustain such a relaxed state for more than a few moments at a time.

Far more than a source of pleasure or physical relief, orgasms can allow you to heal and dissolve all that stands between you and the Mind of Tao itself. They quite literally help you relax into your Being. Chapter 13 introduces the Taoist practice of internal orgasm, which builds on the relaxation orgasm and allows you to let go in ways you most likely have never imagined.

Practice 11: Total Relaxation Orgasm
SEXUAL QIGONG

This exercise is primarily for men, because they are often exhausted after an orgasm, however it can also be used by women to fully release and expand an orgasm to her entire body.

If a man does not want to have a tension orgasm, he has two options. First, as discussed, he can retain his semen and not ejaculate. Second, he can learn to ejaculate with a full relaxation orgasm. To do this is really quite simple.

In preparation for an orgasm while making love, a man will commonly get at least one and possibly several signals that tell him he is about to come. Usually he prefers to allow the pleasure of stroking to continue as long as possible, so he develops an individual strategy to postpone the tense, pleasurable feeling that initiates his ejaculation.

As he rides the edge that leads to climax, even though the tension itself is quite enjoyable, he will now attempt to relax the tension and take the edge off it. By doing this for an indeterminate period of time (longer and longer, ideally), he can begin to develop the habit of simply being willing to relax sexual tension, a skill that he will need to master for a total relaxation orgasm.

When making love, there is usually is a countdown to ejaculation. The old one, two, three …mega-contraction…followed by a feeling of exploding and then…"whoosh!" can be deconstructed with a Taoist perspective where each stage has options.

Option 1: In the one-two-three period, if a man is able to totally relax everything he possibly can—his body, the feeling in his genitals, his muscles and nervous system—he may be able to continue, extending the pleasure a whole lot longer without feeling the need to ejaculate.

Option 2: At the moment the mega-contraction starts, he can fully relax it. If successful, he may lose the need to ejaculate. If so, great—his kidney qi is protected.

Option 3: The total relaxation orgasm, which proceeds in a three-step scenario.

Phase 1

He becomes aware of when the explosion is going to happen. A few seconds before, he allows the pleasure of the impending explosion to grow, but starts to relax everything inside that he possibly can, especially his nerves.

At the moment of the explosion itself, the intensity of the pleasure and ever-increasing relaxation completely commingle. This might change the feeling of the exploding orgasm, sometimes making it better, but sometimes temporarily diminishing the pleasurable charge. Not to worry—within a few weeks the full pleasure usually returns, but in a slightly different way.

Phase 2

When the explosion happens, he relaxes even more. The stronger the explosion, the more he must increase the relaxation that accompanies it.

The pleasurable energy of the explosion does not, I repeat, does not remain in the genitals. Rather, the relaxation enables the orgasm to spread outward from the genitals through the entire body—to toes, fingertips and head, and everything in between. The more he can relax, the more the pleasure wave will spread throughout his whole body. Although this type of relaxation comes easily and naturally to women, men need to practice a bit. The good news is that the tension orgasm is just a habit, one that is actually fairly easy to break.

Phase 3

When the "whoosh!" happens, it's like a wave in the ocean. The wave moves from the ocean toward the shore, crashes, and then pulls back. Following the initial emanation of energy on the explosion, the reverberation of the explosion starts to push out his ejaculate. As the fluid goes out, he should relax as much as possible, until any residual tension release can be completely absorbed into his body with no residue.

After a man comes, and if he doesn't withdraw right away, he will often feel as though he is dribbling out the last bits, whether he emitted semen or not. He may be feeling the fluid itself or simply feeling the effect that coming has generated in his qi and nerves. At this time, before withdrawing, he should relax any tiny bits of remaining tension even more, until they completely dissipate, and only then pull out of her.

While lying next to her, he should continue the spread of the orgasmic release until his body stabilizes the relaxation, and there is no residual buzzing inside. Or, if there is a buzz, it's subtle and pleasurable rather than strained.

Complete relaxation orgasms have several benefits. They prevent the downsides of ejaculation, which includes strain on the kidneys. Over time, they bypass the potential repercussions of dead jing.

If a woman has a full orgasm, the energy will go through her entire body, and she will be recharged. If a woman has only partial orgasms, she can apply the principles in this exercise to enable full-body orgasms. ●

How a Woman Can Help a Man

A woman's attitude can make or break the moment with respect to her man's ability to "perform." Nothing will have him go soft so fast as feeling pressured, criticized or misunderstood. Understand that arousal can occur "between the ears" before it occurs between the legs—or independent of the genitals altogether at certain times in a person's life. That said, it's helpful to look at the basic differences between his arousal and hers in terms of their genitals.

For a man, attaining an erection requires that his kidneys and body cooperate to provide a strong flow of blood and qi to his penis. Getting hard is a bodily function that cannot be replaced or mimicked should it fail. Contrast this with the woman's situation: if she has trouble getting wet, she or he can easily use a little saliva or reach for some lube. Over-the-counter and inexpensive, vaginal-lubricating jellies can be obtained online or at any drugstore.

It may sound obvious or unimportant, but the simple fact that a woman can get herself wet through artificial means at a moment's notice takes the pressure off. Men do not have that advantage. Although erectile support drugs are fairly easy to obtain, they don't always "do the deed" and can cause a variety of side effects.

Here are some natural methods a woman can use to help her man stay hard—or not ejaculate, when he is on autopilot and clearly moving in that direction:

- To aid and increase his erection during foreplay, before or during intercourse itself, or to restore flagging erectile ability, she can stroke and massage the area of his lower back up to his lower ribs. This activates his kidney energy, which is the source of a man's sexual energy.

- Be aware of his breathing. When you hear his breath become rapid, this signals the beginning of a countdown to ejaculation. What you need to do is to shift his physical movement and breathing rhythm. As he withdraws and before he goes back into your vagina, try to get his breath to slow down. Use the muscles of your vagina to slow his thrusts or interrupt his familiar "I'm about to pop!" pace.

- You can interrupt the revving up to a climax by strongly pressing the place where a man's perineum and the root of his penis join. Prostitutes throughout all parts of Asia use this technique. The downside of this method is that pressing too hard in this region can cause excessive pressure to build up in the blood vessels and arteries of the genital area. This can cause postcoital discomfort and even bruising in a small percentage of men.

- Massage and activate the top of his neck and also his occiput, which is important to include. A man who is overly stressed will tend to have his energy stuck in his head.

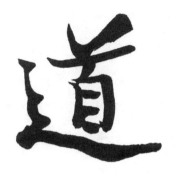

SECTION 3

TAOIST BRIDGE PRACTICES

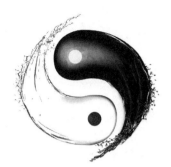

CHAPTER 9

Breathing into Intimacy

In order to move from the ordinary sex methods presented in the previous chapters into sexual qigong and sexual meditation practices, you need to develop a solid foundation for developing and using qi. If you can already feel, move and direct qi, then you are ahead of the energy game. If not, then you can develop the skills to work with qi by learning a variety of practices, including Taoist breathing, qigong, tai chi and energy massage. In this chapter and the next we will look at various bridge practices that you can use to most quickly develop the required skills for the more advanced sexual work.

All the world's great spiritual traditions have precise and systematic methods that usher us into the heart of human consciousness. In many of them, such as Taoism or Buddhism, focusing on the breath is one of the portals to greater internal awareness. Breath can also be a direct path to learning to work with your qi and consciousness.

The Taoists developed precise methods for teaching people how to breathe well. At the foundation stage, these include breathing techniques that show you how to have correct posture, extend the duration and quality of your breath, and use breathing to relax your nervous system, all important components to having more fulfilling and pleasurable ordinary sex.

More intermediate Taoist breathing techniques help create physical, mental and psychic qi qualities valuable in any meditation tradition.[1] More advanced practices, including those considered to be sexual practices, include learning over thirty to forty different breathing rhythms, some of them used in conjunction with sound and vibration. This chapter looks at why the breath is so important in sexual practices and gives an overview of the types of Taoist breathing practices found within ordinary sex, sexual qigong and sexual meditation.

---

1. The basic Taoist Longevity Breathing methods that form a solid foundation for sexual meditation are described in the following of the author's books: *Relaxing into Your Being, Opening the Energy Gates of Your Body* and *The Tao of Letting Go,* as well as in his *Longevity Breathing* DVD and *Taoist Breathing* CD set. Also visit www.energyarts.com for details of online Taoist Meditation programs.

TAOIST LONGEVITY BREATHING

It's a simple fact: most people in the West have never learned the optimal way to breathe and if you were to ask them what creates the breath, they would answer, "The lungs." However, it is actually the diaphragm that does the work. The average person breathes shallowly from the front of his or her chest, taking only small breaths of a few seconds. These shallow breaths never fully reach the whole of the lungs, which includes the back, right, left and top. Furthermore, due to working on computers and holding tension, many people intermittently hold their breath for extended periods of time, depriving the body, lungs and cells of oxygen. It is no wonder that at the end of the day most people feel lethargic and exhausted.

Lastly, many people, because of these bad breathing patterns, have diaphragms that are locked and frozen, with a limited range of movement. A stuck diaphragm leads to a cascade of negative health effects, not the least of which is the general downgrading of the internal organs. On one hand learning to breathe better can improve your overall health and give you more energy; on the other, you can learn how to incorporate specific breathing methods within sexual qigong and sexual meditation.

The author has developed a program to teach authentic Taoist breathing in systematic stages called Longevity Breathing.®

This program teaches you to learn how to breathe from your diaphragm and the whole belly—including the front, sides and back of the belly and all the internal organs connected to these areas.

Learning to breathe from your belly strengthens your diaphragm. This is important, as it is your diaphragm—the muscle separating your lungs and belly—that enables you to breathe. Your lungs do not move independently. As your diaphragm goes down or contracts, you inhale and the lungs automatically fill. When the diaphragm rises up or relaxes, you automatically exhale as the diaphragm pushes the air out of your lungs.

The purpose of learning the initial stages of Taoist breathing is to help you:

1. Learn concentration and focus within meditation and sexual practices.

2. Retrain your nervous system to relax.

3. Extend the duration of your breath in progressive stages.

4. Improve the functioning of your vascular system and internal organs, including the heart.

5. Breathe with your entire belly, into your sides, and lower and upper back.

6. Breathe into the uppermost part of your lungs, which most people rarely use.

7. Increase the amount of oxygen in your cells and maintain a better balance of oxygen and carbon dioxide, part of which is ensuring that the carbon dioxide is fully expelled on the exhale.

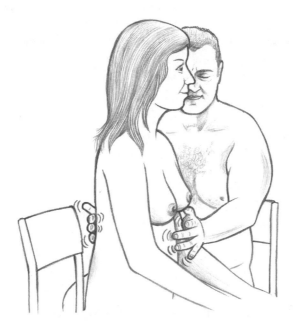

Figure 9-1: Tapping Her Diaphragm to Stimulate Better Breathing

In later stages, Taoist breathing will help you:

1. Build up the levels of qi in your body and improve energy flow through your channels

2. Increase awareness of the energies within your lower tantien

3. Engage the breath with the spine, the soles of the feet, the etheric body and all three tantiens.

This kind of breathing simultaneously gives your internal organs a continuous massage and more oxygen. Once learned, Taoist breathing methods such as Longevity Breathing can be done twenty-four hours a day.

CONTINUOUS CIRCULAR BREATHING

In order to encourage the circulation of qi, the Taoist Water method uses a continuous breathing method that joins the inhalation and exhalation in an unbroken stream. The breath is never held in either direction between the inhale and the exhale. The goal is to have a smooth, continuous, relaxed, circular breath that involves the whole body.

This method of continuous circular breathing and qi circulation is opposite to the majority of breathing methods commonly taught in the West and India. The Water method position is that, although holding the breath is not completely unnatural, it usually creates more structural tension in the nervous system, especially if a person has not been trained in the holding technique from childhood or at the latest by the early twenties.

For example, in Tibetan and Indian yoga, there are techniques that involve holding the breath to control energy movement through the body's channels by moving *prana* (qi) to a place, holding it there in order to absorb the energy into the appropriate channel, then exhaling to move it more strongly and deeply within the same channel or into a different channel, and finally holding the breath for a while to completely absorb the energy into the body and form a bridge to Consciousness itself. The Taoists generally discourage such techniques and instead focus on helping people create a smooth continuous breath that does not shock the nervous system. They recognize that most people already have too much stress locked into their bodies.

EXTENDING THE LENGTH OF YOUR BREATH

In Taoist breathing, another major emphasis is to increase the average duration of your breath by getting your whole body to breathe. The duration of a breath for the average person is commonly less than five seconds. Most people can easily and safely learn to extend the breath's duration to fifteen seconds, including both inhale and exhale. Then over time they can comfortably extend their ability to a thirty-second breath. After being able to practice a thirty-second breath for a while, during times where you are not consciously practicing, a ten-second breath normally becomes automatically sustainable. This doubles the breath of approximately four or five seconds that most people normally maintain.

After this, Taoists found that a two-minute breath was the next major milestone, with the next step being what the Taoists call a Turtle breath, in which a single breath lasts a total of eight minutes. Turtle breathing forms the basis for many advanced Taoist longevity and bodily regeneration programs.

At each stage as you extend and stabilize your breath, the nervous system undergoes a dramatic upgrade that has long-term health benefits. As you work with the various practices in this book, you can learn to completely relax your breath and then later to lengthen your inhales and exhales.

A word of caution: it is important that as you extend your breath you do so slowly. Extending your average breath takes time and is not a quick fix. The principles of relaxation and the seventy-percent rule are always emphasized in Longevity Breathing. If you feel stress or tension arising at any point while learning the basic material in this chapter or while practicing the author's more comprehensive Longevity Breathing program, you should immediately back off and stabilize your system before going further.

BREATH AS A BAROMETER IN LIFE AND SEX

In the Taoist Water tradition, focusing on your breath helps you become aware of when and where you are not relaxed. For example, involuntarily holding the breath commonly happens when people release strong negative emotions, such as fear, anger, loss and depression. If you can notice this contraction and bring your breathing back to a smooth and relaxed state, many of the negative emotions can immediately start to dissipate.

As your body heats up during sex, it is natural for your breath to change. Radical changes in breathing, however, can be barometers of some type of blocked energy. For example, you might be in the midst of a highly charged session of foreplay when your breath or that of your partner breaks from its normal pattern of arousal and excitement. Your breath may suddenly freeze, or sound ragged, weird or strange. When that happens, you may also feel a corresponding general wave of tension in the body or find that a specific place in the body has become tense or contracted. Any sudden constriction of the breath is often an indication of a subliminal physical, emotional or psychic energy blockage. In many cases, your partner may be more aware of this tension than you.

When you are engaged in Taoist sexual practices you can look for changes in the breath to see if they are signals of internal blockages that need to be dissolved within you or your partner. Recognizing these changes and putting your attention on them can easily become an opportunity to locate and release these blockages within your eight energy bodies.

You and your lover can experiment with your breathing patterns during lovemaking, just like jazz musicians improvise with their instruments. This can increase your physical and emotional pleasure as well as releasing tension and giving you a deep sense of relaxation.

Experimenting with your breathing during lovemaking can increase your physical and emotional pleasure and give you a deep sense of relaxation.

Practice 12: Breathing from the Belly
ORDINARY SEX

This method is particularly easy to learn if you lie down and put a book on your belly. Initially you use the muscles of your belly to move the book up and down. When you understand the mechanism of doing so, practice lying down without the book, then sitting, standing and moving.

Many people have either weak or overly tense belly muscles due to holding or sucking the belly in. For both men and women, the modern media culture reinforces the ideal that a flat, tense belly is the ideal. Taoists do not hold this viewpoint and believe that a slightly more protruding belly, resulting from total relaxation rather than muscle contraction, gives space to and energizes your internal organs, providing superior health benefits. Rather than external looks, the focus is on how the contraction influences the flow of qi. If at first you find it difficult to do this primary exercise, be patient with yourself.

Keep your tongue on the roof of your mouth (where it would be if you said the sound "le").

1. Become aware of your breath. Let it become smooth and comfortable.

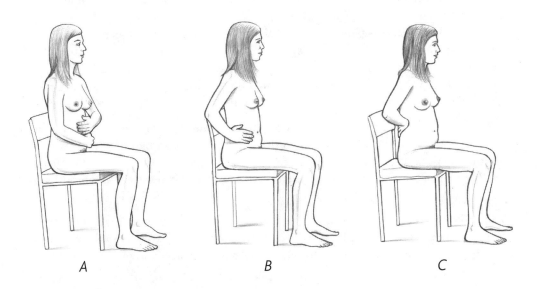

A   *B*   *C*

Placing your hands on the relevant area of your abdomen enables you to feel the degree to which each inhale and exhale is relaxing and energizing your abdominal movements and breath.

Figure 9-2 A–C: Breathing from Front, Sides and Back of the Abdomen

2. Put one hand on your chest, and let the other rest lightly on the book if you are lying down, or on your abdomen if you are practicing without the book or in a sitting position. Ideally, your chest stays relaxed and does not move much.

3. As you inhale and draw in air, gently let the muscles of your belly move forward. As you exhale, relax and allow your belly to return to its original position (Figure 9-2 A shows this done sitting).

4. As you gain sensitivity, if you have been doing this exercise lying down with a book on your belly, remove the book and put your hands on different parts of your belly, that is, on the sides and rear of your abdomen (Figure 9-2 C shows this done sitting) and try to ensure that as you inhale, all the parts move evenly. When people first learn belly breathing, some areas, for example the lower belly, tend to be easier to move than other parts.

Your partner can assist you in this exercise by putting his or her fingers very lightly on a part of your belly and asking you to move those fingers. To help you, he or she might very lightly tap the region to enable the nerves to release and relax.

Begin with two breaths of continuous, unbroken and relaxed awareness, and then rest for a moment. After this, progress to three breaths, four, and so on, all the way up to thirty. How much you want to practice after thirty breaths is a personal decision. ●

BREATHING IN ORDINARY SEX

The potential pleasure and satisfaction of ordinary sexuality can and usually is diminished by poor breathing. If you want to have better sex, Taoists would say, "First and foremost, learn to breathe better." Taoist Breathing is a simple, effective way to learn how to master your concentration, consciously become aware of your personal connection to inner and outer energies and overcome the nervous jumping of the monkey mind.

It teaches you to become aware of when your breath becomes tense, whereby you might gulp air or hold your breath, for example, which blocks your ability to experience increased sensation. In this way, Taoist Longevity Breathing teaches you to relax during lovemaking.

YIN AND YANG OF BREATHING

Any practice affecting the energy flows through the eight energy bodies can be done in either a yin or a yang way. This is true for any action, including how you move energy in sexual relations. You can breathe in either a yin or a yang manner, even though your belly will still go in and out with each breath in more or less the same way.

Yang projects to actualize a task. For example, you can focus your intent to make your breath expand into your internal organs, so everything in these areas moves well. Yang generally has the view to achieve a goal in the most direct way possible. Although this may be good for some purposes, yang energy can bypass the intimate nature of relationships when it meets yin.

Yin goes about a task differently. It is not always as direct, but can be equally effective going through a different route. In breathing, the yin way is that the body accepts, absorbs and makes a relationship with the breath. When this happens, the body will absorb the breath, allow the breath to open naturally and even enable it to sink and soak into the nervous system. This creates a structure that will make it possible for the breath and the body to form an ongoing, softer relationship with each other. Yin loves to absorb and encompass something so that the next step can naturally grow out of it. This is equally true whether working with your breath or any kind of qi work, sexual or otherwise. For yang, it is enough if the task of the moment gets accomplished. For yin the immediate need is less important than the ability for an ongoing relationship.

Practice 13: Breathing from the Belly, Sides and Back
ORDINARY SEX

Basic belly breathing is commonly taught in progressive stages as part of the Longevity Breathing program: first you learn to expand the whole front of your belly evenly; next you add expanding the sides of your belly equally on both sides; then you learn to expand your belly backward. The final stage is learning to expand the belly equally in all directions simultaneously. The following practice is the final stage.

1. During your inhale, do all of the following simultaneously, to the best of your ability: Expand the front, side, and back parts of your belly evenly in all parts, and the back (but not front) of your lungs.

2. As you exhale, do all of the following simultaneously to the best of your ability: Let the back of your lungs and the front, side, and back of your belly return to their original position at the same or slower speed than they expanded (Figure 9-2 A–C).

Be sure not to gulp air, breathe through the mouth (unless your sinuses are blocked) or hold your breath. Again, begin with two breaths using continuous, unbroken and relaxed awareness. Then rest for a moment. Then progress to three, four, and so on, all the way up to thirty breaths. It's up to you how much you want to practice after you reach this point.

During sex, you'll want to use this relaxed belly breath while kissing, sucking, moving, touching your partner in any way and while having intercourse. This practice alone will help you to experience increased sensation without charging your nervous system with tension.

Once you have a stable breath, you might also try breathing even more slowly for prolonged periods of time. This will enable you to draw out every drop of pleasure from the moment. ●

BREATHING IN SEXUAL QIGONG

Breath is not qi, and qi is not breath, although the two are joined in many ways. The awareness of your breath and the ability to direct it is a definite precursor to the following:

- Consciously moving qi, both inside your body and that of your partner
- Finding energetic blockages in the first four energy bodies
- Feeling the energies of the lower and middle tantien.

Within sexual qigong, focusing on breath is one of the easiest ways to develop the awareness of the flows of energies inside your body and that of your partner.

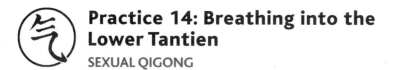 ### Practice 14: Breathing into the Lower Tantien
SEXUAL QIGONG

The following breathing practice can increase your internal awareness:

1. As you inhale, use continuous and unbroken awareness to follow your breath from your nose, down the central channel of your body to your lower tantien. After you are able to do this comfortably, as best you can, inhale qi into your nose from your etheric field until you can finally inhale qi from the boundary of your etheric body, using a series of progressive steps. As before, continue to breathe from your nose and down to your lower tantien.

2. As you exhale, use continuous and unbroken awareness to follow your breath from your lower tantien up the central channel and center of your body to your throat and out your nose. After you are able to do this comfortably, as best you can, let the qi commingle with your breath and continue outward. Carry on till the breath reaches the place from which you originally inhaled, until over time that place is the boundary of your etheric body.

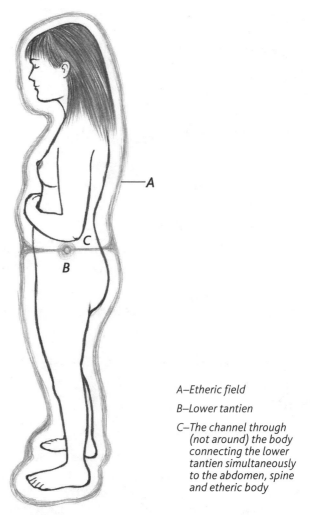

A—Etheric field

B—Lower tantien

C—The channel through (not around) the body connecting the lower tantien simultaneously to the abdomen, spine and etheric body

Figure 9-3: Breathing to the Etheric Body from the Lower Tantien and Vice Versa

As in the previous exercises, begin with two breaths with continuous, unbroken and relaxed awareness, then rest for a moment. Then progress to three breaths, four, and so on, all the way up to thirty. How much you want to practice after thirty breaths is a personal decision.

This practice helps many men to increase the time before they ejaculate and gain more whole-body pleasure from each stroke. Likewise, for many women, it can help them gain better control of qi moving in the body and make orgasms last longer.

Within qigong there are thirty to forty basic energy breathing methods, including those specific to sexual qigong, most of which will not be covered in this book because of space limitations and because they are best learned with a master. Some are for specific situations, while others are more general in nature.

In order to obtain the benefits of any Taoist breathing method, a basic principle is to integrate a specific breathing rhythm into lovemaking only when you can do so without strain. If a breathing rhythm causes tension or makes the task at hand more difficult, then you should shift to a different breathing method or just begin to breathe naturally, coming back to the specific breathing practices later.

These are a few examples of other qigong breathing practices:

- Dragon Breaths to heat and cool the body

- Engulfing and dispersing breaths

- Breathing along specific pathways that activate energy channels and project qi along them, done in conjunction with Outer Dissolving

- Breathing into and out of specific parts of the body, such as the spine, feet, genitalia, erogenous zones, occiput, and points and energetic centers, both physical and nonphysical, within the first four energy bodies. ●

HEATING AND COOLING DRAGON BREATHS

At certain times while making love, either partner may need to heat up or cool down his or her qi or physical body. A woman needs to maintain her internal heat in order to keep her vagina warm and moist (yin). Insufficient body heat can cause the qi within the vagina to become overly cool. Loss of vaginal heat will cause her nerves to lose sensation, at which point her arousal may fizzle out. Then, in a cascading fashion, the blood flow to her vagina slows down, her ability to lubricate diminishes or stops completely, and her orgasms weaken or simply don't happen. The Dragon Heating Breath can reverse this process.

Men have the opposite need. Excessive heat often builds inside a man's head or groin. If he does not cool down, he may ejaculate sooner than he'd like. When a man starts to produce excess yang qi, his brain easily starts to overheat. This can make the whole sexual experience tortuous, which automatically initiates his need to ejaculate to put an end to this discomfort.

Overheating is why many men, especially those whose genes derive from cold climates, simply want to stop whatever activity they might be doing as soon as their internal temperature goes above a certain level. When a man's groin gets overheated, his nerves tend to go dead or weaken and he will lose sensitivity in his penis. For him, the Dragon Cooling Breath is crucial. You can use Taoist Dragon Heating and Cooling Breaths both for sexual and nonsexual purposes.

Practice 15: Taoist Dragon Heating Breath
SEXUAL QIGONG

Aside from sexual purposes, the Dragon Heating Breath may be used when you need to withstand severe cold weather. For sexual qigong, use this method to kick-start the opening of your energy channels and dramatically increase the heat in your lower tantien. You can then send that heat to your internal organs to warm, strengthen and heal them. Once you raise your inner fire in this way, you can spread the heat throughout your entire body.

A woman can use the Dragon Heating Breath to warm her vagina. When doing so, a woman should focus her energy on her legs and perineum as well as her vagina.

There are several variations of the Dragon Heating Breath; the one described here is the easiest to perform.

1. Inhale through the nose, making a barely audible rasping sound by slightly narrowing your air passages and sinus cavity. Simultaneously, focus your qi in the center of whatever area you've chosen as your point of attention (for example, the vagina or lower tantien). Continue breathing until this area begins to ignite, and allow the heat to build to the next level on subsequent breaths. The transition between inhale and exhale should be as circular and seamless as possible.

2. Exhale with a wide-open mouth, expelling the air at least three to six inches from your mouth. Make sure you adjust the angle of your head so the force and heat of the breath does not disturb your lover.

The exhalation occurs in two stages:

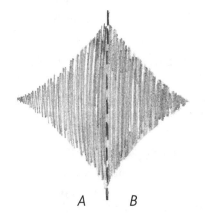

A–First half of exhale
B–Second half of exhale

A   B

Figure 9-4: Taoist Dragon Heating Breath Exhale

A. On the first half of your exhale, begin with your windpipe and sinuses fairly closed and tight (but not tense). Then allow your windpipe and sinuses to relax and open *slightly*. You want the air to escape and spread as if from a funnel whose small end is in your mouth, widening significantly as it moves away from your mouth. Just as a spark in a forest can ignite vegetation (on the inhale) and then spread (the first half of the exhale), this type of breath will catalyze your internal heat to rise to the next level.

B. On the second half of the exhale, with your mouth still wide open, constrict your sinuses and windpipe a tiny bit more as you continue to project air away from your mouth. Only now, in opposite fashion, your breath reverses and narrows so the funnel begins with the big end in your mouth and finishes with the breath almost concentrated to a point at the funnel's small end. As the raspy sound coming out of your throat fades, its sharpness increases and continues increasing until the end of the exhale. This allows your internal heat to both increase the maximum amount and stay contained within your body. Metaphorically speaking, you are fanning an energetic forest fire to become larger and larger with each new breath. ●

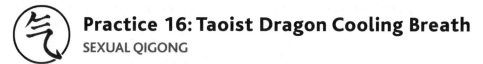 ## Practice 16: Taoist Dragon Cooling Breath
SEXUAL QIGONG

Just as the Heating Breath can help you in cold weather, the Cooling Breath can mitigate unpleasantly hot weather. This breath can also be used to cool down the brain or internal organs overly heated from excessive excitement, stress or overwork.

In the context of sex, a man can use the Cooling Breath to switch his breathing pattern to stop the ejaculation reflex when his breathing speeds up as a natural prelude to orgasm. When a woman does not want her man to come, she can initiate the Cooling Breath, knowing that he will get the signal (consciously or subliminally) to join or mimic her, thereby avoiding going automatically into ejaculation mode.

1. On the inhalation, silently draw air in through the nose. Have the sense of the air penetrating and saturating the areas of the body where the heat buildup feels most intense, usually (but not always) either the head or genital area. Then, use the first half of the Small Heavenly (Microcosmic) Orbit[2] to energetically draw up, move and dissolve the sexual heat building in your groin (see Chapter 11, Figure 11-6). Direct the energy away from your testicles and erection, toward the perineum and tailbone, then up the spine to the neck and on to the crown of the head—the bai hui point.

---

2. The qi pathway known as the Microcosmic or Small Heavenly Orbit goes from the perineum up the spine, over the crown of the head to the mouth and down the front of the body from the mouth to the perineum.

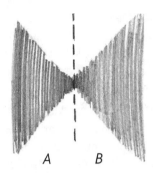

A–First half of exhale
B–Second half of exhale

A   *B*

Figure 9-5: Taoist Dragon Cooling Breath Exhale

2. Once again, you will be exhaling in two stages:

    A. During the first part of the exhalation, your mouth initially should progressively open halfway—do not strain the muscles of your mouth. Then, close your windpipe ever so slightly, but nowhere near to the degree used in the Dragon Heating Breath. The sound you emit upon exhaling is like the sound of a dragon's breath, something like a muffled leaf-blower running at about one third of its full power. Energetically, you should have a sense of cooling qi descending from your lower tantien to your perineum and then from your tailbone rising up your spine and saturating your brain.

    B. During the second half of the exhalation, completely relax your throat and open your mouth wider to release the remaining air. The out breath should disperse in a diffuse, wide stream, as if coming out of a big funnel with the wide end facing outward. The aim is to allow the full volume of air to disperse in a lateral fashion, moving out not so much like stream but rather as a widening estuary that is several feet across at the end. This allows a release of the heat in the brain as it flows out from the crown of the head, ears, mouth and—to a lesser degree—from the eyes. ●

BREATHING IN SEXUAL MEDITATION

There are many sophisticated Taoist breathing methods that can be applied with Outer and Inner Dissolving practices during sexual meditation. Variations and refinements of breathing practices within sexual meditation include:

*   Breathing into specific sites in the body.
*   Moving air in a very diffuse manner (yin) or focusing it like a laser (yang).
*   Humming sounds made at various pitches in general or targeted as vibrations within different parts of the body.
*   Making audible sounds, ranging from almost silent to very loud in order to create strong frequencies of vibration within the body.

Some of these techniques are described in Chapter 16. Most of these practices are beyond the scope of this book and they need to be taught by a living master, who can tailor the information to your particular needs and stages of development, as well as monitor how each practice is affecting your health and your energy bodies. Even in the presence of such a teacher, the practices need significant repetition to sensitize your awareness.

As you progress and integrate different types of breathing into your practices, you will actively embody the central points that allow each breathing technique to reveal itself to you over time. With practice, the subtleties of the method will become evident. This is the way to obtain the maximum benefits. The following is one of many sexual meditation breathing practices that exist.

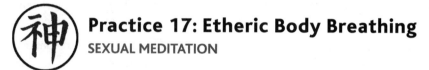

Practice 17: Etheric Body Breathing
SEXUAL MEDITATION

This practice is a bridge between breathing within sexual qigong and sexual meditation. Learning it helps you to become more aware and present to your energy bodies.

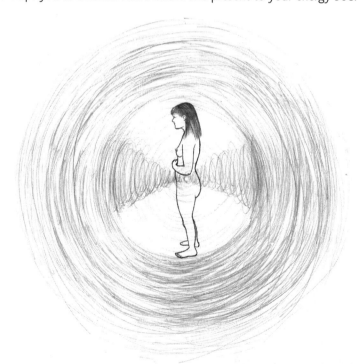

Figure 9-6: Expanded Breathing to and from Etheric Body and Beyond

To start this practice:

1. Inhale from the edge of the etheric body, with the breath consciously drawn into the lower tantien simultaneously from two directions: from the rear, through the mingmen point on the spine and from the front, through the skin of the belly at the lower tantien. The mingmen is also known as the "Door of Life." This energy center is located on the spine, between the kidneys, directly opposite the lower tantien on the dai mai. It is an energetic "belt" that exists on a horizontal plane and circles from in front of the lower tantien around to the spine and mingmen, then continues back around to its point of origin in front of the lower tantien (Figure 9-7).

2. On the exhale, the feeling of the breath is simultaneously directed away from the tantien backward to the mingmen point, located in the lower spine back directly behind the lower tantien, and forward to the skin on front of the body. Then it is moved both forward and backward beyond the physical body to the outer edge of the etheric body.

3. At a very advanced level of practice, after the Inner Dissolving methods of meditation are introduced, the exhale is followed as far out in space beyond the boundary of the etheric body as the energy was originally drawn from when inhaled. ●

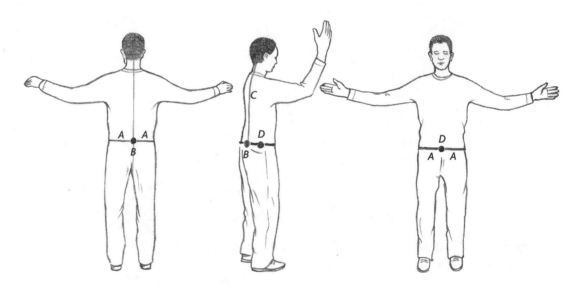

A–Dai mai   B–Mingmen (located on spine)   C–Spine
D–Lower tantien (at core of body in front of spine)

Figure 9-7: The Dai Mai

Taoist Neigong Yoga: A Spiritual Meditation Practice

Traditional Taoist yoga is a powerful system that was taught as a course of study in the Taoist priesthood to which I belonged. It is significantly different from India's Hatha Yoga and the Buddhist forms of yoga found in China and Tibet. Taoist Neigong Yoga™ is the specific method I developed to teach this system. Much like qigong, it is a yin, soft, relaxing and meditative style of movement. It is unlike Hatha Yoga in several ways:

- Taoist Neigong Yoga is fully Chinese and not Indian in origin. It is a complete system because it incorporates all sixteen neigong components (see Chapter 10, "Sixteen Neigong Components"), unlike popularized sub-branches of Hatha Yoga such as Yin Yoga.

- The focus is not on advanced body-bending postures and difficult stretches, rather only simple and intermediate-level postures that observe the seventy-percent rule. This helps energy to flow unobstructed within the body, which is considered the yin fast-track to qi cultivation.

- You relax your insides to stretch; rather than stretching your outsides to relax.

- It is a meditative and soft practice rather than a hard, athletic, high-performance type of yoga with super-stretches. Extreme physical postures in China were traditionally part of the repertoire of Chinese opera and circus where twelve-year-old girls and boys could easily do the most difficult postures of Hatha Yoga.

All postures in Taoist Neigong Yoga are achieved by physical, mental and emotional relaxation. This internal release causes the external physical stretching which enables enhanced, more complete whole-body breathing and the opening up of energy channels. Practice sets are done with circular movement and without deliberately holding. By putting your mind in your body while maintaining the proper physical alignments of each movement, you release the nerves of the body to enable your qi to flow more effectively.

The Taoist Neigong Yoga system I teach is rare in the West. Most yoga labeled "Taoist" that is available in the West does not incorporate the complete range of the sixteen energetic components of neigong including a progression of Taoist breathing methods. When I studied in China, I was taught thirty different Taoist yoga sets of increasing complexity that systematically integrated all the energetic components of neigong.

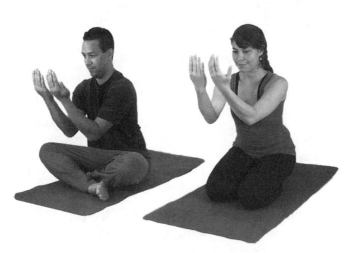

*This posture is included in the first and second sets of Taoist Neigong Yoga.
Each set uses a different method of consciously moving breath within the body.*

Figure 9-8: A Beginning Posture of Taoist Neigong Yoga

Although Taoist Neigong Yoga can make you healthy and strong, it primarily fits into the category of spiritual meditation rather than a physical practice. As such, it is a preparation for Taoist sexual meditation because of its focus on:

- Preparing the body for prolonged periods of sitting or sexual meditation.

- Integrating and teaching the energetics of all sixteen of the Taoist neigong components in a different format from qigong or tai chi.

- Consciously relaxing, releasing and activating energy bodies one through seven.

- Developing and using qi specifically for Taoist sitting and sexual meditation.

In the priesthood training, all trainees were required to do qigong, but only a minority practiced Taoist Yoga as an elective. Historically in China, the ratio of people doing qigong to people doing any kind of yoga was approximately twenty to one. However when my instructors heard of my previous background in Hatha Yoga, I was invited to learn.

I began doing Hatha Yoga in high school during the 1960s, which I continued when I moved to Japan and then in India. This was at a time when Hatha Yoga did not have the same popularity that it now enjoys. Towards the end of my studies, I was able to do the most advanced Hatha Yoga postures. I experienced the awakening of the Kundalini Shakti in India after a three-month period of doing yoga pranayama twelve hours a day (approximately one thousand hours of practice just on breathing).

I originally did Hatha Yoga for three main purposes: to acquire extreme flexibility for martial arts, to run qi smoothly through my energy channels and to sit properly in meditation poses for long periods of time. I had completed all three of these goals before I started training in Taoist Yoga within the Taoist priesthood. My previous yoga training was the perfect foundation for learning it and this helped to further accelerate my meditation path.

I was also glad to have found a gentler yogic practice that focused on internal energy because I was not encouraged about the direction yoga was taking. I had seen too many people injure themselves from excessive Hatha Yoga practices that push the body far beyond what is reasonable given the age, amount of training and general fitness level of many practitioners. I have observed this to be an increasing problem especially since the middle of the 1980s.

Both Taoist Neigong Yoga and Indian Hatha Yoga are valuable for ordinary sex. Good general flexibility in the bedroom makes possible all kinds of interesting movements and positions. Like qigong, Neigong Yoga prepares you to meditate, but unlike qigong, it incorporates the sixteen neigong components in different sitting and lying physical positions that mimic the sexual positions you are more likely to use in the bedroom.

The first two sets of Taoist Neigong Yoga incorporate Taoist Longevity Breathing and the conscious movement of breath through the body, leading to full relaxation. The later, more advanced sets develop the qi techniques and the dissolving work needed to do all the sexual meditation methods in this book, including those found in Chapters 17 and 18. It is my hope over the following years to be able to bring out the complete Taoist Neigong Yoga system that I developed from my in-depth training within the Taoist priesthood.

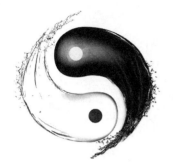

CHAPTER 10

Tai Chi and Qigong— Foundations for Sexual Practices

The practices of tai chi and qigong are the most accessible qi cultivation systems that can be found in the West. They offer a dynamic means to build a solid qi foundation in your body for the sexual qigong and sexual meditation practices presented later in this book.

Traditionally within Taoist groups, students would be taught sexual qigong and sexual meditation only after they demonstrated a degree of competence with qigong, tai chi or another related energy art. At the very least, a student of the sexual arts would be practicing and improving his or her tai chi and qigong forms while going through the sexual training.

Most Western exercise systems focus solely on muscular and cardiovascular strength, often through repetitive linear movements. In contrast, tai chi and qigong focus on moving energy, opening energy channels and on consciously working with circular or spherical flows of energy. Both traditional tai chi and qigong teach you how to build, store and use qi. They can dramatically improve your health and vitality and help upgrade your body's overall energetic system.

In this chapter we will examine how qi is cultivated in these energetic practices. Then we will look at the energetic capacities that are required for someone to do the sexual qigong and sexual meditation practices described in this book.

In the last part of this chapter we will explore a two-person interactive tai chi practice called "tai chi push hands." Tai chi push hands is another bridge practice to help you learn how qi flows between two people. Push hands trains you to be more sensitive and skillful with the different energies you may encounter in a partner, all in a nonsexual setting. That increased sensitivity can then be transferred into better lovemaking.

THE ART AND SCIENCE OF NEIGONG

Most types of training, whether intellectual or physical, start with foundational practices, which are then added to and built upon progressively over time as the skill level of the learner increases. A musician must first practice the scales; a child must first learn the alphabet. Taoist qi cultivation also has a set of core practices called *neigong* which incorporates sixteen internal energy components that can be likened to an energetic alphabet. Neigong is translated in English as "internal energy skill" or "internal energy development."

For many decades in China, the words neigong and qigong have been used virtually synonymously, even though there are technical differences. In recent years the word qigong has become more popular, although you may hear both terms used interchangeably.

Neigong is the Taoist art and science of how to move qi through the body. It is an art, because how you learn the energy components is infinitely varied. It is a craft or science, because this knowledge has been studied and codified for thousands of years into a complete energetic map and system. The beginning stage of qigong/neigong focuses mostly on the first two energy bodies (the physical and etheric). Neigong is the language of qi that becomes embedded in all the subtle physical movement forms of China that are commonly taught, such as tai chi or qigong, and it is directly integrated into all Taoist sexual practices. Tai chi is by far the most popular type of energetic practice worldwide, and it is a specific form or style of qigong or neigong.

It is important to recognize that the forms or outer movements of tai chi and qigong are just containers, like the outer case or shell of a laptop computer. The invisible qi methods and techniques, or neigong, are like the software programs that are invisibly sequestered inside the case. Physical movements alone do not make a practice qigong or neigong. What matters is how the qi flows within them.

SIXTEEN NEIGONG COMPONENTS

The sixteen neigong components are the core energetics within all of Taoism. As you progress in learning each of them, they integrate into all Taoist sexual practices. Each neigong component can potentially be done in a more yang or yin manner. The neigong components are:

1. Breathing methods, in increasing complexity. Your ultimate goal is to coordinate the expansion and contraction of your belly with every anatomical part and energetic function within both your physical and etheric bodies.

2. Moving qi in a specific direction along all the various ascending, descending and lateral connecting channels within your body. The process includes methods to

help you feel your qi, so that you can move it smoothly to where it will work most efficiently. Part of this is concerned with how to transform or dissolve and release felt qualities of the energy that flows within specified channels.

3. Moving qi in specific ways through all your main and secondary channels, including the acupuncture meridians, points, energy gates, Macro- and Microcosmic Orbits, as well as the multitude of other tiny interconnecting channels that cause specific functions to occur.

4. Precise inner and outer body alignments that prevent the flow of qi from being either blocked or dissipated.

5. Inner and Outer Dissolving to release and resolve all blockages within all eight of your energy bodies from the physical to the Tao.

6. Bending and stretching your body's soft tissues both in the direction from the inside out and the outside in and along your yin and yang acupuncture channels to activate, strengthen and balance them.

7. Opening and closing methods (pulsing) that you integrate into your body. Opening means to expand, grow larger or flow outward and emanate like a sun. Closing means to condense and get smaller in an inward direction, like the gravity force of a black hole. Closing carries no connotation of tension, contraction or force in the movement, only a continuous inward flow toward a point of origination. Opening and closing actions can occur within any of your soft or hard anatomical tissues, as well as anywhere within your body's subtle energy anatomy (channels, points, aura and so on).

8. Working with the energies of your aura to connect your physical body with your etheric field and its attendant emotional and mental states. A more advanced stage is to connect the energies of your body and aura to the rest of the psychic and spiritual energies that exist beyond your body and within the universe.

9. Becoming aware of and amplifying the circles and spirals of energy inside your body that may be weak, and strengthening and controlling the flow of the currents that are already operating well.

10. Consciously moving qi to any part of your body at will (especially to your internal organs and glands and within your brain and spinal cord). This includes absorbing or projecting qi from all body parts at will.

11. Awakening and controlling all the energies of your spine and all they connect to. This includes your vertebrae, brain, cerebrospinal fluid, spinal cord and the layers within it, and your entire nervous system.

12. Awakening and using both the physical and psychic left and right energy channels.

13. Awakening and using both the physical and psychic central energy channel, which controls all the others.

14. Developing the capacities and all the uses of your lower tantien, the main energetic center that directly affects all physical functions, as well as your sense of fear, insecurity and death and the sense of being physically and psychologically stable and grounded.

15. Developing the capacities and all the uses of your middle and upper tantien spiritual centers. The middle tantien (heart center) governs all relationships. It is intimately tied to all our most subtle emotions and intuitions and is considered the source of consciousness within the body. The upper tantien, located in the brain, is critical to longevity, because of its ability to activate the pituitary and pineal glands (master glands). It is also responsible for maintaining well-functioning, clear thought processes and psychic capacities. The upper tantien is the human bridge to all of time and space.

16. Integrating and connecting each of the previous fifteen components into one unified energy. Permanent integration is different from a temporary buzz or having a lot of energy that generates strong experiences but ultimately goes nowhere. If you lack number sixteen, it is difficult to absorb and integrate the good qualities of the other fifteen in a stable and comfortable manner that allows you to use them effortlessly to maximum effect.

Each of the sixteen neigong components are interrelated with and organically connected to the rest. Together these components form a circular whole. As a person learns and integrates more and more neigong, his or her ability to work with qi often increases *exponentially*. The human energetic system continuously gets upgraded as each new piece comes online. Each of the sixteen neigong elements is a methodology of qi, not merely a technique. Each component may have hundreds of potential techniques scattered throughout the many groups and schools of Taoism.

Shengong is the fusion of qigong/neigong and meditation, and works with the higher energy bodies—emotional, mental, psychic, karmic and body of individuality.

Energy Arts System of Qi Cultivation

There are many systems for working with subtle energy, or qi, in the world. Some are more complete, others less so. The Taoist system of qi cultivation is renowned for both its completeness and precision. I encourage you to find the most comprehensive system that works for you, whether it is mine or that of another teacher or even an entirely different tradition.

As a Taoist lineage holder, my responsibility to this tradition has been to be a bridge from the East to the West, teaching what I learned in China. I created the

Frantzis Energy Arts® System—a progressive, modular way for Westerners to learn physical and energetic components by breaking them into specific qigong sets. Some of the sets focus on specific neigong components, while others, such as tai chi, bagua and Gods Playing in the Clouds™ Qigong, are containers to hold all the neigong components as they are learned.

Many of the Energy Arts programs are directly relevant to learning the particular neigong components that will help you successfully embody and accomplish the sexual qigong and meditation methods presented in the later part of this book.

Here is an overview:

- Taoist Longevity Breathing, which is briefly explained in Chapter 9 (neigong component 1). These breathing methods can be put directly into all sexual practices.

- Dragon and Tiger Medical Qigong teaches you how to move and clear energy within both your own and your lover's aura (components 2, 3 and 8). Even as a beginner, you will find that this set quickly gives you a recognizable feeling of qi in your body (see "Dragon and Tiger Medical Qigong" section later in this chapter). Its methods applied to sexuality appear primarily in Chapters 11 and 12.

- Opening the Energy Gates of Your Body™ Qigong teaches you all the refinements of Outer Dissolving including how to move energy downward and how to locate and feel key junction points along the energetic pathways, called energy gates (components 1, 2, 3, 5, 10 and 14). You do this first in yourself and then with a partner in sexual qigong. Some of these methods appear in Chapters 11 and 12.

- Marriage of Heaven and Earth™ Qigong teaches opening and closing, or pulsing (component 7), and the pathways of the Small and Large Heavenly Orbits (also known as the Microcosmic and Macrocosmic Orbits) of energy (components 3, 6, 7, 10 and 14) that are used extensively in both sexual qigong and sexual meditation (see Chapter 13, "Opening and Closing: The Pulse of the Universe").

- Bend the Bow and Shoot the Arrow™ Qigong teaches you to feel and activate the energies of your spine, including the spinal pump discussed in Chapters 17 and 18 (Components 3, 6, 7, 10, 11, 13 and 14).

- Spiraling Energy Body™ Qigong teaches you how to instantly jump your energy across distance, move qi upward and activate the left, right and central channels used in both sexual qigong and sexual meditation (Components 2, 3, 5, 7, 8, 9, 10, 12 and 13). Its methods applied to sexuality appear in Chapters 17 and 18.

- Gods Playing in the Clouds™ teaches how to work with the lower, middle and upper tantiens, and how to fluidly move between the left, right and central channels as described in the advanced practices of Chapters 17 and 18 (all 16 components, especially 12 to 16).

- Taoist Meditation teaches Laozi's basic Inner Dissolving method (component 5), a primary technique in all sexual meditation (see Chapters 15-18).

THE PROCESS OF FEELING QI

With ongoing practice and with time, the living qualities of qi can be felt as clearly and concretely as holding an object in your hand. This is not some New Age idea; it is a skill you can develop, as many before you have already done. Your awareness of energy will awaken in subtle stages, layer after layer, as your body, mind and spirit gradually open. Regular practice of tai chi and qigong will, of course, enhance and speed up this marvelous process of discovery.

As your body becomes more alive, you will start to feel and know your anatomy experientially. You'll be able to feel your internal organs such as your liver—not intellectually or visually, but kinesthetically—and you'll be able to sense what they are doing.

The process of opening the body is not linear; energy travels in spirals and, until the body opens, the spirals can be intermittent or weak. For a while a certain part of the body will open; then, later on, a different area will open, while the other part closes again. The process is a bit like a game of "Now you see it, now you don't." Be patient. The time will come when your body opens up and stays open and becomes completely accessible to your awareness.

What happens if you practice qigong for a while but do not feel anything happening in your body? This is the case for many people. Don't get discouraged and give up because it often takes time to become sensitive to your qi. Sometimes a person may actually be getting results but is not aware of them. Some benefits may include: feeling generally more comfortable, being able to do more things without strain, improved health and not getting sick as often as you used to, better concentration and increased sensation during sex.

When you notice these effects, often it is because your qi is growing stronger over time whether you feel it or not. Keep practicing and you will eventually feel the qi in a very real, direct way. Eventually, the movements of the body, the full intention of the mind and the movement of the qi will all happen together.

QI PRACTICES FOR HEALING

In Western countries, qi practices for self-healing are taught as part of qigong training. Using qi to heal others is commonly taught intellectually in acupuncture classes or experientially in qigong tui na (qi-based therapeutic bodywork). However, instruction in any aspects of sexual qigong and Taoist sexual meditation is extremely difficult to find in the West, as there are very few adequately trained masters and severe constraints on teaching this material in a public setting. Learning qigong or qigong tui na practices would thus be extremely useful for anyone who wants to incorporate healing techniques into their sexual activity or have sexual qigong practice enhance their healing abilities.

BUILDING BLOCKS FOR QI CULTIVATION

There are hundreds of qigong, tai chi and other internal martial art forms. Whichever of these you take up, you will first learn rudimentary physical components of the movements, together with physical principles such as not locking your joints, protecting your knees and getting your body to move as a whole. The goal of all energy arts practices is to have qi strongly flowing through the body, mind and spirit in a smooth, balanced, connected and fluid manner through all the energetic pathways, without blockage.

Photos by Mark Thayer

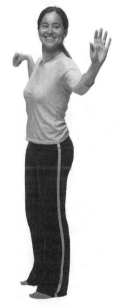

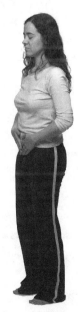

Qigong practice cultivates vitality, relaxation and a sense of well-being.

At the conclusion of qigong practice, qi is stored in the lower tantien.

PHYSICAL FOUNDATIONS

Correct physical alignments allow the energy channels to flow properly and are often required before energetics can be integrated. This is so that you know the correct body positioning to avoid blocking or dissipating your own qi or that of your lover in sexual qigong or sexual meditation. Understanding these physical components is also the key to avoiding injury from all kinds of physical activity. For many students, learning the correct physical movements can take a long period of time and is the primary focus.

The core physical building blocks for qi cultivation may include:

- Basic postural alignments.
- Learning how to shift weight.
- Turning movements that are initiated from the hip joint, or kwa.
- Loosening and relaxing the shoulder blades, neck and back, which are often locked in place and stuck because of computer work or bad posture.
- Protective principles, such as how not to lock your joints or put excessive weight on the knees.
- Determining what your personal seventy percent is given your body, age and whether or not you have any injuries.

Learning the core physical movements can be likened to building a strong container. It is important that the container you build does not have any structural problems or leaks. Once you have the basic physical movements, then the next step is to put more of the energetics into the container.

ENERGETIC FOUNDATIONS

The energetic components are the primary reason to practice tai chi and qigong. They are what make these practices ideal for health and healing. Each energetic component that you integrate is like a new software program that upgrades your nervous system and makes your body more conscious.

The core energetic building blocks for qi cultivation may include:

- Learning to tune your mind inward, commonly done initially with breathing, to put your consciousness directly into different parts of your body.
- Feeling energy between the palms of your hands and pulling and projecting this energy between them.
- Feeling major energetic junctions, called energy gates.
- Feeling the qualities of blocked energy, starting with the physical energy body, and learning to dissolve blockages at progressively deeper layers.

As you practice a tai chi or qigong form and incorporate the physical and energetic principles, your nerves gradually let go and you naturally begin to relax. You are able to feel and discover where your body is tense, and over time, with practice, you learn to release that tension more or less permanently. As you do this, your body becomes softer and more sensitive. Your qi builds and flows freely.

Your focus and concentration gets better, helping you to turn inward without as many barriers. You become healthier in all ways: the circulation of all the fluids in your body becomes stronger; your joints become more flexible; your physical balance improves and your internal organs are strengthened. This helps people feel more alive and naturally increases energy, flexibility and overall longevity.

INTEGRATING THE SIXTEEN NEIGONG COMPONENTS

At this stage, the training becomes more complex, but also far more interesting. The components of neigong are progressively taught and layered into the forms. You will be taught increasingly sophisticated physical and energetic components, with either yang or yin qualities, which you then layer and seamlessly integrate into the forms you are learning, as well as other practices, such as sexual qigong. As you progress, the physical movements of the form improve and so does your ability to feel qi internally. This may include learning such physical skills such as:

- More precise internal alignments, which may include correcting back and joint problems.
- The ability to precisely coordinate movements of the upper and lower body, for example, moving the elbow and the knee together.
- Making movements flow smoothly, without stops and starts.
- Not slowing down or speeding up from one movement to another.
- Matching your range of motion to the least capable or weakest link of your body—not your strongest.
- Using and directing qi for specific healing purposes.
- Accessing your higher energy bodies.

Your qi and your physical body are intimately linked, like the water of a river and the riverbed in which it flows. Your qi flows through your body, mind and spirit in all layers of the eight energy bodies. The best approach is to develop the body first and then cultivate your qi. If a river swells to be larger than the channel through which it flows, it becomes unstable and overflows, to no useful effect or even causing destruction.

Conversely, if you build a large enough riverbed, it can handle any amount of water with no turbulence or destructive effects. The same relationship holds between qi and your physical body. Learning physical movements and the related physical principles mentioned above will prepare your body's energy channels to handle more qi with comfort and stability.

TAI CHI AND QIGONG

Tai chi and qigong are renowned as practices that can make people incredibly healthy and reduce stress by upgrading the flow of qi. Both practices also reduce anxiety by relaxing the nervous system, which is an extremely important issue for enjoyable sex. There are hundreds of different styles of qigong and many major and minor styles of tai chi, some more effective than others. There are also many teachers, each with varying degrees of ability. Generally, what style people learn and with whom they study is dependent upon what is available in their local community rather than what might be the best or most appropriate for their needs.

Although it is beyond the scope of this book to go in detail about the various forms of tai chi and qigong, what follows is some basic information that may be useful on your path.

SELECTING A QIGONG OR TAI CHI STYLE

There are five primary branches of qigong available in the West: Taoist, Buddhist, Confucian, medical and martial art qigong, with the Emei and Kunlun styles being less common. Each branch can have many individual styles with separate names. Within these major categories, there are hundreds of qigong sets, which may contain as few as 5 movements or up to 150 movements. Some are medical qigong sets that specifically address common health problems, such as liver ailments, cancer or nerve disease. Others are designed to upgrade the overall health of the body and still others focus on enhancing the intellectual functioning of the mind. Some qigong sets cultivate internal power for martial arts. Depending on your fitness levels, your time available to learn and the local availability of teachers, you will have to find a qigong set that is the best match for your specific needs. Many qigong teachers teach some energy work, but two crucial issues are important: how well they do so and, perhaps more importantly, how long it will take for you to learn the physical movements that underpin the energetic work.

Tai chi was originally developed as a martial art and it had two goals: to make practitioners very healthy and at the same time teach them physical self-defense through using both yin (called soft in Chinese) and yang (called steel) qi methods. The five primary styles, mostly named after the teachers that developed them, are Yang, Wu, Chen, Hao and combination styles. Each style has short forms (typically 16 to 24 movements), which are easier and quicker to learn, and long forms (up to

128 moves). In the West, the most popular form of tai chi taught is the Yang style. Within the last few decades simplified forms have been developed primarily from the Yang style and have been applied to specific health problems, such as mitigating arthritis or improving balance. The Wu style of tai chi is a smaller style that is excellent for health, meditation and integrating neigong components. The Chen style, which is growing rapidly, is the most overtly martial style and the most physically demanding on the body, due to stomping, twisting and spiraling movements—and thus this style is best for those without health problems or injuries.

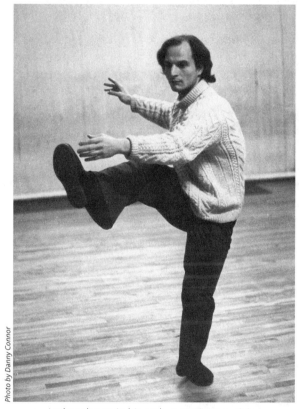

Photo by Danny Connor

Author shown in his early twenties practicing
the Chen Pan Ling combination style of tai chi.
This form has over one hundred movements.

Although qi development is critical in tai chi, few teachers go beyond teaching the physical movements. This is because for longer tai chi forms, it can take up to a year just to learn the physical moves. Some teachers may know a few energetic principles, but not much more. The description of neigong presented in this chapter can help you better assess whether a teacher is just teaching external movements or is also integrating the internal energy components.

TEACHER CONSIDERATIONS

To learn techniques that can be incorporated into sexual qigong, you will want to find a practice that teaches you how to relax the body, mind and emotions as you do the physical movements of whatever form you learn. The teacher should also be able to show you how to feel, activate and strongly move energy in your body.

If you want to learn how to link your energy to that of someone else, then practices such as tai chi push hands, described later in this chapter, will accomplish this if the teacher's emphasis is on feeling and being sensitive to qi and not just on developing muscular skills or better physical movement.

If your primary interest is practicing sexual meditation, then your qigong or tai chi teacher must help you learn how to go very deep inside yourself and relax the mind and spirit. This can be done either in sitting meditation or by using tai chi or qigong as a moving Taoist meditation practice.

Unfortunately, in the West, there are no clear standards for teachers, and their marketing claims can sometimes be misleading. Currently there is a large influx of new qigong and tai chi teachers with little or no experience other than a weekend seminar or two. Also it is advised not to automatically assume that because a teacher is from the East, he or she knows the inner workings of these arts. In fact often learning from someone whose native language is different from your own can make learning tai chi or qigong more of a challenge.

Here are some other questions you can ask yourself when looking for a teacher:

- What is his or her primary emphasis in teaching? Is it cultivating qi, martial arts, improving general health and/or specific health aspects, and does he or she also teach healing techniques?
- How much emphasis is placed on developing such physical foundations as correct alignments or proper turning techniques? Without this, your ability to develop qi may be severely hampered.
- How much of the internal components of neigong does he or she know?
- What methods are used to teach neigong?
- Does the teacher embody the techniques, and how well are they transferred to students? Some teachers may be good practitioners but poor at teaching or vice versa.
- What is the teacher's training history?

After that, it comes down to what is actually available where you live and whether you are comfortable with the teacher. There is a very old Taoist saying: "A teacher can take you to the gate. Only you can decide to pass within." Qigong and tai chi can be gates into the world of qi. But you must put in the regular practice to build the energetic foundation you need for sexual qigong and sexual meditation.

Dragon and Tiger Medical Qigong

While in China, I was fortunate to be passed the lineage of Dragon and Tiger Medical Qigong, a powerful qi cultivation system. It activates and balances the energy that travels through the major acupuncture meridians of your body, giving you more vitality, boosting your immune system and reducing stress.

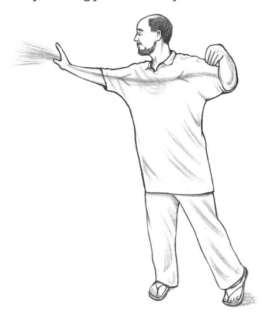

Energy is drawn across the body through the heart and discharged from the palm. This movement loosens the upper body, energizes the heart and balances the right and left sides of the body.

Figure 10-1: Dragon and Tiger Medical Qigong, Movement 4

Dragon and Tiger uses only seven movements, each repeated twenty times, and takes just fifteen minutes to do. Other qigong systems that provide these medical benefits can include twenty, fifty or more than one hundred movements and thus take far longer to learn and to practice.

Besides providing the basic benefits of all medical qigong styles, Dragon and Tiger's specialty was for use in cancer therapy, particularly to help reduce the side effects, both physical and emotional, of chemotherapy and radiation treatment.

Dragon and Tiger Qigong originated from the Chan (called Zen in Japanese) Buddhist tradition in the Shaolin monastery about 1,500 years ago. It was used to keep the monks within the high clergy in optimal health. I learned Dragon and Tiger from Zhang Jia Hua, a niece of one of the Chan Buddhist high priests.

After the Communist revolution, this priest decided to allow Dragon and Tiger to be released into the secular world. Since he had no living male relatives, he decided to teach Zhang all his qigong and Chinese medical knowledge. This was rare because classically in China, family secrets (especially those relating to qigong or martial arts) were only passed down to male relatives. The traditional rationale for this was that a woman would marry out of the family, and the family's patent secrets would then belong to the new family. This would in effect destroy the family's privileged position and potentially impoverish future generations.

Extremely proficient in the use of qigong for medical purposes, Zhang became a doctor of Chinese medicine and vice president of the All-China Qigong Association. She also became the private physician to some high government officials and, as a result, was able to propagate this form of qigong for medical purposes during the chaos of the Cultural Revolution and its aftermath in the 1960s and 1970s, when most other forms of qigong were temporarily suppressed.

During fifteen years of active teaching during that period, Zhang taught and qualified more than twenty thousand instructors. According to Zhang and many others within her field, these instructors spread the healing art to twenty million Chinese people.

Zhang agreed to accept me as a student after a meeting with Liu Hung Chieh. A vigorous, seventy-year-old woman when I first met her, Zhang was an impressive teacher. She taught me privately in her home and at her clinic. It was her hope that I would teach and train teachers in this wonderful healing art when I returned to the West.

The foundational qigong set within the Energy Arts core qigong system, Dragon and Tiger Qigong can enable you to:

1. Feel the qi along the acupuncture meridians on the skin and, as a next step, strongly move it with your hands at the level of the wei qi (wei chi), located just beneath the skin.

2. Sense how tension and stress in the body and mind impede the ability to feel and move qi. Conversely, the quieter and more relaxed your mind, the greater becomes your ability to strongly activate qi, and push and pull it.

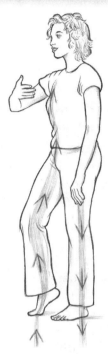

In this movement, qi moves down the outside of the leg into the ground, and earth energy is brought up the inside of the leg, along the left or right channel to the shoulder's nest. This relaxing movement energizes the lungs and liver and increases breathing capacity.

Figure 10-2: Dragon and Tiger Medical Qigong, Movement 1

3. Feel where qi is weak and strengthen it.

4. Use qi to help heal injured parts of your body, such as knees or shoulders, as well as many illnesses.

5. Use the breath to help release stagnant qi.

6. Feel and activate your etheric field (aura).

7. Use the movements to speed up qi circulation in the body, much like a water turbine, and super-charge it.

This form of medical qigong uses hand and foot movements to clear and move qi within the body along the acupuncture yin and yang meridians by stimulating the qi of the etheric body or aura. The skills learned within Dragon and Tiger provide an excellent foundation for sexual qigong.

INTERACTIVE PRACTICES—TAI CHI PUSH HANDS FOR SEXUAL SENSITIVITY

For millennia Taoist qi practices done with a partner—often termed "dual cultivation" or, in modern language, "interactive" practices—have been used as a relatively easy and direct way to contact another person's consciousness and cultivate greater awareness of qi. When the inside of your body heats up, when everything starts cooking and you get really hot, the capacity to become aware at the physical, energetic and psychic levels can dramatically open up.

The term dual cultivation has been typically used in literary works for well more than fifty years to refer primarily to sexual practices, however it includes more than that. Dual cultivation practices don't have to be sexual and include talking, tai chi push hands, sharing energy with trees or other living things in your immediate environment, and even linking your qi to that of the moon, planetary bodies or stars.

Ordinary tai chi movements by themselves increase your personal sensitivity to the potential range of sexual sensations that you are capable of feeling. Push hands, the two-person practice within tai chi, goes much further. It gives you a pragmatic training method for enabling you to recognize and feel the energetic sensations happening in a partner. Push hands can provide an effective jump point from just feeling qi inside yourself to working with the energy flows of a partner—a key part of sexual qigong. The qi cultivation skills learned in push hands can be directly transferred into sexual practices. Because sex is such a kinesthetic activity based on sensation and physical touch, the distinction between visualizing qi and actually feeling it is not a minor point. Through specific push hands methods you learn to distinguish different energies in you and your partner. You learn to develop sensitivity and to fluidly respond to energetic changes, moment by moment.

Push hands is an art of working with both your own energy and that of your partner. In this practice, two partners follow the flows of energy to try to unbalance or "push" each other off center while their arms or hands remain in continuous contact as they move in a variety of ways. The practice is the bridge between tai chi form work and martial arts sparring. Yet when practiced in a playful, non-threatening manner, push hands can be a wonderful antidote to stress, as well as developing the qi sensitivity necessary for sexual qigong and later sexual meditation.

When practiced in a playful manner, push hands can be a wonderful antidote to stress and develops the qi sensitivity you need for sexual qigong and sexual meditation.

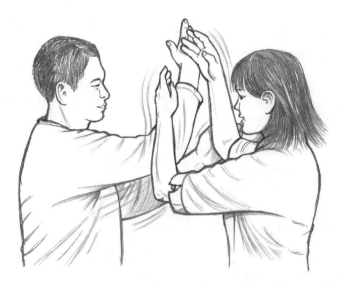

Figure 10-3: The Interactive Tai Chi Practice of Push Hands

STICKING TO YOUR PARTNER

In tai chi push hands, partners maintain continuous contact with one another, called *sticking,* which involves hand, arm and waist sensitivity. The skill trains you to be sensitive to the ever-changing qi of another human being in unpredictable, fluid circumstances, while never losing contact.

This skill is extremely relevant to sex where you must really connect with and influence your lover's qi by continuously sticking to the flow of that person's subtle qi at progressively deeper emotional, mental and psychic levels.

This puts the idea of "contact" on an entirely new level. When rolling around in bed, you are not just pleasuring your lover's physical body, you are consciously contacting and merging with the deeper levels of his or her mind, bodily energy and emotions.

When you learn to transfer this skill to lovemaking, you'll never tire of each other because each moment will be extremely alive. What makes any lovemaking more exciting is the element of unpredictability. In contrast, overly predictable, scripted sex can get rather boring. Learn to "stick" with your partner and you open a sexual feedback loop that has infinite possibilities.

When you apply sticking to sexuality, you go through three stages. First you make contact. Next there's a sexual buildup, in which you stay connected and ratchet up the pleasure and excitement, and finally, you tip over into orgasm by using Outer

Dissolving to release the blockages or by receiving a serious bolt of energy from your partner or projecting qi yourself.

LISTENING

Another primary technique of push hands is "listening" and interpreting what you energetically hear. Until a student learns this technique, it is difficult to sense what a practice partner is doing or about to do. Learning to listen involves a lot of experimentation and sensing into the eight energy bodies to get a feel for how they influence the movement of qi.

In a sexual context, this form of listening lends itself exceptionally to opening up your ability to access your own and your partner's energy bodies, including the deeper layers. When this listening involves the psychic, karmic and essence energy bodies you can achieve a depth of intimacy that is unavailable in ordinary sex. Lovemaking is no longer just about physical sensations and body parts. You go deeper to touch and connect to your lover's higher energy bodies. At the deepest levels you may suddenly feel into the whole of their soul.

The skill involved is not that different from ordinary push hands skills, in which you seek, through bodily touch, to skillfully destabilize another's feet, his or her root. The direction you point your awareness and the purpose are different, of course, but the actual subtle tactile and energetic ability is essentially the same.

Both sticking and listening can train a practitioner to overcome one of the major obstacles in meditation, the perception syndrome, "It's happening, it's not, I have it, I lost it..." that can go on ad infinitum. The direct experience of actual qi in motion is not ambivalent.

STAGES OF PUSH HANDS PRACTICE

As you practice tai chi push hands, you will progress through three levels that relate to ordinary sex, sexual qigong and sexual meditation:

Push Hands Skills Applicable to Ordinary Sex

Ordinary sex improves for both sexes when partners increase their sensitivity and ability to feel one another. Push hands abundantly cultivates the ability to feel your lover. It also teaches you to be totally present during sex, and this greatly enhances sexual play and contributes to better orgasms. As briefly mentioned earlier in terms of learning the sticking techniques of push hands, when you integrate all the skills of push hands into ordinary sex you do the following:

- **Stage 1:** You find your partner's sexual center. In each moment, you are seeking that point at which his or her sexual energy is bottled up and ready to be released.

This enables you to know where and how to touch him or her to elicit the greatest possible response. If you don't make contact with this ever-changing sexual center, his or her sexual response can be mediocre. In contrast, if you can track and land on your partner's sexual center, pleasure will naturally start to release.

- **Stage 2:** The buildup—you endeavor to continuously recognize, track and release whatever new sexual centers or reservoirs of sexual energy spontaneously appear. Sexual energy tends to pool in certain areas that are bottled up, and they yearn to be free. If you can feel, locate and open these areas during foreplay and intercourse, you eliminate the internal resistance to orgasm.

- **Stage 3:** The parallel to sending someone flying in tai chi push hands (using a powerful discharge technique known in Chinese as *fa jin*) is sending your partner over the edge into orgasm. Besides the purely physical rubbing, the agent of the orgasm is your energy and intent being suddenly directed toward the orgasmic site, which may be external or internal.

Push Hands Skills Applicable to Sexual Qigong

Incorporating skills from push hands into sexual qigong can make you a better lover in a number of ways:

- In addition to physical sensitivity, you go beyond to cultivate nonphysical energetic sensitivity, eventually developing a concrete ability to recognize the ever-changing qi of your lover's body, emotions, mental and psychic energy. This allows you to recognize where qi is healthy and flowing and where orgasmic and any other energy may be blocked and in need of release.

- By using the Outer Dissolving method, blockages in the first four energy bodies can be released and potentially resolved in three stages during sex that are progressively more difficult: releasing only your own blockages, releasing only your partner's blockages and finally releasing blockages of both of you simultaneously.

Spiritual Push Hands and Sexual Meditation

Spiritual Push Hands is where martial arts, meditation and sex can combine. Tai chi done with just physical movement and even with qi techniques cannot fulfill the full spiritual potential of the art. This merely builds the technical foundation that tai chi with meditation, or spiritual tai chi, requires.

The primary reason for using tai chi for meditation, as in all Taoist meditation, is complete spiritual awakening by resolving blockages in the eight energy bodies. Spiritual purification is a fundamental part of most major religious traditions and Taoism is no exception. Within Taoism, both tai chi push hands and sexual meditation use Laozi's Inner Dissolving methods to accomplish this.

Although the idea of spiritual purification is not and has never been a significant part of the tai chi martial arts tradition, there is in China what is called *wu de* or martial arts morals. This refers to using martial arts to build moral character according to ordinary Confucian or Buddhist principles.

Spiritual tai chi can be looked at from three levels, each using more specific and refined methods. The first level is practicing tai chi with meditation, or Taoist spiritual tai chi. This type of tai chi can be found but is still rare. The second level, even rarer, is combining tai chi push hands with meditation, or spiritual push hands. At the third level, the rarest and most specific application of tai chi push hands, you work with spiritual tai chi push hands as a training method for sexual meditation.

At the current time, there is virtually no written material in the West regarding the first two levels of spiritual tai chi, that is, meditation combined with either tai chi or tai chi push hands. The author learned these methods over several years in Beijing as a disciple of the Taoist Immortal Liu Hung Chieh.[1] Both are complex subjects that demand direct hands-on instruction and transmission from a teacher. A brief summary of spiritual tai chi follows.

Combining tai chi, including push hands, with meditation has several defining characteristics. Similar to sexual meditation, it uses Taoist Inner and Outer Dissolving, the core methods of Laozi's Water tradition, alternating between sitting practices and moving push hands to access the blockages within and resolve them.

All the defensive and offensive push hands techniques that deal with the opponent's physical energy body are included in spiritual push hands, but it goes beyond to include the energies within each of the remaining seven energy bodies. One of the terms used in ordinary push hands to describe the extremely subtle, soft and defensive yielding technique is "the opponent falls into emptiness." The ordinary and energetic meaning of this is when the opponent attempts to land their power on you, you move your body or manipulate your qi in such a way that the opponent's force seems as though it has fallen into a bottomless black hole. It cannot contact any solidity. The result is that the attacker's force is totally neutralized.

In spiritual push hands, very powerful yin defensive techniques are created by releasing into the actual state of emptiness, wherever the energy is blocked within you and your partner in any of the eight energy bodies. As the basis for its yang offensive techniques, push hands uses moving into or exploding into emptiness, called *fa shen* in Chinese. In spiritual tai chi push hands, energetic *fa jin* and spiritual *fa shen* now becomes a method to resolve your own and your partner's deeper energetic blockages all the way up through the eighth energy body.

---

1. Within the Taoist tradition the title "Immortal" refers to someone who has actualized all eight energy bodies. An Immortal's consciousness has merged with the Tao.

The most advanced methods of using spiritual tai chi and push hands cross over into sexual meditation and can be done in several ways:

- Having your partner release his or her blockages and fall into your emptiness, when you detect the resistance at whichever energy body it occurs.

- Helping both partners to gain experience so they can continuously fall into, fall out of, re-enter and continue to stay in emptiness. This provides a context for you to stably remain in emptiness while meditating. This provides important training to avoid and overcome doubt, a standard obstacle for many meditators, where a person wonders ad infinitum, "Is emptiness happening? Do I have it? Did I lose it? Is it back?" Being able to listen to and stick to emptiness is a fairly advanced form of sticking, whether in bed or in tai chi push hands. This is especially so after a third neo-central channel is created in the later stages of sexual meditation (see Chapter 18).

- Gaining experience in creating and using emptiness with *fa shen* to aid or cause your sexual partner to have internal orgasms or at least increase or spread them more easily into an ever-expanding quality of emptiness inside one or both of you.

Many paths can realistically lead you to the bedroom of either sexual qigong or meditation. Learning tai chi, you move through several progressive stages, where the next stage or layer depends on the one preceding it. First you learn the physical tai chi movements. Next the subtle energetics fuse into the movements. Then comes the tactile and energetic sensitivity training of tai chi push hands. You are now prepared for sexual qigong. Next you reach an even deeper stage where you do spiritual tai chi as Taoist meditation. Finally, you seamlessly combine spiritual tai chi, push hands, meditation and sex practices together and you are well prepared to delve into sexual meditation.

Spiritual Martial Arts

Since the early 1960s, I have been intimately involved with tai chi chuan and other internal martial arts such as bagua and hsing-i. Ordinary martial artists can obviously become great fighters without being engaged in spirituality. They can become confident, relaxed, easy going and competent in the midst of physical combat.

The quest for spirituality is highly optional in martial arts. Spiritual practices develop the potential for a martial artist to become a great spiritual warrior in the battlefield of life. I was very fortunate to be taught spiritual martial arts by the

Taoist Immortal Liu Hung Chieh, who held direct martial art and meditation lineages. I have never found anyone else in the West who knows or teaches spiritual martial arts to a similar depth.

Spiritual martial arts are not for the faint-hearted. Believing in spirituality is easy. The test beyond lip service is to honestly embody spiritual qualities in daily life. Taking the path of spiritual martial arts means the following four things:

1. The martial artist must deliberately seek to encounter and then dissolve and overcome his or her inner demons. This can take more inner courage than that needed for the most severe physical combat.

2. Spirituality must fundamentally shift a martial artist's innermost identity to focus on the good of the whole with universal love and compassion, rather than a view that is primarily centered on the self-interests of winning and losing either as an individual or for his or her tribe. A path is not spiritual if it creates someone who becomes confused or fixated primarily on acquiring and using psychic or other forms of power and control.

3. Spirituality must make the martial artist genuinely moral—a sincere, developed, strong moral awareness that naturally comes from inside one's core. To live by moral principles means to deeply investigate, understand and agree with the rules by which one wishes to live. It means recognizing what is spiritually relevant and valuable to one's inner decision-making processes.

4. Spirituality must awaken the innermost nature or core essence of the soul or Being. At the core, a person is fully alive and awake rather than half-asleep. From this point, the innermost essence or soul can make a direct personal connection to the natural forces and energies that permeate the Consciousness of the universe.

Genuine morality and sensitive intelligence enables people to sanely navigate the complex and often contradictory moral ambiguities of living through complex and unpredictable situations. In my book *The Power of Internal Martial Arts and Chi,* I have devoted an entire chapter to Spiritual Martial Arts.

As other advanced teachers from the East either migrate to the West, or teach Westerners who have travelled to train with them, it is my hope that perhaps there will be some with advanced skills in both martial arts and meditation who can begin to beneficially transmit this specialized spiritual knowledge to their martial arts students.

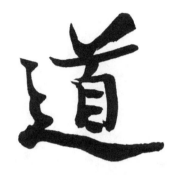

SECTION 4

TAOIST SEXUAL QIGONG

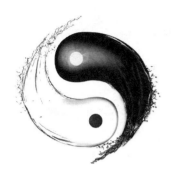

CHAPTER 11

Energy Clearing and Dissolving

At the very heart of Laozi's Water method is the assumption that you can develop the ability to feel and be fully conscious of whatever is happening inside the body, mind and Spirit. This is done through consciously feeling and using qi, which is the emphasis of Taoist sexual qigong.

At the most basic level of sexual qigong, the Taoists developed many practices to expand the whole arena of sexual arousal and pleasure, beyond what ordinary sex techniques offer. These energetic practices enable you to feel and move energy in the bodies of both you and your lover more strongly.

When you start feeling deeply inside yourself or your partner, you will find places where your energies or that of your partner have become frozen—where either person's physical body, qi, emotions, thoughts and so on have congealed in some way. These dense areas, in turn, close down the channels and points through which energy would otherwise flow freely through your entire system (including your entire multidimensional Being), or that of your lover.

To quote the classic Taoist text *The Secret of the Golden Flower,* as translated by Thomas Cleary, "If you can operate yin and yang, turning them suitably, then naturally all at once clouds will form and rain will fall, the plants and trees refreshed, the mountain rivers flowing freely. Even if there is something offensive, it still melts away all at once when you notice it. This is the great cycle."[1]

All energy inside a human being, if free (that is, unblocked), is like a flowing river. Due to innumerable conditions and circumstances, however, we commonly do not retain the free-flowing energies that should naturally be ours at birth (aside from karma and birth traumas). Condensed or blocked energies assume an actual form or shape. Instead of flowing freely, the energy gathers and stagnates, as if in a putrid pond.

These condensed energetic shapes block the normal flow of qi in your various

---

1. Cleary, Thomas, *The Taoist Classics: Volume Three* (Boston: Shambhala, 1991), 311.

energy bodies, causing all manner of illness, dysfunction and diminished capacity. With training, these blockages can be recognized and resolved. This is why the practice of sexual qigong begins with techniques to dissolve blocked physical energy and move it outside the body.

The level of sexual qigong, or subtle energy sex, initially progresses in four stages, each increasing in difficulty:

1. Becoming generally aware of moving energy in yourself and your partner.
2. Externally activating your partner's energy channels using touch or by stimulating their etheric fields or aura to cause energy to move within their body.
3. Using the Taoist practice known as Outer Dissolving (described later in this chapter) to free energetic blockages in yourself and to energetically penetrate your partner's body to release their blockages, open the flow through his or her energy channels and enable his or her energy field to have greater ranges of sexual sensation.
4. Replicate, especially in foreplay, all the same techniques done with Outer Dissolving but now do them with the methods of Inner Dissolving as explained in Chapter 15.

In any long-term process, some aspects and practices will be easier than others at different points in time. Ideally in sexual qigong you begin doing foreplay first with Outer Dissolving because this is how you are going to move energy inside yourself and your partner when your genitals meet. However, this presumes you have the skill to use your consciousness to penetrate and move energy within your and your partner's body. If you have not yet developed this skill, you have another easier option—to externally work with the etheric body.

EXTERNALLY ACTIVATING AND CLEARING QI

The starting point for many in sexual qigong is to learn to awaken your partner's energy by externally stimulating and clearing his or her etheric body, which will mimic where the qi in the channels of the physical body are stuck. You do this by running your hands through your partner's etheric field or by stimulating and touching their skin. This turns on the energy in various ways, often leading to sexual arousal and igniting the dance of lovemaking.

Sexual arousal naturally makes your energy more fully activated, vibrant and alive at levels that might not otherwise have been readily apparent. Your ability to feel and experience areas of your consciousness that were previously numb or hidden increases, because your subtle senses become more alert and fully capable when you get turned on. As your physical energy becomes flush, your mind expands, making it easier to contact and gain influence over your tissues and subtle energies.

Over time and with practice, you can learn to tune into subtle energy flows and feel you and your partner on many levels, both inside your bodies and in the energy fields surrounding your physical selves. This allows you to directly experience the energies—sexual and beyond—that exist within your partner's multidimensional Being. This amounts to quite a radical shift from the foreplay methods commonly used in ordinary sex. Foreplay takes on whole new meaning when you are making love to an energy being rather than just a romantic partner or a sex object.

ENERGY CLEARING FOR LOVERS

In Taoist sexual qigong, your first priority when making love is to make sure both of you have a clear qi field that is free of negative or competing energies. The reason for this is simple: you want to be with your partner and not have other people's subliminal or psychic energies in bed with you. The energetic presence of others can cause either or both of you to freeze up when your bodies touch and your sexual energies begin to merge. This is true even when the energies within your field are not sexual in nature. For example, a slave-driving boss who gave your partner hell before he or she left the office may still be lingering in his or her field. Even the energetic presence of one of your lover's platonic friends can cloud the field between you.

The aim is to remove any energy stuck in either of your auras (i.e., the qi or etheric body) that does not specifically belong to the two of you. This allows for complete privacy and intimacy between you. The unique nature of the energy field that the two of you create can be especially hampered at the psychic energy body level if other people's energies are present in either of your energy fields.

Depending upon the nature of these energies, they can have an array of effects from bodily pain to inhibiting emotional feeling and expression. In fact, what many experience as *inhibition* is often related to these subtle "foreign" energies. It doesn't much matter if the competing energies are from a prior sexual encounter or just the normal, daily congestion that accumulates in the energy body. The point is that during sexual activity, you want only your energy to fill your partner's energy field (and vice versa), so you need to clear whatever is lingering there.

In addition to clearing his or her field, when you do this as a preliminary practice before lovemaking it helps your lover's nerves to unwind. Commonly utilized in nonsexual contexts, the practice of clearing the etheric body is a fundamental qigong method, particularly for increasing health and vitality. In a nonsexual context, aura clearing doesn't generally tend to generate as intense a response. However, when done in a sexually charged atmosphere, with both of you oozing sexual heat, more dramatic effects may occur. Again, it is crucial to accept and simply be present to whatever arises, no matter what comes up for you or your partner. Remember, however, the rules of sexual noninterference; if you are working with your partner's energy and you ask him or her to participate in the sexual qigong techniques, he or she must agree to join in the energetic practices.

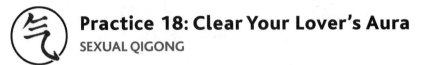

Practice 18: Clear Your Lover's Aura
SEXUAL QIGONG

This practice clears any types of energetic blockages in you or your partner. Any blocked energy or baggage you carry into lovemaking will inhibit your ability to feel and move qi. It will also decrease your sensitivity and pleasure.

While clearing your lover's aura, feel free to look in each other's eyes, engage in whatever playful and seductive amusements you both enjoy, or—with eyes closed—simply relax and feel. The main point is to play around and become sensitive to your lover's nonphysical energy before you move to putting your hands or anything else on or into your partner's body.

This exercise describes a woman clearing a man's aura. A man clearing a woman's aura would go downwards first, from her head or belly to her feet, before going up her body.

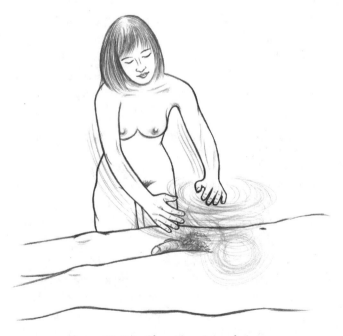

Figure 11-1 A: Clear Your Lover's Aura

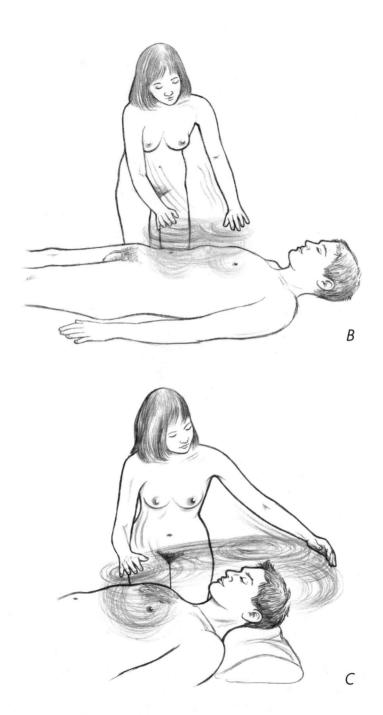

Figure 11-1 B–C: Clear Your Lover's Aura

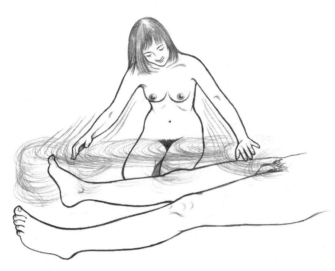

Figure 11-1 D: Clear Your Lover's Aura

The woman first goes up her lover's body from his groin to awaken his yang energy (Figure 11-1 A–C) and then down from above his head (Figure 11-1 C–D) to awaken his yin downward flow until the up-down energy circulation of his entire body is fully activated.

Begin by using your open hands and feel the area above your partner's skin with your palms. Become aware of different energetic pressures that exist in layers, every inch or so above his or her body. Tune into these pressure fields and notice what you feel, for example:

1. Heat or cold

2. Relatively uneven pressure buildups

3. Dead zones

4. Bloated areas

5. Irregular or blocked spaces.

You may feel the blockages as energetic sensations in your hands, such as little balls like pieces of paper or sponge, a sensation similar to what you feel when you put two magnets next to each other, irregular sensations, holes, condensations, or odd obstructions.

Clear the energetic fields around your partner's body with stroking, pushing, pulling, throwing or sweeping movements to move the blocked energy. Continue stirring the energy until it becomes smooth and you no longer get a sense of any energetic obstruction.

This has two effects. First, it helps your partner's energy come back to life (like the energy equivalent of taking a weight off them or receiving a blood transfusion). Second, it eliminates some or most of the residual energetic impressions of all the people your partner has been in contact with that day.

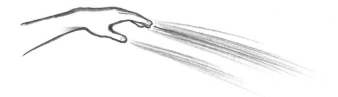

*Use your hands to pull out any blocked qi in your partner's field and
discharge it away from his or her etheric body with your palm or fingers.*

Figure 11-2: Discharging Blocked Qi

Ultimately, you want the space of his or her field to be clear, unblocked, smooth and regular, so that your hand passes easily through the air around the body. As you do the clearing, keep in mind the variety of sexual positions you might want to enjoy. It's best to clear the whole of your partner's aura, but at least clear your partner's energetic aura as far above, below, and to the side as you are likely to touch one another at any point during lovemaking.

Keep in mind that the etheric fields extend anywhere from four inches to many feet beyond the skin. Be sure to clear as best you can above and to the side of your partner's body. If one partner is significantly taller than the other, clear the full distance. Be sure to clear above each other's heads, which is especially important if you like to enjoy oral sex. The distance you clear should be far enough to extend past the field of your legs to the end of your aura past your feet in any position your bodies may assume.

As long as you are not beginning from a point of nervous exhaustion, this energetic body foreplay can be as sexually exciting as any other form of sex play. If the sexual charge in the room is strong, you may even induce sexual undulations and strong contractions, giving a foretaste of a highly-charged lovemaking session. ●

SEX DRIVE AND LIBIDO

Sexual appetites are far from static in any one person. For short or extended periods of time, we may find ourselves feeling:

- Highly wild and sexual
- More neutral or sexually ambivalent
- Uninterested and yet compliant, when we are willing to engage even though we really don't want to.
- Not interested even in the slightest.

Not everyone has a high sexual drive and, in fact, a surprising number of people find it very difficult to get turned on. The degree of arousal can vary, depending on any number of factors, including compatibility and which yin-yang qualities are predominating in each of the energy fields of each partner at any point in time.

When dealing with arousal difficulties or a reluctant or low-libido partner, Taoists frame it as an opportunity. They use the old expression, "Let's get the teapot water boiling!" Most people begin foreplay by kissing, hugging, nuzzling and groping each other. This is sufficient if both are in a sexual, raucous mood and easily turned on. For a lover in a neutral, ambivalent or outright uninterested state, a more sensitive, attentive approach is needed to get him or her aroused.

First, understand what mental or emotional space your partner is in so you can adapt Taoist hands-on sexual techniques accordingly. Spend time talking and checking in with your partner. Listen attentively and reflect back what they say. Listen, too, for what is not being said. Getting in synch emotionally and mentally is part of foreplay, even if you are not yet making physical contact.

Many Taoist sexual qigong practices can help get your partner aroused and in the mood, even more than ordinary sex techniques. For example, a man who focuses on learning to get the sexual energy moving in a woman can really turn her on. A man can stimulate the etheric qi in the lower part of her body below her pelvis until her qi powerfully exits her feet (Figure 11-3). When working with the qi in a woman it is always best to initially move her qi downward toward her feet in the lower yin part of the body.

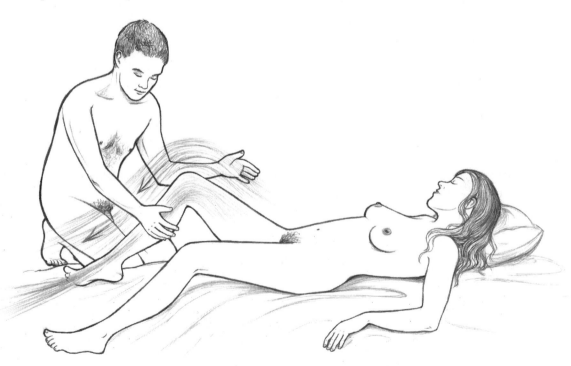

Figure 11-3: Moving Yin Sexual Energy to Arouse a Woman

YANG FIRE OF THE EYES

The eyes have it, as regards a man's attraction to a woman. His visual cortex is directly linked to his genital region. A minor visual cue, such as a certain curve to a woman's waist or the roundness of her hips, can trigger a sexual response. In this respect, he's a bit like one of Pavlov's dogs,[2] because his sexual response is biologically automatically conditioned to a stimulus (a feminine curve) that doesn't always signal "time for sex!" His animal nature is hard-wired. Rather than try to change it, women can learn to leverage it. Taoist women would use the direct connection between a man's eyes and his sexuality to activate his emotions, because they understood that his subtle anatomy includes a direct channel linking the heart center and the eyes.

If a woman wants to activate the emotional side of a man's sexual response as opposed to the physical side, she should activate his heart center fully and then raise that heart energy right up to his eyeballs. There is a direct channel of energy that links the heart center to the eyes and upper tantien. If a woman can help a man activate this channel and thereby reduce his "yang fire of the eyes," she can significantly increase his emotional response during and after lovemaking.

Suppose foreplay does not culminate in intercourse and the man falls asleep. If the woman has activated the channel from his heart to his eyes, he will be more predisposed to sharing emotional yin energy when he wakes up. This may or may not cause a man to bond with a woman emotionally, but for many women this can enhance the emotional experience. Taoist men used a similar approach to increase a woman's receptivity to sex; if he activated her lower body, she would more easily become sexual upon awakening, sometimes assertively initiating sex.

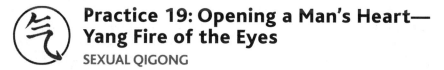

Practice 19: Opening a Man's Heart— Yang Fire of the Eyes
SEXUAL QIGONG

The purpose of this practice is for a woman to link a man's heart center to his eyes. First, activate his heart energy with a light use of the fingers or fingernails on the skin near the region of the heart or, even more effectively, move and trace the energy above his skin in the etheric body. This is similar to how you would move energy in your own etheric body when doing any of the movements of Dragon and Tiger Qigong.[3]

2. Pavlov, I. P., *Conditioned Reflexes: An Investigation of the Physiological Activity of the Cerebral Cortex,* trans. and ed. G. V. Anrep (London: Oxford University Press, 1927).

3. Frantzis, Bruce, *Dragon and Tiger Medical Qigong: Health and Energy in Seven Simple Movements* (Berkeley, CA: North Atlantic Books, 2010).

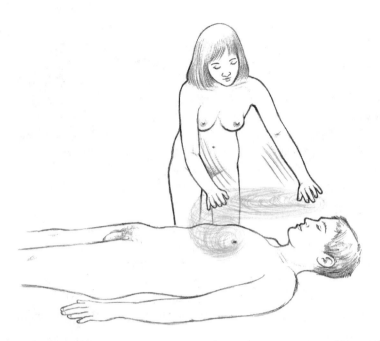

She stimulates his etheric body to move energy from his heart to his eyes.

Figure 11-4: Activating a Man's Heart Energy

You may feel two kinds of flutters in a man's heart. One will have a spasm-like quality of holding something in. Keep playing with the flutter until it softens up and releases. This is where learning finger and hand sensitivity really pays off (see Chapter 7, Practice 7, "Cultivating Finger Sensitivity with Tofu").

The second type of flutter will feel as if something wants to flow and move upward but is on the edge and it just can't move yet. For this type of flutter you just add a bit of encouragement and keep moving it along till the energy goes to his eyes. How? Be creative in every way you can. You might, for example, focus on either his physical or etheric body with your mind and intention; you might creatively use sound or other body parts—eyes, hands, tongue, breasts—to encourage this link to occur. At or above his skin, you move energy through his etheric body to make the link, or dissolve any blockages in the channel between the heart center and the eyes until the energy in it flows smoothly.

Be aware that your lover may resist having his energy moved from his heart to his eyes and may find a way to stop you. He might suddenly change positions, start talking or otherwise shift the dynamic without even realizing why. Any significant change to the way he knows himself as a sexual being can trigger a response. This isn't about you; it's a natural homeostatic mechanism within the human mind-body. ●

OUTER DISSOLVING MEDITATION METHOD

Taoist Water method practices define challenges, diseases and illnesses that reside in any of your eight energy bodies as blockages. Dissolving methods begin when you consciously use your awareness to focus your mind on any specific condensed energy shape or pattern within yourself or, in the context of sexual practices, within your partner. The objective of dissolving is to release and resolve any energy that has congealed, metaphorically, into a specific shape. You want to make such energy release its shape so it becomes neutral and without boundaries, so that it no longer obstructs your mind, body or Spirit in any way.

The dissolving meditation methods of the Water tradition are a practical way to release blockages in the whole mind-body complex, so you can fully transform and ultimately experience conscious harmony with the Tao right down to your bone marrow. Then you naturally act according to principles expressed in the *Tao Te Ching*.

The Taoists have developed two distinct approaches for using the mind or awareness to release blocked energies in the body—Outer Dissolving and Inner Dissolving. Sexual qigong primarily utilizes Outer Dissolving, while sexual meditation uses Inner Dissolving, which will be explained in Chapter 15. Sexual qigong prepares you for the Inner Dissolving methods of sexual meditation. How Inner and Outer Dissolving methods merge during Taoist meditation is described in Chapter 18.

Both dissolving practices have a fundamental principle that whatever you do must ultimately feel comfortable. You learn to exert full effort without strained force, which almost sounds like a contradiction in terms. Doing so means refining and relaxing the tendency of the mind to strain for a goal. To employ all your effort and yet not use force or contravene the actual limits of the body, mind and Spirit is the gentle way of Laozi's Water tradition.

> *To employ all your effort yet not use force*
> *is the gentle way of Laozi's Water tradition.*

ICE TO WATER, WATER TO GAS

For millennia, the Taoists have used the phrase "ice to water, water to gas" to describe the Outer Dissolving process. "Ice" refers to blocked or congealed energy. "Water" refers to the acceptance and relaxation of your internal blockages until they no longer cause tension. And "gas" refers to the *complete release* of all the original bound energy moving *away* from your physical body. If not completely released, the energy may revert to ice. Outer Dissolving is a core practice of sexual qigong.

The primary concerns of qigong—physical health, healing and strength—are best served by Outer Dissolving, which is applied to blockages in the first and second (physical and qi) energy bodies. Outer Dissolving, by reducing stress and clearing the energies of the body will also have secondary beneficial effects on emotional disposition (the third energy body) and mental performance (the fourth energy body). Trapped energy is released externally, away from the body, into the space outside the body to finish and be fully resolved only once it reaches the boundary of the etheric body or aura.

An important note of caution: while dissolving can be done from top to bottom (downward), from bottom to top (upward), or in any number of other directions, you must initially learn to allow energy to flow downward first. This is a necessary safety precaution that prepares you to handle upward and other directional flows in a way that avoids the potential of possibly causing harm to your central nervous system.

Outer Dissolving methods release qi blockages in the physical body and help restore its optimal functioning. The techniques can clear the energetic blockages that repress the physical body's ability to fully relax during sex. When the body releases stress and relaxes, this enables the emergence of maximum pleasure, bliss and joy.

The physical bliss that results from using Outer Dissolving in sexual qigong can be extremely mood-elevating, making sex better for both partners, and can create an ongoing afterglow that improves day-to-day life outside the bedroom. Moreover, these elevating effects of sex-derived bliss can act as an antidote to the stress that builds up from the trials and tribulations of life and can, at times, mitigate such stress for several days.

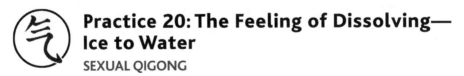

Practice 20: The Feeling of Dissolving— Ice to Water
SEXUAL QIGONG

CAUTION ADVISED: If you have heart disease or very high blood pressure, you are advised not to do this exercise as it may cause your body too much strain.

This practice describes a simple way to understand and feel the beginning of the Outer Dissolving process. First, clench your fist as tightly as you can, causing your energy to contract, until your knuckles turn white. Then feel your hand; feel yourself seeping into the bound energy inside it and expand your contracted energy. Do so until without opening it you completely relax your fist (ice to water).

The best way to do this is the yin way of concretely feeling it, rather than the yang way of only imagining it in your mind. Then continue to focus your awareness on your closed fist until it feels empty of all solidity, with a completely amorphous quality indicating that your energy has expanded out of your hand into the air (water to gas). This is one example of what a blockage might feel like in your body. Again, this dissolving technique must be accomplished in a yin way by feeling it, not merely picturing it as visualization in your mind's eye. Although visualization is the yang way a Taoist Fire school might do a practice, this is not the case for the Water tradition.

Next, with your hand remaining in a fist, again put your intention on it. Let your mind focus on your fist, and then let it relax until all the feeling and blood comes back. This process can take a while. The more you hold on, the less you can let go and the longer it will take. The more you let go, the faster your hand will relax and regenerate.

Keep your hand in a fist. It's easier to relax your hand when you open it up, but the sheer act of making a fist is hardwired into people to cause tension. It is that kind of deep tension you are trying to release in this exercise. When people get really angry they don't open their hands, they close them. If you were to try holding a fist for half an hour, you would see how exhausting it would become. It takes a lot of energy and stamina to maintain control and tension, yet people do it all the time.

Now open your hand very slowly. See if you can let go of control and just let it open of its own accord. Don't try to control the movement of your hand—just let all the crinkles release on their own. As you let your fist release and the blood slowly comes back, your hand will open up. It may open up very slowly, but even so, let it happen of its own natural accord. Let go of your need to control. If you can do this consciously, in time you'll find you can let go of the things you didn't even know you were holding on to, and you'll notice that you are more relaxed. ●

THREE STAGES OF DISSOLVING IN SEX

- In the first stage of dissolving, you learn to use the super-charged energy that is naturally generated during sex to access and release all your personal energy blockages. As you practice, you will get better and better at finding and then dissolving your personal blockages. You learn to feel different types of blockages.

- In stage two, in addition to dissolving your own blocks, you now learn to go into your partner's body to seep into and dissolve whatever blockages you find. This takes a much higher level of sensitivity.

- In stage three, both partners learn to link their own energy and Spirit with that of their partner. Once linked, it is possible to consciously move into the partner's Mindstream, the deep subtle stream that underlies a person's awareness, usually hidden unless explicitly sought. At each stage of practice, all personal blocked energies encountered can be released and resolved in this way. Initially these three stages are done with Outer Dissolving and later by using Inner Dissolving, a deeper, more advanced practice.

SCANNING AND DISSOLVING BLOCKAGES

As you start the Outer Dissolving process in sexual qigong, to locate a blockage you initially learn to scan your physical body to feel and find one or more of four internal conditions present in your body. Different people may feel and experience these conditions in a variety of ways. In particular, a man's perception of these conditions will tend to be very different to that of a woman. Later you use the same Outer Dissolving process to locate blockages not just in the physical body but in all of the first four energy bodies.

THE FOUR INTERNAL CONDITIONS

As you practice sexual qigong and later sexual meditation, you will find various energy blockages. All energy blockages can be experienced in one of four ways:

1. Strength
2. Tension
3. Something that doesn't feel quite right, even if you don't know what it is
4. Any kind of contraction

1. Strength

Everybody wants to be strong in a variety of feminine (yin) and masculine (yang) ways. Nobody would really like to be weak, impotent and useless in the world. So in the West there is a lot of emphasis on developing strength. In meditation, however, strength has a completely different meaning.

Taoists don't typically use the word "ego," but there's a kind of a strength that produces every kind of yin and yang ego. It's the voice that says, "This is what I will do: I will make the world be the way I want it to be, quietly or loudly, no matter what obstacles must be overcome." This creates a lot of pressure and stress.

Strength can be stubbornness, which leaves you with the inability to change. When you are too stubborn, you feel strong. Psychological strength has many faces that can look anywhere from soft yin internal collapsing to fierce yang hyper-pushing. Strength can also be connected to anger. Who doesn't feel strong when they get angry? Likewise, when people get incredibly fixated on thoughts and ideas, on what they believe and think is true, they are acting from strength. Everything then becomes rigid rather than flexible.

The Taoists say that when you really have it, you don't notice it. What this means is that, generally, when everything is working well, you aren't aware of it and it does not bring you a feeling of strength. You just feel at ease and natural. When your energy is flowing smoothly, you don't feel strong; instead you simply feel comfortable and naturally have what you need to get the job done.

When you feel strength, it's usually because you are relentlessly pushing and straining. Eventually you snap or you get sick. Take the classic yang type-A, driven personality who is highly successful, but suddenly drops dead from a heart attack caused by overwork, or someone who strongly and stubbornly holds onto his or her extreme yin sadness and despair. Do you have high blood pressure? If you train yourself to become more sensitive, you can feel when your blood is forcing its way through your system.

You want to able to recognize when you're feeling a blockage of strength. Where are you trying too hard in your life? Where are you forcing your body or mind too much? In what life circumstances are you finding yourself continuously frustrated, angry or overwhelmed?

2. Tension

The second of the four conditions indicating blocked energy is tension. Tension always involves a fight. Something is pulling and seeking dominance over against something else. It could be something as small as the question of how you are going to make a deadline or how you are going to accomplish the task in the amount of time you have to do it.

Being angry or depressed are examples of emotional tension. Someone or something is breaking through a boundary, and you want to it to remain intact. Those two things are pulling in opposite directions. Depression is a type of inward or yin emotional tension; being angry is a more yang emotional tension, but depression is just as powerful as anger.

Can you recognize if you have any tension inside you from other emotions, like greed or grief? What causes tension and pulls you in opposite directions in your life? You are here, but you want to be there. You don't know if you should be with this person or that person. You are ready, but an opportunity hasn't presented itself. Don't overlook these fights that might be occurring inside your body. Maybe your tissues are constantly tense—knots pull your muscles in opposite directions, while nerves twitch.

3. When Something Doesn't Feel Quite Right

The third of the four conditions is tricky. Our inner worlds are filled with an amazing amount of congestion. Most people are not even aware of what's there. As infants, we have many experiences before we understand and can use language. When we were in our mother's womb, we picked up everything that happened to her. If she was yelled at, if she was beaten, if she underwent stress, if she drank, if people around her were putting out incredibly negative vibes that she was soaking up—any of these situations disturbed us. Conversely, if she was incredibly happy, content and peaceful, we picked that up too.

There are trillions of connections between neurons in the brain. Experiences get wired with a cornucopia of input. All you know is that something doesn't feel right. It is one thing to know what bothers you, but quite another when you haven't got the faintest clue. You may never get to the bottom of it, but something that doesn't feel quite right will become a nagging part of your real, ongoing experience. When people can't figure out what is unconsciously bothering them, they get frustrated or feel helpless, which may lead to lashing out, running away or getting depressed.

So you must be present to these feelings even if you can't seem to identify where they are coming from. These feelings account for the malaise and confusion in the world. Some people appear to have everything anyone could ever want, yet life just doesn't seem to flow for them.

You have to be present to what you are feeling. When you become present, you can apply your intent to get rid of what holds you back using the dissolving process.

4. Contraction

The fourth condition is contraction. The primary difference between someone who is very awake and someone who is sleepwalking through life is that someone who is awake is not contracted. Someone who is closed down or contracted is half asleep. What people call "ego," "stress" and the "fear of living" are examples of contraction. Likewise, blood vessels closing down and organs malfunctioning are also examples of contractions. Rather than being open and operating fluidly, certain parts of the body start to contract and eventually shut down.

The Taoists call contraction the "hallmark of death." A thousand diseases can be described as nothing more than something in the body closing down. For example, a heart attack results from the interruption of blood supply in a main artery when it becomes clogged to the point of shutting down. You use the dissolving process to find contractions and then gently relax them.

All energy blockages will make you feel one of four conditions—
strength, tension, some kind of discomfort or contraction. A thousand
diseases are contractions—something in the body closing down.

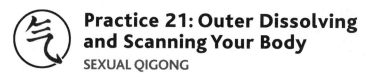

Practice 21: Outer Dissolving and Scanning Your Body
SEXUAL QIGONG

This practice takes you through the Outer Dissolving transformation of ice to water to gas. It is easiest to do this practice either sitting or by standing. Start by using your mind to scan your body downward from head to toe until you locate a place in your body where your energy is blocked or frozen, identified by one of the four conditions of strength, tension, undefined discomfort or contraction. As your awareness becomes more sensitive, you can begin to feel or experience the outer contours of any blocked or frozen energy space that your mind contacts.

Next, your awareness begins to feel and enter into the obvious solid mass, causing the frozen energy to begin to soften, until you reach the center of the blockage. This is the transformation of ice to water. In the same way, if you put an ice cube in a pan and heat it on the stove, you will observe as you should feel in your own body, that the outside of the ice cube melts first, with the melting progressing slowly toward the center of the cube. Upon encountering a blockage, you should always stay alert for the slightly more subtle energy that exists inside and behind the energy that is felt clearly—that is, a layer which is deeper or beyond whatever you are currently dissolving.

As the frozen energy in your body becomes and feels soft or flowing (like the water in the pan), you keep your attention on that place and your awareness continues to cause that energy space to expand until there is a sense of the trapped energy expanding out beyond your skin—perhaps as much as a foot or two outside the surface of your skin to the boundary of your etheric body (also known as the aura). This is the transformation of water to gas.

Like the water in the pan, which will not turn to gas (steam) until the ice cube is entirely melted, the dissolving of an energy block also moves in stages. It is best to practice dissolving while sitting, standing and or lying down and to become familiar with the process in a generic context before dissolving in a sexual context.

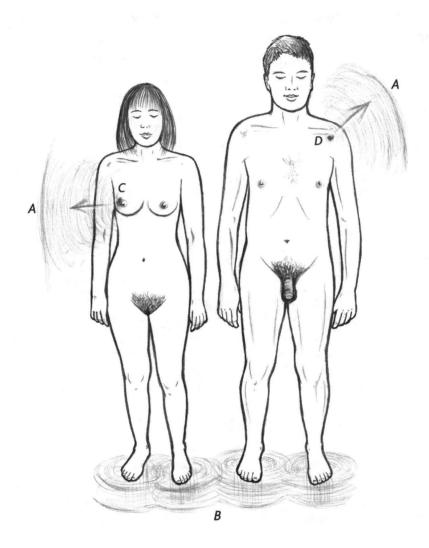

A—Boundary of the etheric body to the sides
B—Boundary of the etheric body below the feet
C—Blockage in the breast
D—Blockage in the shoulder

She dissolves and releases a blocked energy point in her breast.
He does the same with a blockage in his shoulder.

Figure 11-5: Scanning and Outer Dissolving Standing Practice

For example, a woman can use Outer Dissolving to dissolve a blockage in her breast, as shown in Figure 11-5. When going from water to gas, the blocked energy goes outward from her skin to release in the corresponding place at the boundary of her etheric body where it resolves. This can also develop her ability to experience more yin sexual pleasure from her breasts.

Likewise, as also shown in Figure 11-5, a man can dissolve a blockage in his shoulder[4] to release in the corresponding place in his etheric body. This can improve his health and make his arms more sensitive to yang sexual energy and pleasure. ●

RESOLVING AND DEALING WITH REPRESSION

The Taoist meditation method of Outer Dissolving can release and resolve the energies that bind sexual repressions inside you. You can then be free of these repressed energies rather than merely wishing you could be.

Repression is usually thought of as bottled-up negative emotions. This is especially so as regards trauma, the roots of various emotional and mental dysfunction, repressed memories and post-traumatic stress disorders, and of course sexual repression. When yang energy is repressed, as the old saying goes, "repression leads to violence." When yin energy is repressed, then this often makes a person feel collapsed, diminished, depressed and just plain miserable.

What is not often talked about is that when people repress the negative they very often equally repress the positive. Qualities such as pleasure, peace, happiness and joy also get repressed and locked away inside. The repression of the positive emotions doesn't get as much press, but it is equally draining. Many people are subject to this pervasive form of positive repression, and it prevents them from being blissful as a natural state of being. When observing infants, you can see the natural bliss state in action. At times infants will playfully gurgle, becoming incredibly happy and blissful with virtually no provocation except the naturalness of their Being.

The feeling of natural bliss is quite unlike the usual happiness we feel in response to some external cause; it is a natural wellspring that—in an ideal world—would be easily accessible, rather than as a rarely experienced exceptional state. It's a sad state of affairs when natural qualities get repressed during sex, which is supposed to be a sanctioned time for pleasure and ecstasy.

The process of releasing repression begins with Outer Dissolving. However, later it is Inner Dissolving that gives you a method to clear the most powerfully repressed negative emotions and to free positive emotions in your inner world in both yin and yang energetic ways.

---

4. For more details on the location and functions of the shoulder and breast energy gates, see Frantzis, Bruce, *Opening the Energy Gates of Your Body: Qigong for Lifelong Health,* rev. ed. (Berkeley, CA: North Atlantic Books, 2006), pp.133–34 and 136–37.

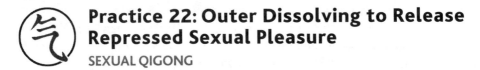

Practice 22: Outer Dissolving to Release Repressed Sexual Pleasure
SEXUAL QIGONG

Outer Dissolving can be used to enhance your ability to give and receive pleasure. To do so, first locate a spot where you are blocked—where your sense of receiving or giving pleasure with your partner can go only so far and no further. Some find it is easier to give than receive. Others can receive but tend to withhold rather than give, while some just need a bit more in both directions. Blockages can be located in many places, many of them quite counterintuitive.

People are different and experiences will shift over time. Maybe for you it always seems to be located in a specific spot or spots in your physical body, which may stay constant or constantly shift. Or it might be that the pleasure blockage is attached to some emotion or background thought, or just a general nonspecific feeling. Maybe there are several ways it shows itself, moving from location to location.

Recognize what this blocked energy feels like, regardless of whether it is a discrete location or just a large, vague and amorphous feeling of something blocked. Next, as you continue to make love, use the Outer Dissolving process of "ice to water and water to gas" to release the blockage and physical barrier to your feeling more pleasure, joy and bliss. Later on, you can apply the methods of Inner Dissolving, as described in Chapter 15, to go beyond the physical obstacles and release the deeper blocked emotional, mental, psychic, karmic and essence barriers to gain an even greater sense of spiritual sexual pleasure and bliss. ●

THE SMALL HEAVENLY OR MICROCOSMIC ORBIT

As your practice of sexual qigong deepens, you are going to start working directly with the flows of energy in the body along specific pathways or orbits. Taoists view the human body as a microcosm of the entire universe or what the Chinese also call "heaven," in contrast to planet earth. According to Taoism, there are two ways that this microcosm of the universe manifests in the human body. One of these manifestations is called the Small Heavenly Orbit, also known as the Microcosmic Orbit, which is only within the body's torso and head. Second is the Large or Great Heavenly Orbit also called the Macrocosmic Orbit, which includes the arms and legs. Both are primary energy circuits in the body. The Microcosmic movement inside a human being has many functions.

The standard pathways of these orbits work through two of the extraordinary meridians in acupuncture—the governing and the conception vessels. These go upward from the perineum, along the spine to the top (crown) of your head and

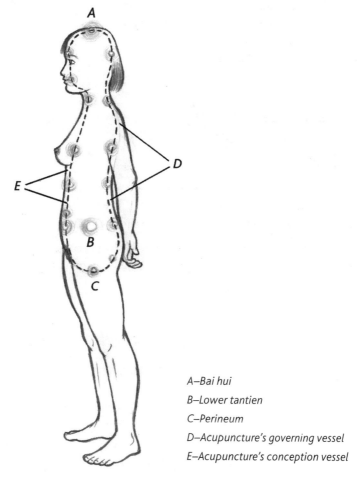

A—Bai hui

B—Lower tantien

C—Perineum

D—Acupuncture's governing vessel

E—Acupuncture's conception vessel

Figure 11-6: Microcosmic or Small Heavenly Orbit of Energy

downward from the top of your head along the centerline of the front of your body back to your perineum again.

In acupuncture, each different point along the governing or the conception vessel directly attaches to a whole series of acupuncture points inside your body. So theoretically, if all the acupuncture points along your governing and conception vessels—the Microcosmic Orbit—were one hundred percent fine, then the energy in your body should work reasonably well.

The Taoist Fire or yang tradition strongly focuses on the Microcosmic Orbit right from the very beginning in all its qi practices, not just sexual ones. Within the

Taoist Water tradition, the Microcosmic Orbit is not prominent initially as regards ordinary sex, sexual qigong and sexual meditation. This is due to the Water method's initial emphasis on Inner and Outer Dissolving meditation practices. It only begins using the Microcosmic Orbit extensively in advanced sexual meditation practices as described in Chapters 17 and 18.

Practice 23: Transfer Sexual Energy around Your Body

SEXUAL QIGONG

This preparatory solo sexual qigong exercise replicates energy movements you can use when engaged in intercourse. Figure 11-7 shows how this exercise would be practiced by a woman, Figure 11-9 depicts a man doing the practice.

Place your hands lightly on your genitals. Women need not physically penetrate the vagina (or can do so very lightly), but should use just enough pressure to feel the energy of the hand going into the vagina.

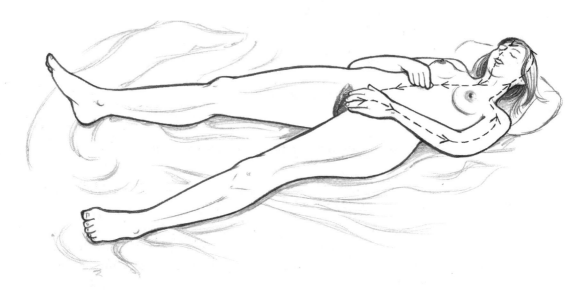

She moves energy from her vagina up her arm to the top of her head and down the front of her body back to the vagina. She may also bring energy down her body back to her hand using either the Microcosmic Orbit or the central channel.

Figure 11-7: Woman Transfers Energy from Vagina around Her Body

Using your mind, take the energy from your hand and do this exercise in three progressive stages.

1. With your mind, dissolve any blockages in your hand in a yin, soft way, until it feels smoothly energized and relaxed.

2. Without force, start opening and closing your inguinal region, or kwa, as you pull and push the sexual energy in and out of your hand (Figures 11-7, 11-8 A–B and 11-9). When transferring energy around your body you may choose to use one of two pathways:

   • Either the Small Heavenly or Microcosmic Orbit (Figure 11-6) up the spine and down the front centerline of the body

   • Or up and down the central channel. See Chapter 3, Figures 3-2 and 3-3 for more information on the location of the energy channels and the kwas.

   Pull your dissolved energy from your hands into your genitals in one of two ways: either into and up your spine (that is, from your genitals to your perineum, to your tailbone, and up your spine), or from your genitals to your perineum, up your central channel, and into your lower tantien.

3. Push the qi from your spine or lower tantien to your genitals and from your genitals pull the energy back into your hand.

4. Move your dissolved energy rhythmically back and forth between your genitals and your spine or lower tantien until it flows smoothly, with minimal effort.

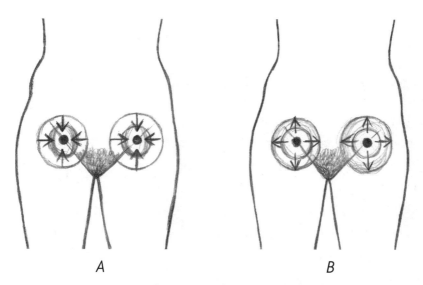

A   B

A) Kwa closes. B) Kwa opens.

Figure 11-8 A–B: Opening and Closing the Kwa

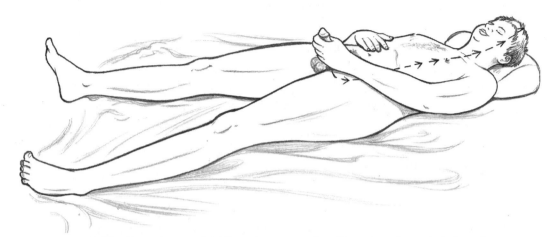

Holding his penis, a man initially projects energy from his penis up the central channel (inside the center of the body) to the crown of his head until the flow becomes stable. He may bring energy down his body back to his hand either using the Microcosmic Orbit or the central channel.

Figure 11-9: Man Transfers Energy around His Body

5. Use the tip of the penis or opening of the vagina (not shown) to push the energy

    •   Either from your hand into your genitals and up the central channel to the tantien and crown of the head

    •   Or from the perineum and tailbone through the mingmen point (see Chapter 9, Figure 9-7) on the spine, and up the spine to the crown of the head.

6. Then continue to pull energy down

    •   Either using the Microcosmic Orbit down the conception vessel on your body's front centerline, down in front of your lower tantien, and return it back to your genitals and into your hand

    •   Or, for a more advanced practitioner, down along your central channel.

7. Push your lower tantien's qi out from your genitals into your hands, and project that energy up your arm. Move it from the wrist to the elbow, to the shoulder, and up to:

    •   Either the spine and neck, to the top of your head

    •   Or through the armpit to the central channel to the crown of the head.

8. Then down from the crown of the head

    •   Either from the central channel to your perineum, continuing up to your genitals, where you complete the circuit in your hand

- Or to the perineum via one of two routes: a) the front (anterior) part of the spine to the tailbone and up to the genitals or b) down the Microcosmic Orbit's conception vessel on the front of the body's centerline and continuing up from your perineum to your genitals, where you complete the circuit in your hand.

It is very important that you move your energy gently, without force. If you force your energy or your mind during sex, your nerves can become exhausted sooner rather than later. When sex becomes a forced exercise, it becomes more of a power trip—very different from something sensual, erotic or meditative. ●

Sexual Qigong Is Not Inherently Spiritual

Although sexual qigong can be extremely powerful, it is not in and of itself spiritual; neither is the sole act of being able to deliberately direct and move qi inside your own body or that of another.

The qi you acquire from sexual qigong can definitely make you feel more alive and vibrant, with more "oomph" to get things done. However, by itself, running or consciously directing energy is not inherently spiritual unless and until combined with spiritual awareness. Qi, like fire, is a neutral force. Just as fire can cook food, it equally has the potential to burn human flesh.

Many stories within Buddhism, Hinduism and Taoism make the point that "demons" can move energy inside themselves just as well as "saints" or "angels." The difference rests in their motivations and actions rather than the energetic capacities themselves.

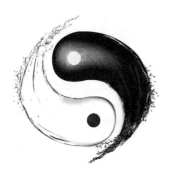

CHAPTER 12

Energy Foreplay and Sex

Any activity, physical or energetic, that sparks your lover's interest before intercourse or generates sexual arousal falls under the umbrella of foreplay. With ordinary sex, foreplay usually involves a wide array of external enticements to get the sexual juices going, including dancing, a light brush of your lips to the deepest French kiss, oral play to finger play to fantasy role-playing. Lovers do whatever it takes to create desire and arousal in their partner.

Energy foreplay, rather than focusing on physical touch and sensation, revolves around moving energy within you and your partner. It also focuses on using Outer Dissolving practices to free blockages and open up your energy fields, which gets the qi circulating and moving.

The previous chapter presented the initial ways to move energy externally and introduced the basic method of Outer Dissolving. This chapter builds on that knowledge to show different ways to work with energy, such as targeting specific yin and yang surfaces of the body, and explains how to direct energy to different erogenous zones.

As you move past foreplay to intercourse, you learn sexual qigong methods that can extend lovemaking and expand your ability to experience different types of orgasms. You also learn the art of moving energy for specific purposes and how use the energy generated in sex to clear deeper energetic blocks.

YIN AND YANG IN SEXUAL QIGONG

Understanding how yin and yang energies operate within human beings, both sexually and in other respects, is important for students of Taoist energy arts. Yin and yang qi circulates in several ways inside the body, including the following flows:

1. The body has yin and yang acupuncture meridian surfaces. Energy moves along these surfaces in specific directions (see Figure 12-1 A–B).

2. The lower part of the body below the lower tantien is yin, going from the pelvis to the bottom of the feet. It is from this area that the natural sexual energy of a woman is derived. Above the pelvis and lower tantien, going to the fingertips and up to the head is yang. It is from the upper part of the body that the natural sexual energy of a man is derived, rather than originating in his genitals.

3. Yang energy moves up the body, and yin energy drops down the body.

The Taoists recognized that massive polarization could occur as the forces of yin and yang mixed within a couple and during sex. Within sexual qigong, they developed various balancing practices to bring awareness to and use these energies while making love. One notable example of this is that Taoists found that circulating qi along the yin and yang acupuncture meridian surfaces and energy lines could dramatically increase the flow of energy during sex.

YIN AND YANG SURFACES AND ACUPUNCTURE MERIDIANS

If you want to hyper-charge the energy in either a man or woman's body, one of the exceptional ways of doing this is by moving energy through the yang and yin meridian surfaces. By energizing the yang and yin surfaces you also energize and balance all the yin and yang meridians that are contained within them. The yin meridian surfaces are on the front of the body and along the soft interior sides of the limbs. The yang meridian surfaces are on the back of the body and along the outer sides of the limbs.

Whether you're stroking his or her legs or arms, your touch will tend to have a greater effect if you stroke in the direction of the yang and yin meridians as indicated by the illustration. Stroke your partner down the outside of his or her legs or arms, up the inside of the legs or arms, up the back and down the front. The effect can still be quite considerable even if you go in the opposite direction.

Where you start makes a big difference: a man begins on the lower part of a woman's body, and a woman begins on the upper part of a man's body.

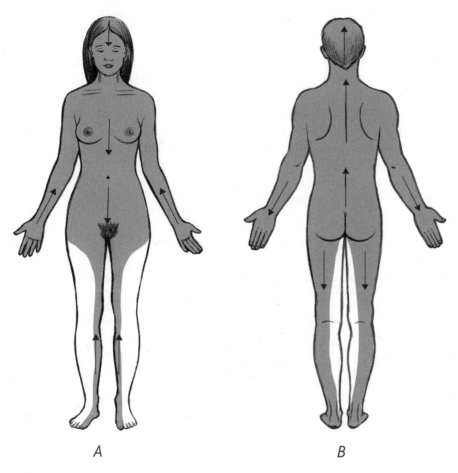

A) Shaded area shows yin meridian surfaces. B) Shaded area shows yang meridian surfaces.

Figure 12-1 A–B: Yin and Yang Surfaces of the Body

As a general rule, a woman wants to initially work on the man's torso, neck, head and arms. It is best to start sexual play moving upward from the base of the spine with the yang (posterior/back) surfaces of a man's lower and upper back, neck and head first, and then continue on to his arms. Rub, stroke or gently caress the back of his neck and head. Then work down the outside of his arms to his fingertips and massage his back before moving toward his buttocks and the outside of his legs. Next, turn him over and work on the yin (anterior/front) of his body, from the face to the pelvis and including the yin inside surfaces of his arms and hands.

Next, turn him over and work on the yin (anterior/front) of his body, from the face to the pelvis and including the yin inside surfaces of his arms and hands.

Conversely, a man works on the yin (anterior/front) side of the woman's body first. Begin at her feet. Spend plenty of time here, because the feet are energetically alive and sensitive in a woman, and the degree of arousal may surprise you. Then work up the inside of her legs to her pubic region, then on to her belly and breasts, and up the front of her throat, face and up from the inside of her fingers and arms. Then turn her over and work on the yang parts of her body, starting from the outside of her feet and working your way up to her head as previously done with a man.

Be creative and attentive in how you touch your partner. Energy flows within the subcutaneous tissue, just below the surface of the skin. Use your fingertips or nails to lightly stimulate and excite your partner's skin and the area just below it. Vary the pressure and speed of your strokes, always listening, feeling and watching for your lover's response. Most often, the yin surfaces require a lighter touch, whereas the yang surfaces may require a firmer touch.

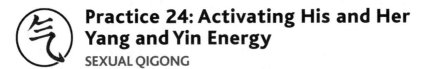

Practice 24: Activating His and Her Yang and Yin Energy
SEXUAL QIGONG

There is a major difference between clearing energy (see Chapter 11, Practice 18), which is primarily an external phenomena, and hyper-charging energy within the body. You initially do clearing so your or your partner's sexual libido is not diminished. In Practice 24 the focus is on moving qi to get the yin energy of a woman and the yang energy of a man fully online. Hyper-charging the movement of qi in the body creates more energy for the sex act itself and also can dramatically increase your pleasure.

Part 1: Activating His Yang Energy: Her for Him

Use the following to pattern your man's energy so he can maintain an erection longer without the usual strain that results in loss of feeling. It also helps him stay connected and sensitive to your energy.

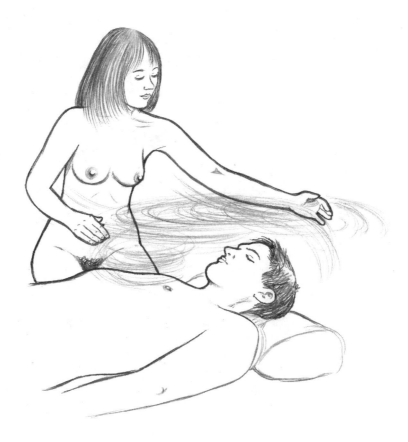

To help him maintain an erection and increase his emotional sensitivity,
she boosts his yang energy by clearing his blockages from his lower tantien
(not shown), through to the heart center and then above his head.

Figure 12-2: Clearing His Energy from Heart to Head through the Etheric Body

1. Begin with the man lying on his back. With your hands slightly above or gently touching his body, move the energy up from his lower tantien to his heart area, clearing any blockages you find along the way. When blockages are cleared, it frees his qi to naturally begin moving upward. After you feel his heart area open, continue to clear the energy to the top of his head. Then continue and move the energy above his head to the end of his qi or etheric body (Figure 12-2).

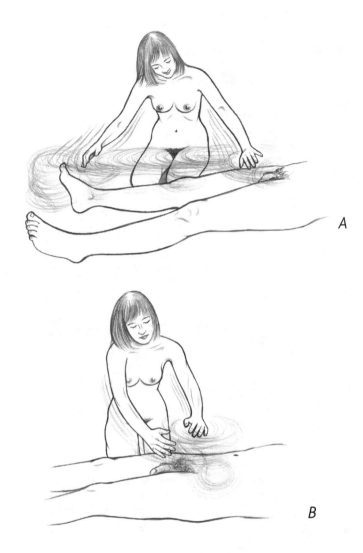

A) From lower body to genitals. B) From genitals to lower tantien.

Figure 12-3 A–B: Clearing Blocked Energy from the Feet to Tantien

2. Next move to his lower body. Begin below his feet to clear and raise the energy upward
    to his genitals (Figure 12-3 A). When the energy in his genitals begins to come alive,
    clear and move the qi from the genitals to the prostate (located in a man's lower pelvis
    under the bladder) and then to the lower tantien until it stabilizes there and activates
    his yang energy (Figure 12-3 B). Next move the energy up to his navel and then to his
    heart center. Once it stabilizes there, continue moving his yang energy upward to his
    crown and finally to above his head (Figure 12-2).

Part 2: Activating Her Downward Yin and Upward Yang Energy: Him for Her

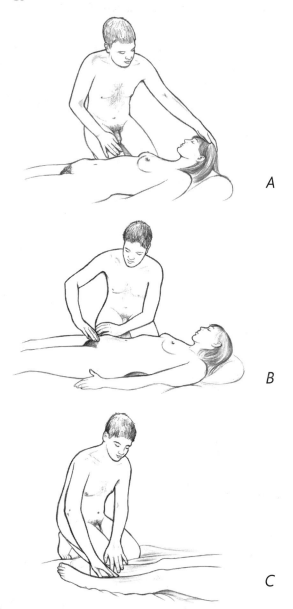

A

B

C

He clears her energy downward from her head to energize her hips, legs and feet where the yin sexual energy is most powerful.

Figure 12-4 A–C: Activating Her Downward Yin Energy

When the yin qi of a woman condenses in the lower, yin part of her body, especially in the feet and yin meridians on the inner ankles, calves and thighs, it becomes easier for a woman to achieve either outer or inner orgasms. Follow this procedure to sexually activate and awaken her yin qi.

1. Have her lie on her back with the yin part of her body facing you. Begin by clearing from the end of her qi body above her head to below her feet (Figure 12-4 A–C). You can do this with your hand above her skin to stimulate the qi of her etheric body, or alternately by moving your nails or fingertips along her skin. Once you feel her begin to stir, gradually move up from her feet to her ankles.

2. Once the energy in her feet has relaxed and cleared, progress upward to the calves, knees, thighs and perineum before moving to her vagina (Figure 12-5 A–D).

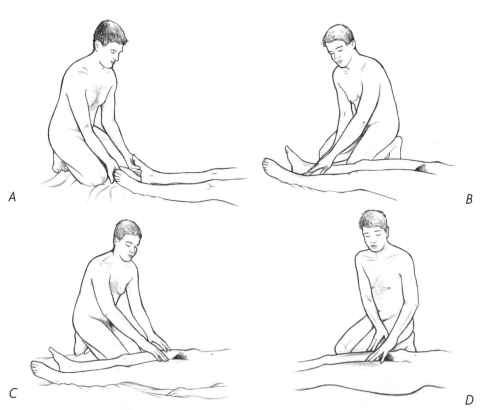

A

B

C

D

He activates the yin energy of her legs by moving her qi from her feet to her vagina.
He either may do so with his fingertips, or by stimulating her etheric body.

Figure 12-5 A–D: Activating the Yin Energy of Her Legs

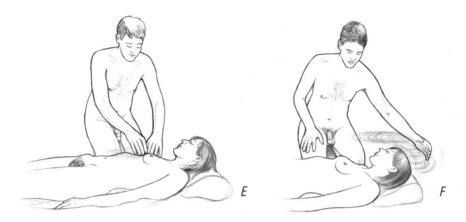

To activate her yang energy, he moves her qi from her lower tantien to her head or beyond.

Figure 12-5 E–F: Activating Her Upward Yang Energy

Do not progress up her body beyond her vagina until you feel her vagina fully come to life (Figure 12-5 D), as all or most of her dead or constricted energy clears. If necessary, you can move down and up between the vagina and feet several times before moving further upward. When you are successful in this exercise, the bottom of her vagina will feel as if her qi has fallen out from it and her sexual energy will begin moving down her legs, exiting from her feet and into the earth.

3. Once this happens, you begin to clear her energy from her vagina upward to her lower tantien and stabilize there. Then from the lower tantien, move the energy upward to her breasts and middle tantien—the spiritual heart center. This begins to activate her yang energy (Figure 12-5 E).

4. Again, wait to stabilize and linger here for a while. You might say encouraging words or give her a few light kisses. Only then should you begin clearing her upper torso toward and above the head, in any way you like, such as using your fingers or palms to move qi through the etheric body (Figure 12-5 F).

When upwardly clearing etheric energy above the heart for either sex, especially focus on your partner's throat notch (see Figure 12-9), mouth, tip of the nose, ears, eyes, third eye, the occiput where the spine joins the skull, the crown of the head, and even above the crown of the head to the end of her etheric body.

Part 3: Projecting Qi into Your Partner's Body

The following practice builds on the hand and finger sensitivity you have begun to develop from practicing the Taoist methods for enhancing ordinary sex described in Chapter 7.

In the back and forth flux of lovemaking, it may be either a lighter or heavier pressure that will stimulate the nerves of the genitals more deeply or more toward the surface. A fundamental sexual qigong skill is to gain the ability to touch the surface of your partner's skin, project your physical qi and conscious awareness into your partner's body and then, with subtle physical pressure, penetrate right to the center or bottom of the penis or clitoris, or target specific rings of the vaginal walls.

Once your preliminary qigong practices are cultivated and your ability to control the projection of your qi is refined, in addition to using finger pressure, you can project energy from your fingers to activate the deeper internal energies of the penis or vagina, rather than only their sexual nerves.

Again, using the tofu hand-training technique (see Chapter 7) will help you develop the smooth, continuous touch this method requires. It also teaches you another key asset of a skillful lover: sexual patience. When engaged with a partner, use very light hand and finger pressure, especially for the vagina (the penis generally responds more easily). A man can stimulate the woman's clitoris by applying physical pressure or by projecting qi both into her clitoris and the associated rings of sensitivity spreading outward from it.

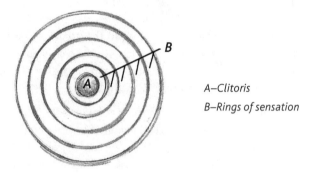

A–Clitoris
B–Rings of sensation

The epicenter of the clitoris has two qualities associated with it: depth and width. Depth is the vertical distance from top to bottom. Width begins from the center of the clitoris and extends sideways into or beyond the vaginal walls as much as the circumference of an American quarter.

Figure 12-6: The Clitoris

Eventually, you can take the sensitivity skills learned by practicing on tofu and use them to project waves of energy through your lover's body. This is a wonderful way to get sexually warmed up. For example, a man can put his hands on a woman's foot and project a wave going through her calves and up to her knee. When you have mastered this, you can continue the wave up to her vagina, adding an interesting sexual dimension to the ever-popular foot rub. This wave naturally induces the yin energy of the earth to aid a woman's orgasmic ability. Many women naturally clench their feet just before or during climax—this is related to earth energy. In a similar fashion, a woman can put her hand on a man's belly or lower back and project a wave to his chest, neck or head, thereby awakening his yang energy. ●

Ancient Texts Describe How to Maintain an Erection

Tian Xia Zhi Dao Tan ("Discussion of the Highest Way under Heaven") from the Ma Wang Dui series, tells men to do the following simple sitting qigong practice upon arising in the morning, not only to improve general energy and blood circulation but also to cultivate better erections:

"Raise your spine, relax and lift your anus, letting your qi drop to your lower tantien. Then swallow your saliva, draw in your buttocks, raise your spine and lift your anus a bit more and from your tantien make your qi drop to the penis."

During sexual intercourse, a man is advised to move his tailbone and waist. In doing so, he must relax his back and lift his anus. He should move slowly, so that the woman can lubricate; it's best that she has copious water-like sexual secretions.

Following sexual intercourse, to retain qi, the man should remove his erection after ejaculation before it gets soft. Once he has withdrawn, he should lift his anus, bring his qi to the upper back and then let it return to his penis. This allows the man to rest and regenerate more effectively. He should take a shower after having rested a little, rather than immediately after ejaculating. He should allow his qi to become smooth before becoming active again.

The texts also give men the following warnings:

- Avoid sexual movements that cause pain to either your erection or her vagina, they can cause the small blood vessels to shut off.

- If your sweat comes out during sex, it means your yang qi is leaving you.

- Avoid further sexual activity if, through excessive sex, your sperm dries up.

- If not in the mood, don't have sex or, alternatively, give your lover manual or oral sex. If you don't want to have sex, but the partner insists, this damages the body, makes for tense sex, and, in a man, can instill a propensity toward premature ejaculation.

Ancient texts from China tell the reader that a man's erection should be long, wide, hard and hot. A woman's face and body should be hot and her vagina should produce lots of secretions, then, when the man penetrates, he should go in slowly. These texts also talk about Chinese herbs that support better erections, tighten up the vagina and improve the functioning of the genital areas. Clearly, in the days before erectile dysfunction drugs and modern medicine, the Taoists gave men and women plenty of options for improving their sex lives.

ENERGETIC FOREPLAY TECHNIQUES

Once you start touching your partner, a very important consideration is where to start. Just as in the previous practice for activating his yang energy and her yin energy, your approach is gender specific—different for a man than for a woman. As a yin yang technique you were also instructed to trace your lover's aura over his or her main energy channels and yin and yang surfaces.

The Taoists have an old phrase that says, "If you haven't touched every part of your lover's body with your energy in the weaving back and forth between foreplay and intercourse, then you haven't completed the experience." At some point in the process of making love, if possible, you want to deliberately touch every single part of your partner's body, allowing your mind to go into their body-mind and theirs into yours. This allows you to have a whole experience of your lover rather than just leaping on top of him or her. Obviously, if you've been with your partner for years and years, you may not do this every time, but strive to do it more often than not.

In the previous practice of moving energy around your lover's body you were instructed to use your hands, both physically and energetically. After doing one cycle you can switch your technique. On the second or third pass, you might use your mouth and kiss your way up or down your lover's body, or use any combination of kissing, nibbling, nuzzling and rubbing that your lover enjoys. Your aim is to explore, stimulate and make contact with every inch of your partner; this is usually more than sufficient for the body to fully turn on for intercourse. The following section explores other Taoist foreplay methods.

KISSING, DISSOLVING AND MERGING

The Taoists have a different take from most people in the West on kissing, one of life's sweetest pleasures. When kissing, Taoists would use the Outer and Inner Dissolving methods to dissolve each other at any point of contact between body and mouth. Since you'll be kissing almost every part of your lover's body during foreplay and intercourse, this allows you, over time, to dissolve into a sea of blending energy.

The Taoists have a unique take on kissing, one of life's sweetest pleasures. They use methods when kissing that allow the two lovers to dissolve into a sea of blending energy.

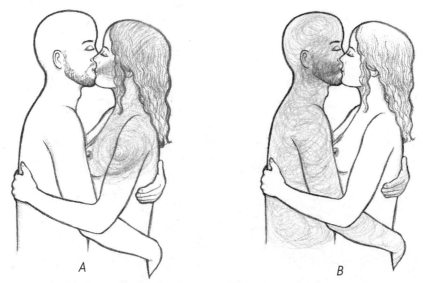

A) While kissing, he first dissolves everything in her body from the top of her head to her heart before moving down to her feet. B) She does likewise to him.

Figure 12-7 A–B: Dissolving during Kissing

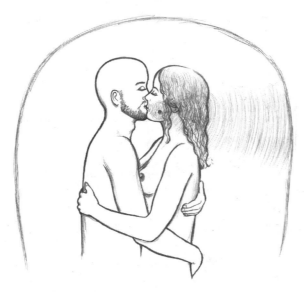

He dissolves a specific blockage in her body, for example in the jaw, until the blockage releases to the boundary of her etheric field. She could do likewise with a blockage in his body.

Figure 12-7 C: Dissolving Specific Blockages by Kissing

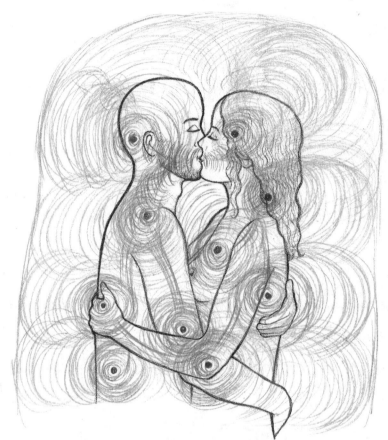

Etheric fields of both lovers interpenetrate and merge with each other naturally after sufficient energy gates or blocked points have been released and resolved.

Figure 12-7 D: Merging Etheric Fields When Kissing

At any point in a kiss, from either the mouth or tongue, it is possible to dissolve every part of your partner's body and, from there, to move into the Mindstream (see Chapter 15, "Connecting with the Mindstream"). Since kissing can be very electric, it is a good way to exponentially increase your ability to feel qi and eventually psychic sensations. You can kiss along the right, left and central channels to open these critical energy pathways. Likewise, you can use your kisses to open up all the secondary energy channels in the body, including the acupuncture meridians that are commonly closer to the surface of the skin.

In mouth-to-mouth kissing (both with and without tongue involvement), there are specific, important energy gates that need to be dissolved in both lovers.

Familiarize yourself with the following energetic connections and be aware of them next time you are kissing your partner:

1. The point where the yang and yin meridians change over on the acupuncture governing and conception vessels—where the tongue connects to the roof of the mouth when you say any word with a strong L sound (Figure 12-8). This is a critical junction for both the Microcosmic and Macrocosmic Orbits; dissolve this energy gate fully in order to release these two circulations of qi. Kissing is the easiest way to mutually join and dissolve your orbits and, in so doing, connect with the whole of your partner's energy system.

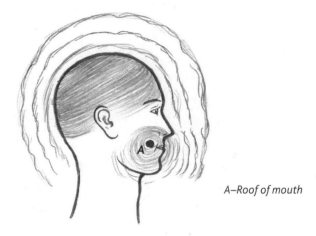

A–Roof of mouth

Figure 12-8: Dissolving the Roof of the Mouth and inside the Brain

2. From your mouth to the whole inside of your lover's brain. Throughout the entire time you spend making love, the brain is constantly emitting all sorts of energies and brain waves. It becomes important to dissolve from your lips and tongue upward into your partner's brain, so that when you're kissing with the lips you're actually kissing with the whole of your brain, into the whole of your partner's brain.[1] Smoothing out the signals coming from the brain will make it easier for both of you to telepathically register moods and feelings that emanate from one another. This practice also helps remove any subliminal tensions or "ghosts" that remain in your individual or shared thought streams.

---

1. Work with the whole of the brain only. Specific points in the brain may sometimes be felt in qigong practice. It is important to avoid trying to use your intent to forge connections between them if they are not naturally and spontaneously occurring on their own. This is because deliberately connecting certain configurations energetically may have dangerous consequences. Learning how to work with these points safely requires you to find a master with the appropriate knowledge.

3. The channel that extends from the root of the tongue through the notch underneath the throat and down to the heart center or solar plexus, which is one of the most commonly blocked pathways in human beings. This energetic channel influences your ability verbally or non-verbally to tell the truth and simply say what is in your heart without any deception (Figure 12-9).

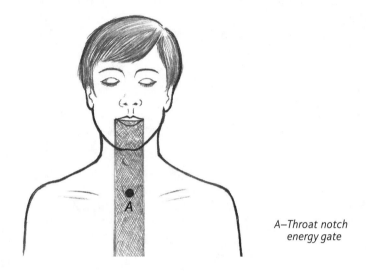

A—Throat notch energy gate

Figure 12-9: Channel between the Throat and the Heart

4. Slightly underneath the throat notch and behind the sternum is another especially important energy gate that you want to open (Figure 12-9, point A). This gate corresponds to the throat chakra of yoga. If it is closed, your capacity to produce sounds will be inhibited, and the words and internal vibrations that want to flow while making love will be shut down. A blockage here can stifle your ability to express yourself, such as by making sounds of pleasure, saying "I love you," letting your lover know what you want and don't want him or her to do, and so forth.

5. While you are kissing, activate the energy channels from either or both legs to the perineum, genitals, tantien, up the center of the body to the heart and, most importantly, from the heart to the mouth. After dissolving blocked energy gates, qi will next immediately flow more strongly between any two connected points. The activation occurs through your mind's intent. This is extremely important if you and your partner wish to have complete emotional expression, both overt and subliminal, with each other. Eventually, this allows you to transcend selfish motivations and naturally harmonize your energy with that of another.

NUZZLING, TONGUING AND RUBBING

You can use your head for erotic play. Wherever and whenever you rub your head on your partner's wonderfully alive body, clearly dissolve your own body and head first. Then continue dissolving into the area of your partner's body that you are contacting. You may want to nuzzle, kiss or rub with genitals, noses, or whatever. At the point of contact, using your awareness, you simply dissolve and move into your lover's body, penetrating with your consciousness and dissolving his or her bound energies, creating an ocean of qi between and within both of you.

In the Water method of Taoism, this penetrating and dissolving is done in a very yin, soft, unforced way. You do not want to encourage the psychic defenses and the closing-down of your partner. You want to come into his or her energy field as a psychic nurturer, not an invader. At the psychic level, your clear intent is seduction, not rape. That may sound strong, but having someone energetically force his or her way into your energy field can feel like a subtle or not so subtle intrusion for both men and women.

When you are first learning the foreplay dissolving techniques, you should start with the less sensitive zones, such as energy gates on your partner's body, and save the highly erotic areas for later in your lovemaking session. In other words, don't go straight for the nipples, genitalia, back of the neck, or ears. The natural high arousal that occurs in these areas will distract you from focusing on effortlessly dissolving and enjoying the slow buildup of erotic pleasure. Start with legs, arms or other places that are less likely to lead to overexcitement when dissolving your partner. In this way the entire body will be turned on.

When dissolving is the primary focus of foreplay, you can expect a very strong effect. Rather than the two of you becoming highly aroused in a "hot and bothered" way so common with ordinary sex, dissolving brings you into a deeply relaxed and connected state before you begin genital intercourse. This may seem counterproductive in a culture that places so much emphasis on a strong erection, and in which sex is often equated with penetration. But the fact is that people can make satisfying love for long periods of time once they discover the energetic dimension of lovemaking, even if the man doesn't get hard (or is hard only some of the time) or the woman is not already buzzing and hot.

From the Taoist point of view, a truly skilled lover can give a woman a completely satisfying sexual experience even without an erection. Likewise, a woman can satisfy a man even if her vagina can't get particularly wet. Even the most sexually active man or woman will occasionally find that on some days his or her genitals just won't cooperate. Who knows why? Maybe it's the food you ate, or some disturbing event has happened or overwork has taken its toll. Rather than shut down, it is helpful to remember that performance isn't nearly as important as the simple pleasurable exchange of sexual energy. At the end of the day, it's usually not actually the orgasm or spurting fluids that is the major reason for sex. Rather, it's the deep satisfaction that comes from simply exchanging energy and becoming relaxed enough to release the contents of your consciousness.

Understand this and you can shift the focus from the normal tension orgasm pattern of "ah...aah...aaah...whoosh!" to exchanging sexual energy back and forth. The point is to take the pressure off the situation and allow the sexual exchange to unfold in all its ways, many of which are not intuitively obvious at all.

BLOWING

Blowing light puffs of breath is another delightful addition to foreplay. If you can't dissolve the breath you give and receive, do your best to project and receive qi using relaxed intent. Here are five basic considerations for using this technique to sexually stimulate your partner:

- Move the air with a variety of pleasurable pressures and rhythms.
- Dissolve your own blocked qi as you blow and project it.
- Have your intention and energy move outward with your breath and into your partner; at the point of contact, penetrate and dissolve whatever blocked energy you experience there.
- When you inhale and suck in air, pull and dissolve your partner's energy from his or her body into yours and when you exhale project your dissolved energy into that of your partner.

Modulate the circularity of the breath going back and forth until the sea of energy between you becomes like the undercurrents of the waves lapping the shore. This can cause your partner's body to start writhing and reacting in other ways that will give you feedback that makes his or her sexual pleasure obvious.

POSSIBILITIES, NOT A COOKBOOK

Another favorite saying among the Taoists is, "You want to have all the vegetables in the pot before you start making love." Each of the vegetables is one of the physical and energetic sexual techniques mentioned in this book, or those you might find elsewhere or spontaneously invent. Play with each one until you get to know it intimately. Then combine them fluidly and creatively to make the particular dish you fancy. An unimaginative cook will follow a recipe to the letter, whereas truly great cooks will view that same recipe as a jumping-off point, an invitation to experiment and express their own unique flair.

Making love is an alive, fluid, ever-changing experience rather than a fixed protocol with a specific sequence of steps. Going with the flow with affection is the essence of spontaneous lovemaking. Over time, your sexuality itself will undergo a change. Eventually, your higher emotions will move out to the whole of your life and into everything you do. Sex will no longer be an encapsulated event that remains separate from the rest of your life. The rich, emotional connection experienced there will allow for more emotional intimacy in nonsexual relationships.

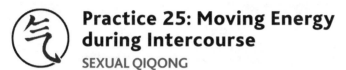

Practice 25: Moving Energy during Intercourse
SEXUAL QIGONG

This is the partner version of the exercise you learned in Practice 23, "Transfer Sexual Energy around Your Body," from Chapter 11. You and your partners can do this energetic exercise with or without clothing, groins touching, or legs entwined around one other, as you prefer. With sexual qigong, if both partners do the practices together, you can now have double the energy available so the process can go considerably further than is possible in the solo versions.

Part 1: Manual Stimulation

In the first part of this practice you move energy while manually stimulating your partner. In this case, touching the genitals becomes more than a matter of simply moving your hands—it enables partners to energetically link.

Begin with the same steps as in the solo exercise, and then project your qi until you get a really clear sense of the energy going from the genitals (yours or your partner's) to the lower tantien, through the torso, up to the shoulders, down to the elbows, wrists and out of your fingers.

When the man is pleasing the woman, the man pulls her vagina's qi into his hands and through his arms and torso into his lower tantien. He then pushes or projects that energy from his lower tantien back through his torso, into his hand and fingers, and then back into her vagina. The same energetic pathway applies for a woman as she plays with his perineum, scrotum or penis. She can pull his energy through her body, channels and into her tantien, and then from there push it back to his genitals.

Part 2: Moving Energy from the Genitals

The next progression of this partner practice involves actively dissolving, pulling and moving energy directly from your genitals into your lower tantien. Later you can move the energy from your genitals to a specific targeted area of the body, perhaps an injured or devitalized place (see Chapter 14).

Once you begin sexual meditation, you can also use this process of moving energy back and forth from your own and your partner's genitals to deliberately get your mind inside your partner's blocked emotional, mental or psychic energy. In these more advanced practices you change from Outer Dissolving to using Inner Dissolving in order to resolve any blockages you find. Progression into these more advanced practices depends on making and stabilizing the first major link—moving energy between your perineum and genitals to the lower tantien. ●

Cautionary Note: Opening to the Psychic World

When you go beyond dissolving your own blocks and learn to go into your partner's body and mind to dissolve the blockages inside him or her, you can often spontaneously tap into the psychic level fairly quickly. Sex provides an ideal gateway into the watery psychic world, which is easier for some people to handle than it is for others.

Sometimes ignorance is bliss. Many people don't want to know about the subtle levels of life beyond the ordinary. Once you open the psychic door, you no longer have the option of a conventional life. Go slowly and remember the seventy-percent rule. If you are experiencing significant discomfort of any kind, it's best to back off and stop practicing. Working with the psychic world is not recommended for anyone with mental health issues.

ENERGETIC EROGENOUS ZONES

The body has an infinite number of energetic erogenous zones. They magically appear when one is both sensitive enough and the energy is just right. All the zones can be powerful sources of sexual arousal and excitement and in the right circumstances generate all kinds of wonderful and delicious orgasms.

For example, there are erogenous zones on the sole of the foot, especially at the three energy gates (see Figure 12-11). There are also erogenous zones almost anywhere from the feet to the thighs, on the back of the knee and spine, at each kwa, and at the ears and neck. Other arousing areas include breast and nipples (Figure 12-12), the center of the armpit (Figure 12-13), and the midriff (Figure 12-10) which controls the up and down flow of energy along the spine in the middle of the torso. Qi dripping from the fingers indicates that the body's energy is fully online (see Figure 12-10).

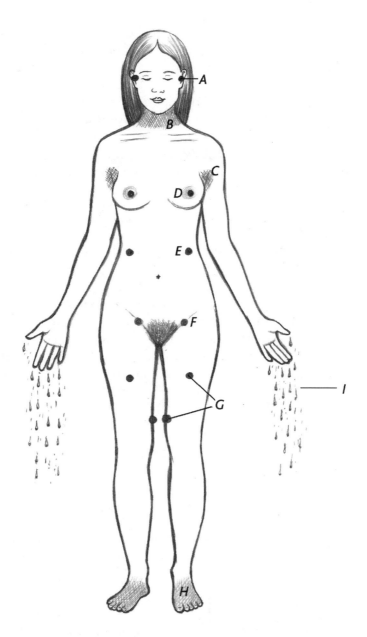

A–Ears

B–Neck

C–Armpits

D–Breasts

E–Midriff

F–Kwas

G–Inner and mid-thigh points

H–Feet

I–Qi drips from fingers

Figure 12-10: Some Energetic Erogenous Zones

With every form of touch discussed in this chapter, you have a wide range of variations to play and be creative with. Whatever foreplay technique you use, you want to dissolve and energetically open up your partner's left and right channels before you start on specific erogenous areas. When working with the left and right channels within the torso, start on the yin (front) side of a woman's body first, and on the yang (back) side of a man's. Then, continuing on the same yin or yang side of your partner's body, reverse the up or down direction of your movement. While moving between one body area and another, be sure to kiss and dissolve everything on both sides of either the left or right channel, both up and down and on the opposite corresponding yin or yang side.

PRIMARY SEXUAL AREAS IN THE BODY

The following is a summary of the primary energetic erogenous zones:

Feet

While all of us love a good foot rub, in a sexual context the feet are extremely important for women, for reasons already discussed. Begin the process initially along the inside of either foot and move on until you reach every part of her foot by first stimulating (kissing, rubbing and so on) and then dissolving her feet. Put special focus on the bubbling well point on the ball of her foot (Figure 12-11, point A), her toes, and the inside edge of the sole of her foot between the big toe and the beginning of the heel along the arch of her foot (Figure 12-11, E).

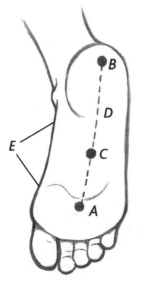

A–Bubbling well point which causes energy to rise in the body and connects to the three tantiens

B–Heel point which causes energy to descend down the body

C–Center of the foot which balances the body's up and down energy flows

D–Line down the center of the sole of the foot which directly connects to the central channel

E–Inside edge of foot

Figure 12-11: Erogenous Zones of the Foot

Knees and Thighs

Progressively going up a woman's body, the next area to enjoy is the back of her knees. This will stimulate her kidney energy and increase her vitality in general. Thighs and inner thighs are incredibly sensitive and arousing in some women and significantly less so in others. You should be aware of two important points on the thigh: the first is about one-third of the way up the inner thigh from the knee to the hip, and the second about half-way up on the front of the thigh (see Figure 12-10, G). Both of these points are not only sexually arousing but also are an energetic gateway to the left and right channels located in the hard part (cortex) of the thigh bone (not the bone marrow inside it).

For both men and women, these two thigh points can be helpful to mitigate knee problems. Although sexually it is not instantaneously a particularly arousing point, this can over the course of a few minutes change, because focusing on this point stimulates the energy of the kidneys, which is directly connected to sexual energy. As a result, commonly you'll see the benefits to lovemaking within a few minutes as your sexual energy revs up, even if this doesn't happen immediately.

The Kwa (Bikini Cut Area)

Most men are naturally drawn to the kwa, where the fold of the hip joint is located, because it feels very soft and pleasing to the touch. This area is a conduit through which energy transfers both up and down between the legs and torso. You want to play with the kwa area until you feel the effect of your dissolving, as your partner's genitals begin to release and heat up. Use mouth, tongue, head, nose, penis, or whatever feels good to both of you.

Midriff

The midriff area, where the "love handles" are, is located between the top of the hips and the bottom of the ribs and goes from each side of the body to the left and right channels (see Chapter 3, Figure 3-3). This area is a major energetic floodgate that helps to control the energy transfer between the upper and lower body and prevents the middle of the spine and the diaphragm from collapsing. Kissing, rubbing and nuzzling actions are particularly recommended in this area.

Breasts and Nipples

The breasts are another major erogenous zone. Although women tend to be more sensitive than men, there is no general rule. It's important to remember that not all women's breasts are erotically sensitive, just as some men get extreme pleasure from being stimulated in this area. During foreplay, awakening the breasts and nipples is a critical point in the movement of energy between the torso, arms, neck and head along the left and right channels. On a woman's body, midway between the nipple and ribcage there is an energy gate that regulates a woman's whole glandular system (see Figure 12-12). Be sure to dissolve this gate. The prostate gland has a similar effect on men.

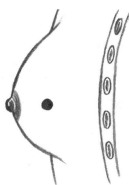

*The energy gate in the center of the breast can be very arousing for some women.
It also regulates a woman's hormonal system and is used therapeutically as
part of qigong treatments for breast cancer in China.*

Figure 12-12: Breast and Nipple

For the Love of Breasts

Above and beyond the tremendous aesthetic beauty of breasts and the concentration of nerve endings in them, their significance—and the enduring love we feel for them—cannot be underestimated. During infancy, the mammary glands are the life-giving source of milk and qi. Breasts are also a potent reminder of mother's heartbeat, a primary anchor in the world of the fetus. These are powerful influences that can condition any child's nervous system and internal rhythms for life. These factors alone would account for the tremendous power and allure that women's breasts have for human males.

Interestingly, in *Bonk: The Curious Coupling of Science and Sex,* Mary Roach reports, "One of the less prominently known similarities between pigs and men: They both fondle breasts. No other males on the planet regularly do this."[2]

For those who experienced poor mother-infant bonding, or in cases in which mother and child remain "tethered" in a way that is harmful to one or both, a woman can dissolve her own breasts to release negative blockages, or a man can dissolve his partner's breasts.

2. Roach, Mary, *Bonk: The Curious Coupling of Science and Sex* (New York: W. W. Norton, 2008), 93.

Due to the concentration of nerves in the nipples, they are, like the clitoris, particularly prone to overstimulation. If overstimulated, a nipple can lose sensitivity and become deadened. Some women's nipples are so hypersensitive that strongly stimulating them can be painful and is a real turnoff. To reawaken sensitivity, simply shift your focus and play with the excitable rings that emanate away from the epicenter of the nipple (similar to the rings of sensation around the clitoris), including the areola and the breast tissue itself. This gives the nerves of the nipple time to release tension and regenerate their capacity to become erotically stimulated again.

Keep in mind that every woman is unique in terms of how much pressure she likes when you squeeze, tongue or suck on her breasts. Also, the amount of pressure that hits her "sweet spot" or turnoff zone may change depending on her level of arousal. Likewise, some men, when highly aroused, can handle a woman sinking her teeth into his chest or biting his nipple, whereas this same amount of pressure might be a major turnoff earlier or at another stage of his arousal.

Armpits: A Crucial Nexus

Perhaps one of the most overlooked of all the erogenous zones are the armpits (Figure 12-13). Many of us like to play with our partner's arms and neck, but we rarely nuzzle into our partner's armpits. This is a real mistake, energetically speaking, because the armpits are a critical nexus that completes a major circuit of energy flow in the body. The energy that flows through the left or right channels and branches off from your head and neck needs to then flow through your armpits and into your upper extremities. If you don't open the energy through the armpit, the circulation of qi can't flow properly down the arms to the fingertips and then complete itself by returning up the arms in order to rejoin the torso. This will significantly downgrade the energy flow through your entire system.

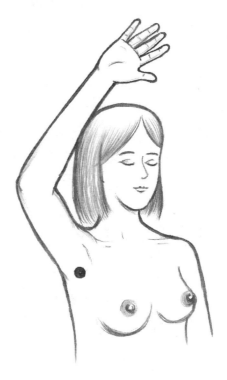

This point controls the flow of energy from the torso and heart to the arms and fingers.

Figure 12-13: Center of Armpit

A lack of qi flow through the arms can cause secondary insufficiencies. For example, it can reduce the energetic effectiveness of cuddling, during which your arms are used to the utmost. During intercourse, it can cause increased strain when one partner uses his or her arms to balance or hold his or her body above the other person. Aside from the practicality of energy flow, the Taoists discovered that stimulating your lover's armpits can be quite a turn-on, stronger, in some cases, than what occurs with the breasts. So don't let conditioned aversion or lack of experience stop you. If hygiene is an issue, draw your partner a hot bath or take a shower with him or her before you slip into bed together.

Neck

The neck is the gateway for the left and right channels reaching the head. A saying in Taoist sexual qigong states, "Wait to begin really playing with your partner's neck until your own qi is dripping off your fingers." During lovemaking, when the circulation of energy in your own body is going strong, you will feel a powerful flow of energy from your toes to your fingers to the top of your head. The clear and present sign that this is happening will be the sensation of qi dripping from your fingers. The stronger you feel energy dripping off your fingers, the stronger your qi circulation, and the warmer your hands, feet and mouth will feel. If your qi is not opened up sufficiently—if it doesn't get all the way to your fingers and start to drip—you will tend to subliminally feel very cold. This can induce an automatic sympathetic response which can make the other person contract rather than open up. So if you feel like your qi is dripping from your fingers, it's time to go for your lover's neck in the friendliest way you can.

Ears

Lastly, let's talk about ears. In addition to the naturally stimulating and erotic nature of the ear, your ears have tiny acupuncture points that correspond to every major body system related to your health. So powerful are these ear points, that some acupuncture methods needle only the ear and no other points on the body. During lovemaking, try kissing, rubbing, lightly tonguing or blowing on the ear. In addition to arousing your partner, you can activate his or her internal organs, glandular secretions, and energy gates. As well as sexually stimulating the ear, you can dissolve into these areas, healing and releasing trapped energy.

If your partner has exceptionally sensitive ears, the "touch and let go" technique works very well. Whether stimulating the ears by kissing, biting, blowing or touching, go as gently and lightly as possible at first, then suddenly separate or let go of contact. Touch and let go, touch and let go, touch and let go and so on. Vary the rhythm and pressure, keeping it unpredictable so that your lover is on the delicious edge of anticipation and uncertainty. Especially with the ears, vary your touch and let go—sometimes slower, sometimes faster. Letting go gives the nerves a chance to release, tremble, and then regenerate and get stronger. Continuous overstimulation often causes the sexual response to shut down. Many men are particularly responsive when a woman uses her breasts to fondle his ears. And both sexes respond very well to gentle, light raking of the ears and neck with fingernails or tongue.

Dissolving from the ear into the brain can help overcome the "I have a headache" syndrome (see Chapter 14, Practice 28, "Relieving a Lover's Headache"). This can also help your partner let go of continuously churning thoughts that have nothing to do with what's happening in the moment. As mentioned before, dissolve the whole of the brain only. You must avoid trying to work with any specific points in the brain energetically as connecting certain configurations can be dangerous.

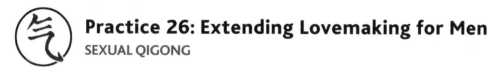

Practice 26: Extending Lovemaking for Men
SEXUAL QIGONG

Part 1: For the Man

A basic sexual qigong practice can help a man delay ejaculation. When a man is about to ejaculate, he withdraws the energy from his penis and transfers it to some other spot inside his body. Using his intent, he then transfers the qi from the genital area to other parts of his body including but not limited to his butt, chest, nipple, head, or even to a specific energy gate.

A man will find that moving the energy that is generated by sex to different parts of his body results in radically different sensations. A useful strategy for many men is to vary the kind of sensations by varying the location where the energy is directed. When a man wants to rest, he should find a place inside his body that does not easily excite him. Then when he wants to delay an orgasm he can shift his energy to that place. Likewise, when he wants to rev up, he finds the place inside his body that easily excites him and directs energy there.

Another sexual qigong technique a man can use if he wants an erection to last longer is to completely relax and dissolve tension in the mons pubis, also known as the pubic mound region. This is where the nerves and the blood vessels that pump blood into the genitals are located.

Part 2: For the Woman to Help the Man

A woman can help a man delay an orgasm. When she feels he is going to come or he indicates he may do so, she brings the qi up his spine. Using her energy, she will want to get the qi to stabilize in the area between the middle of his spine up to the top of his head. If the qi stays in his upper back rather than his lower back and legs, this will slow down or prevent his ejaculation.

If a woman wants to aid a man so that he can maintain a harder erection, she can massage his spine. By massaging his back, she plays with moving his energy so it to rises up through his yang pathways. The occipital region at the back of the head is the doorway for the energy to flow to the crown of the head. Directing qi upward along the back, through the occipital region to the crown allows his body-brain connection to open up so his energy can then travel downward into his body to the lower tantien which will help his erection stay hard. ●

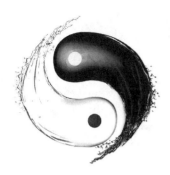

CHAPTER 13

The Power of Internal Orgasms

In ordinary sex, external orgasms allow us to deeply relax the body, mind and Being. They release and balance emotional energy, thereby creating satisfying sex. With sexual qigong, you learn how to activate "internal" orgasms in your body to channel, store and put more qi to use.

Very few people even know what internal orgasms are, much less how to create them because they are a function of knowing how to work with qi during sex. Once you start to become more sensitive to qi and as you learn to work with Outer Dissolving within sexual qigong, the world of internal orgasms opens up.

This chapter and the next explore how you can use internal orgasms for four specific purposes that overlap, yet remain distinct:

1. To gain significantly more pleasure from sexual activity than normally possible.
2. To open up the energy channels of your body.
3. To facilitate Outer Dissolving in the first four energy bodies.
4. To achieve specific healing ends, both for yourself and for your sexual partner.

In later chapters that move into sexual meditation, you will learn about how the energy generated by both external and internal orgasms can be used to supercharge the Inner Dissolving process. This can allow the resolution of the deeper energetic blockages in the fifth (psychic), sixth (karmic) and seventh (essence) energy bodies.

GENERATING INTERNAL ORGASMS

The level of bliss and ecstasy that is created from an internal orgasm is beyond imagining and opens a door to entirely new sexual experiences. As your energy releases and permeates the nerves, you feel a tremendous sense of relaxation. None of the physical tension or bodily contractions that commonly accompany external orgasms is present. An internal orgasm leaves you with a completely relaxed body and mind, regardless of sexual position.

An external orgasm, as spectacular as it can feel, is a physical phenomenon that occurs by building tension and then releasing it. Internal orgasms are primarily an energetic phenomenon. They require that you energetically link your genitals to the place where you wish to have an internal orgasm, while keeping your mind relaxed and open as you do so. Both men and women are equally capable of having internal orgasms. The cultivation of qi for internal orgasms can be used within all the practices in sexual qigong and sexual meditation.

OPENING AND CLOSING: THE PULSE OF THE UNIVERSE

Pulsing, or opening and closing, is the key that unlocks the ability to have internal orgasms. It is one of the primary neigong or internal energy components of all Taoist practices (see Chapter 10, "Sixteen Neigong Components"). Pulsing occurs naturally during lovemaking. The pulsation that occurs in your genitals is part of the pleasurable writhing and undulations that move through the body in waves, as well as more subtly inside your tissues. In more ways that words can possibly express, the ultimate power of sex comes from the relationship between the pulsing that occurs in orgasms and the natural pulse of creation and, in fact, the entire universe.

The ultimate power of sex comes from the relationship between the pulsing that occurs in orgasms and the natural pulse of the entire universe.

Opening and closing is the universal rhythm of life. This natural pulsating energy can be found everywhere: in organic life, human cells, the heart, as well as in the inorganic world. Pulsing can be detected and measured in the oscillating energy of the earth, in stars and even in sub-atomic particles. Our own sun constantly erupts and then the plasma returns to itself via magnetic and gravitational fields in a constantly alternating expand-condense pattern.

Specific areas of the body have a subtle pulse. Pulsing happens with the opening and closing of the mouth, joints, muscles, soft tissues, internal organs, glands, blood vessels, cerebrospinal system, as well as the body's subtle energy anatomy. In order to precipitate an internal orgasm, you use your internal energy to amplify the pulse in specific tissues, organs and energy gates. The pulse is used to isolate the energy at a specific point.

In your body, this expansion and condensing occurs continuously within all your energy gates. These absorb and discharge qi, both externally away from your body and internally between the energy gates and places inside your body, such as joints, organs, and so on.

In your body, this expansion and condensing occurs continuously within:

- Your sexual anatomy.
- Your brain.
- The internal organs, which have continuous energetic rhythms that cause each organ to alternate between getting slightly larger (expanding), then slightly smaller (condensing) in both yin and yang ways.
- Your spine as a whole and every single spinal vertebra—on a micro-level this continuous pulsing enables your spine to maintain its integrity.

When you are actively engaged in sex, the opening and closing actions that occur between the energy of a male and a female has a major impact on the human energetic system. Mixing yin and yang during sex is a powerful form of pulsing, because it so accurately mirrors the fundamental pulse of the primordial energies that make up everything within creation. Most people never notice their condensing and expanding nature. Nor do they connect their inner pulsing to the natural rhythms that exist throughout the universe.

Whereas normal exercise stretches the body, what is commonly neglected in the typical stretching of yoga or gymnastic routines are the natural springs of the body—the source of its elasticity. These springs, or subtle "shock absorbers," are part of the constant rhythm of opening and closing.

For Taoists, openings and closings are one of the most important qualities as regards human energetic anatomy. When you reach an extremely high level of qi development, you can learn to synchronize your internal pulsing rhythms with the pulsations of the universe. While moving qi inside your body, you learn to match, mesh with and then use the pulsations of the earth. This involves first accessing the earth's energy, then merging it with your own until you can use it to boost your own personal qi. The goal is to generate that pulse or frequency inside you in a ratio that matches the pulse of the earth. This requires that you speed up or slow down (whichever is easier) the movement of your own qi until you can feel and access that proper ratio.

WHAT MAKES AN ORGASM INTERNAL?

There are two key characteristics of internal orgasms. The first is your intention—the mind actively directs your qi to a specific point. This means you will be able to unambiguously feel specific qi pathways and use Outer Dissolving practices to release energetic blocks. You must have practiced enough to have built a stable foundation for directly experiencing these pathways, not as an idea but as a felt reality. This will lay the foundation for your mind to be able to direct qi through these pathways to a specific area to achieve an internal orgasm.

Second, an internal orgasm requires that your intention comes from a deeply relaxed mind and body, with no use of force or willpower. This may sound a bit paradoxical, especially for more yang-orientated Western readers who equate intention with a goal-directed, "make it happen" approach that immediately generates internal tension in the body and mind. Although you can achieve an external orgasm in this state, it is highly unlikely that you will achieve an internal one. Why? If you tense or close down your mind, you cut an internal orgasm off at its energetic roots.

The mind is like a double-edged sword. The same mind that can cause your qi to move through the required channels and create an internal orgasm somewhere inside your body can also block and prevent your qi from moving. Most people simply don't have the subtle awareness of how their mind affects and, in some cases, sabotages their energy system.

HOW TO HAVE INTERNAL ORGASMS

Skilled practitioners learn how to use their qi to transfer sexual energy from their genitals to any specific location in the body and experience their orgasm there. There is no sudden contraction, no shock to the system, just an accelerated pulsing or opening and closing that leads to a profound release and relaxation. For a man, developing the skill to direct qi to a spot away from his genitals also eliminates the downside of semen loss, which is extremely important.

Internal orgasms are accomplished in a seven-stage process:

1. Build up the energy in your genitals

2. Relax your mind and body completely

3. Direct energy to the desired site of an internal orgasm

4. Release your qi into the chosen site

5. Start pulsing the qi in that site

6. Dramatically speed up the energetic opening and closing (pulsing) until...

7. It takes on a life of its own and eventually leads to an energetic orgasm.

This type of orgasm leads to a profound release in the chosen site. Afterward, partners can choose to contain the orgasmic energy in that site, direct it through the system, do it again or store the energy in the tantien. Relaxation is essential to generate an internal orgasm. Without a deep level of relaxation, the practitioner won't be able to dissolve or, in the later stages, pulse.

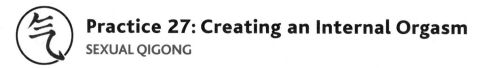

Practice 27: Creating an Internal Orgasm
SEXUAL QIGONG

Using the following practice, you and your partner can experiment with the basic method of generating an internal orgasm:

1. Regardless of sexual position, energetically link your genitals to the site where you would like to have an internal orgasm—you may find this site either by intuition or by feeling and locating a blockage that you wish to liberate.

2. With your pelvis moving, feel, find and dissolve an energetic channel linking your genitals and the place where you wish to have the internal orgasm until you arrive at the chosen site.

3. Dissolve and thereby energize the blockage. Relax and let go as you let the energy build.

4. Allow your qi to grow with a relaxed yin force. Wait until you begin to naturally pulse at the chosen site. This will happen only intermittently at first.

5. Next, spontaneously allow your consciousness and Outer Dissolving to go to a higher level, which will cause the site to start pulsing strongly of its own accord.

6. Energetically dissolve the space and accelerate this internal pulsing, until it takes on a life of its own, in much the same way as the prelude to an external orgasm.

7. When the energetic pulsing at the potential internal orgasm site takes on a life of its own, its speed escalates until a tipping point is reached and the internal orgasm spontaneously and energetically explodes.

To sum up, the energetic acceleration of pulsing takes on a life of its own in an internal orgasm in much the same way as do muscle contractions and sensory pleasure in an ordinary external orgasm.

In sexual qigong, internal orgasms are characterized by an incredible release of pleasurable energy, bliss or ecstasy inside the body. This energy permeates all your nerves and, for many, especially those who are more energetically sensitive, internal orgasms can be more pleasurable than an external orgasm. When you and your lover become sensitive and skilled, this type of internal release is satisfying and relaxing beyond measure or description.

At more advanced stages of sexual meditation, pulsing is combined with the Inner Dissolving methods and this leads to internal orgasms that release into emptiness. Emptiness moves you toward realizing the Tao; extreme pleasure alone does not. ●

ADDITIONAL GUIDELINES FOR INTERNAL ORGASMS

As you start to play with generating internal orgasms, it is extremely important to follow some general guidelines for using and directing your qi energy. When energy flows naturally and is not directed by the mind and intent, it will flow where it needs to. When you consciously direct energy, you need to take precautions so that you do not force energy where it is not meant to go.

It's always best to work directly with a teacher who is experienced in these methods. However, since few suitable teachers of this material are available, it's important to take note of the following precautionary guidelines and considerations for men and women.

CONSIDERATIONS FOR MEN

To create an internal orgasm in a man—regardless of which partner directs the energy—it is especially important to pull the energy upward first within his body before sending it down. If the energy is initially sent downward, he will probably ejaculate before an internal orgasm has a chance to happen. If a woman is giving a man an internal orgasm, she should also follow this pattern by first moving his energy up and only then down his body. Likewise, if a man wants to have an internal orgasm in his knee or assist his woman in giving him one there, the man shouldn't just send the energy from his genitals to his knee directly. Instead, he should initially send the energy up through his upper body, ideally to his head, before it goes down to his knee.

After a man has an internal orgasm in his lower body, he can then bring the released energy to the upper part of his body and crown of his head. He can either hold and stabilize the energy at the crown, specifically the bai hui point, or bring the qi down to his lower tantien, completing the full energetic circuit. If he fails to do this, he'll ejaculate too easily. After the first internal orgasm and when having subsequent internal orgasms within a session, once a man's qi has been stabilized in the lower tantien, he can now go directly from the genitals to the knee without a mandate to go up his body before going down.

Once a man has had an external orgasm, it becomes exceedingly difficult, if not impossible, to have an internal orgasm shortly thereafter, even if he immediately can produce another erection.

Pregnancy and Internal Orgasms

A more advanced technique that Taoist practitioners can use when making love during pregnancy is either or both lovers can deliberately nourish the fetus by directing energy inside it. The woman can target the qi of her orgasm so it occurs inside the fetus, and the man can project the qi of his penis inside the baby. According to the Taoists, it's generally good enough to be natural with this technique and unnecessary to be excessive or methodical about using your sexual energy for this purpose. However, if parents who were Taoist practitioners learned that their baby had potential problems, either through energetic feeling, pulse diagnosis or scientific testing, they would target her internal orgasms and his penile energetic projections to strengthen the baby in the womb.

According to the Taoists, the energy from a man's penis should generally be used to penetrate through the fetus and then continue onward. Generally this is the most beneficial for the fetus. A man should not direct his energy to lock onto a specific part of the growing baby unless there is a significant and compelling medical or karmic reason to do so. Unless there is a very specific situation with the baby or mother, Taoists are very much in favor of circulating energy throughout the mother's entire energy system.

Generally speaking, the parents' sexual enjoyment will nourish a developing fetus, so Taoists view sex during pregnancy in a positive light. However, on any given day, should either partner feel resentment, anger, or other strong emotions, those agitated and negatively charged energies can literally imprint and become embodied within the child. To avoid this negative imprint, Taoists advise clearing energy or meditating before sex to dissolve any negative energy that has built up during the day. This ensures that the negative energy does not transfer to the fetus during intercourse. Without this type of conscientious practice, babies can and do come out of the womb with all sorts of negative imprints that impact them later in life, even though they haven't the faintest clue as to the original cause.

Taoist women before labor use internal orgasms to train themselves to reduce the time they spend in labor and ease the process of giving birth. A highly skilled woman can actually induce labor by making love deliberately and directing internal orgasms into the cervix. This method can be especially helpful when she is close to her due date or when the baby is late.

CONSIDERATIONS FOR WOMEN

When creating an internal orgasm in a woman's upper body—regardless of who is directing the energy—her energy must first come into the legs and feet before bringing it upward into her lower tantien and then to anywhere in her torso or head.

A woman will also find that creating a calm space so that she can relax with Outer Dissolving and later Inner Dissolving as she's having orgasms is more beneficial than if she just has a tension orgasm based solely on contractions. Using the more advanced technique of Inner Dissolving can allow her to enter a space of emptiness. The space of emptiness causes her orgasmic energy to flow back more strongly into her glands and enhance the positive effect on them. Although multiple orgasms without the space of emptiness won't cause the woman harm, it also won't necessarily benefit her glands either. This is an important consideration.

Unlike men, women can have an internal and an external orgasm either simultaneously or in very close succession, for example, an external one in her genitals and an internal one in her legs or upper body. If a woman has an internal orgasm exclusively, usually it will be dramatically stronger than if it is combined with an external orgasm.

LEARNING TO HAVE AN INTERNAL ORGASM

As you may have noticed by now, the process of learning Taoist energy arts and sexual qigong is not linear, nor is it a simple matter of mastering one skill and then moving on to the next. Learning involves a continuous spiral of self-discovery and exploration. As you spiral from one learning opportunity to the next, you learn something new and, simultaneously, have a chance to revisit, rediscover, and integrate previous material at progressively greater, more powerful depths.

This relearning occurs not only because more information is directly stated, but also because deeper levels of your mind have been prepared and opened, enabling you to experience various aspects of the Tao more completely, which can be indirectly hinted at but not overtly stated. New insights will come upon you suddenly, although the "why, when and how" is an organic process completely unique to you. While there are no guarantees that you will be able to gain a specific body-mind skill, just remember that millions have succeeded in doing so throughout human history. So you can rest assured that these skills are attainable.

Don't be discouraged if it takes some time to learn the practices that enable new and different type of orgasms. You can only allow and encourage an internal orgasm to occur; it can't be forced. Allow what is meant to happen to emerge naturally in its own time.

Willpower alone usually cannot hold the sexual energy at the orgasm site long enough to make the internal orgasm occur. This is because the amount of tension you invoke by exerting willpower gets in the way of your ability to relax into a space of inner stillness. Energetic (nonphysical) pulsation, which comes only from a relaxed intent, is needed to seed the possibility of an internal orgasm in the first place.

It takes time for your body and mind to integrate many of the progressive stages you will be learning in sexual qigong and sexual meditation. Here is a common path:

- Sensing the subtle energy, or qi, that fuels, supports, animates and underlies every function of your very alive body. Qi responds to intention, and time is needed to learn to effectively direct it.
- Mastering and applying pulsing (opening and closing).
- Developing Outer Dissolving practices. You must learn to bring awareness and intention to areas that are blocked and frozen so that energy can once again become fluid and start to move, eventually dissipating like vapor once released from your system. This is part of sexual qigong.
- Developing the Inner Dissolving practices of sexual meditation, where the goal is to reach emptiness. Internal orgasms achieved through this method will not be the same as those derived from Outer Dissolving.

Once these skills are learned, it is possible to have a very different experience of orgasm. Instead of the typical tension release, you use a total relaxation orgasm and learn to completely relax at the moment of internal orgasm. This avoids any possible sudden shock that, for example, can come from shattering the delicate energetic lattice generated by the rev-up toward the ejaculation of an external orgasm. The new experiences that occur when you release blockages and have internal orgasms will take time to integrate into your body and mind. Once integrated, they become a stable, natural part of your Being.

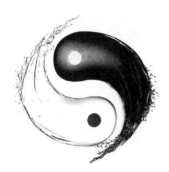

CHAPTER 14

Sex as
Energy Healing

Taoists were fairly unique in that they figured out how to use sexual energy for healing. This chapter describes how internal orgasms can be used for healing purposes. The mechanism is a deliberate transfer of energy to an area that is injured or diseased. Once you learn to heal your own pain and illness, you can begin to use those skills to help heal your lover with his or her permission.

The Taoists are justifiably renowned for their energetic healing practices, which include acupuncture, qigong and qigong tui na (therapeutic energy massage). According to Traditional Chinese Medicine from which Taoist energetic healing practices derive, when a person is optimally healthy, qi circulates through the entire body and mind without disruption. This happens in a smooth, powerful fashion, like a river with unimpeded flow. Conversely, when your life force is blocked, you have pain and disease.

HEALING WITH INTERNAL ORGASMS

It bears repeating (especially for men) that you can have five, ten, fifty or a hundred internal orgasms for every time you have a single external orgasm. If a man wishes to use orgasmic energy to heal a damaged part of his body, he must not ejaculate during internal orgasms. He may do so only after directing the energy of multiple internal orgasms to the needed location.

The four-stage process of a healing internal orgasm is like heating water in a teakettle. For example, here's how this energetic process might work in the case of a woman who wants to help heal a knee injury:

1. Get the water hot. When heating up the water, you will initially move energy down from your tantien to your knee.

2. Bubbles start to appear; this is the buildup stage. Let the excitement that is building in your genitals feed the line between your lower tantien and knee until you feel your knee getting very energized and excited.

3. The kettle makes a loud whistling noise; this is analogous to the strong energetic pulsing sensations that precede an internal orgasm. These sensations, if prolonged, can potentially provide the greatest physical benefit for the knee—even more than an internal orgasm itself. While moving into but not yet arriving at the orgasmic phase, you take the building sensations happening in your genitals and energetically move them down into your knee. Transfer the experience of the orgasmic buildup from your genitals into your knee.

4. Now concentrate the internal orgasm within the knee itself. You could say that this is in effect centering the energy explosion of the orgasm in your knee. Unlike the negative connotations of a physical explosion, this energy explosion can have very beneficial effects.

HEALING ORGASM PROCESS

Here are more details on how a woman might do this practice to direct healing energy to her knee.[1] With or without the aid of a partner, a woman dissolves her energy and clears it on a downward energy pathway to her knee. Then, beginning from the lower tantien, she moves the energy to the vagina, perineum, and—if she is able—right through the center of her bones and bone marrow until she reaches the center of her knee.

She then lets her energy continuously move back and forth between her lower tantien and the injured knee. Simultaneously she dissolves any blocked energy she encounters in both directions. After a while she may start getting into the energetic opening and closing rhythm that normally leads to an internal orgasm, such as the buildup of a wave or contractions. When this starts happening, she maintains the connection between the knee and her lower tantien and she keeps transferring the buildup of orgasmic energy from within her vagina to her knee in a continuous stream.

The process is somewhat similar for a man, although a man must activate his yang energy by initially moving the energy up toward his head before directing it down toward the knee.

COOLING DOWN AFTER HEALING SESSIONS

Be very intentional in what you are doing. Once you've directed the energy of multiple internal orgasms to the specific body part, give yourself time to rest. The

---

1. The author can personally attest to the effectiveness of this method, as he often used it to heal knee injuries sustained in martial art competitions.

man will want to pull out of the vagina or wind down in some other manner while his own or his partner's damaged body part absorbs and stabilizes the energy. Then he can continue making love and ejaculate in a relaxed way without causing secondary problems.

If you don't take the time to rest, absorb, and stabilize the energy of the healing orgasm, it will dissipate and go to waste. When an internal orgasm occurs in a part of your body other than your genitals, the practice can be a lot of fun, or it can be very intense. You never know what effect a transferred healing orgasm will have. Sometimes it can be incredibly satisfying, while at other times it can produce experiences you don't like. You might get a sense of the injured area or your entire body melting; this can be quite pleasurable or quite unpleasant. Sometimes you'll have a sense of light filling your body, or expanding outward from the part of your body where you've generated an internal orgasm. Regardless of whether this happens, you're likely to have a strong sense of expanded qi when you trade a normal genital orgasm to make it happen internally within your knee instead.

HEALING QI AND THE LOWER TANTIEN

All sexual practices to heal physical problems are initiated from the lower tantien, which controls the physical energy of the entire body. Regardless of where a bodily injury is located, always start and finish with the lower tantien to make the best use of its strength.

Let's say you have a thyroid problem. While engaged in lovemaking, a man can deliberately project energy from his genitals into his lower tantien and, from there, move it into his throat. Or, while engaged in kissing or oral sex, he can use this same pathway, genitals-tantien-throat, to bring more qi to the thyroid gland. Women, as mentioned in the previous chapter, need to bring energy down to the feet before going upwards to the throat via the tantien. Equally for both sexes during oral sex and intercourse, projecting and concentrating energy into the throat and thyroid increases the normal orgasmic potential. The weakening of qi from any illness diminishes the overall energy flowing through channels. Strong overall body qi produces stronger orgasms, while weak overall qi circulation diminishes either the possibility or the strength of any potential orgasm.

Most qigong practices teach you to stabilize the qi storage capacity of the lower tantien. Spiraling Energy Body Qigong™ in particular, is an advanced program that teaches you to dramatically increase your energy level and master how energy moves in circles and spirals throughout your body (see Chapter 10, "Energy Arts System of Qi Cultivation"). One technique within this qigong form, which should only be learned through live instruction from a master, teaches you to store and project energy from your tantien instantaneously to any place in your body.

When either partner has an internal orgasm, circulate energy around either or both bodies, making sure some of it remains stored in the lower tantien. Before ejaculating, men need to set the pattern of returning qi to the lower tantien, which becomes a storage battery for their energy. You are storing your qi to be used later. Over time, you can gain a clear sense of the storage capacity of your lower tantien and "bank" quite a bit of energy while making love. When you become proficient at storing qi, you'll have an easier time transferring energy from your tantien to a damaged part (or multiple parts) at will. The key is to practice!

INTERNAL ORGASMS IN SPECIFIC LOCATIONS

When applying the techniques of healing through internal orgasms, it's helpful to be aware that some bodily locations are better to practice on initially than others, just as some are best avoided altogether. It is also important to remember to send energy in the right direction depending on who has the injury.

For example, if a woman has an injury in her upper neck, the man would first send energy down from his tantien into her legs and feet. Then he would return qi upward to her injured neck to have an internal orgasm. For a man with the same injury, the woman sends her qi from her lower tantien to the crown of his head and down to his upper neck.

LOCATIONS TO CONSIDER

The following are areas that can be utilized for internal orgasms. They include points where some of the energy gates of the body are to be found (see Figure 14-1).

1. Bai Hui—the point on the crown of the head (A).

2. Ears—anywhere (B).

3. Nipples—including the energy gate halfway toward the breastbone in women (C).

4. Lower tantien—an orgasm here can produce significantly stronger contractions than genital orgasm only. You can get some contractions like you wouldn't believe, often causing the toes to curl (D)!

5. Kwa—not inside it, but the two points near the surface of the skin in the center of the bikini crease (E).

6. Feet—anywhere that is not too ticklish (F).

7. Upper back—anywhere except the area just behind the heart as this is too strong for some, especially those with a heart condition or whose blood pressure is excessively high or low (G).

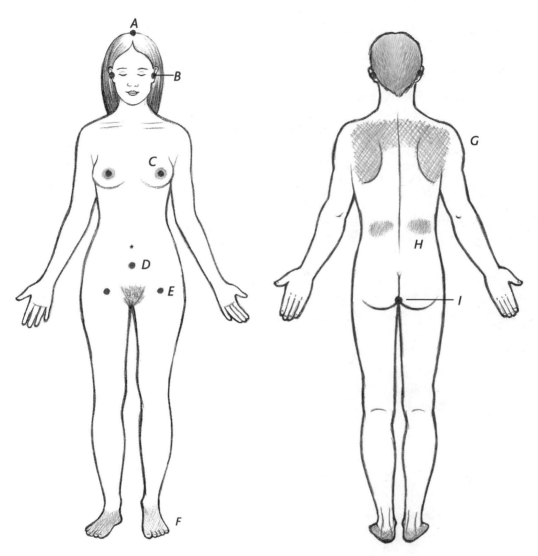

Figure 14–1: Locations of Energy Gates to Utilize for Internal Orgasms

8. Kidney—this organ is directly connected to the overall vitality of the body (H). Stimulating the back of the knee can also activate the kidneys.

9. Anus—not very far up as a related energy gate is maybe only an inch or two in from the entrance to the anus. This benefits the health of your whole digestive system, especially the elimination system for which the anus is the exit point (I).

LOCATIONS TO AVOID

Unless personally directed by a master, internal orgasms should be avoided in the following locations:

1. Brain centers—do not try to use your intent to link and forge an energy channel between any points in your brain that may appear in your awareness. There are over thirty brain centers that in aggregate comprise the upper tantien. Connecting brain centers is one of the most potentially dangerous qi techniques, and one that should only be done under rigorous supervision.

2. Eyeballs—having internal orgasms in the eyeballs can cause weird visual aftereffects (similar to the effect of watching too much television or working on a computer for too many hours) or, in a few cases, even potentially destabilizing visual hallucinations.

3. Heart or pericardium—having internal orgasms in the heart area is best to avoid especially if you have even the slightest possibility of any sort of heart problem. The actual process that causes orgasms to happen in the heart or heart centers involves working only with the middle tantien, which is beyond the scope of this book.

4. Lower back—an internal orgasm may cause people with back problems to gyrate and writhe around, possibly throwing their back out or straining the lower back muscles and ligaments, so use great care in this area.

5. Spinal cord and spine—Taoist masters are exceptionally clear on this point: a practitioner should not attempt to have an orgasm in the spinal cord unless specifically taught this extremely advanced technique in person by a highly qualified master. Orgasms in the spine generally involve intermediate techniques that require guidance from a competent meditation master and should not be attempted by anyone with serious back problems.

6. Liver—if the liver has excessive heat, strong internal orgasms in this area are contraindicated, although you can have very mild ones. Within Traditional Chinese Medicine, a liver that has been taxed by heavy drinking or hepatitis is considered both physically damaged and severely depleted of qi. This leads a person to anger easily or be exceedingly passive-aggressive. Only when an overheated liver is on the mend and the excess heat has radically diminished can a strong orgasm in the liver can be beneficial.

7. Kidney—although normally beneficial, never have an internal orgasm in your kidney if you are exhausted, burned out or tired. The energy you expend will be pulled from your kidneys and eventually weaken your health. The weaker your constitution, the more detrimental this becomes. If you're really exhausted, you're better off getting some rest rather than having sex. Have your lover massage your feet or body then cuddle up and get some sleep.

LOWER BACK PROBLEMS

Cautionary note: Those with back injuries should consult their physician before trying the exercises in this section to make sure that they are appropriate. If anything you are doing makes your pain increase, back off and seek medical advice. This section is included for those who are intermediate or advanced practitioners of sexual qigong and is not for beginners. As stated previously, directing an internal orgasm to the spine should be avoided for those who are new to these practices and for those with serious back pain.

Back pain can make any sexual experience—normal or meditative—unpleasant and possibly even harmful, as pelvic thrusting tends to exacerbate lower back problems. Add to that the psychological stress of a realistic fear that you might hurt yourself, and you have a double whammy. To help address this problem, it's important to become familiar with one of the eight extraordinary channels known as "the great meridian" in acupuncture, the dai mai (see Chapter 9, Figure 9-7).

Rather than worsening the condition with each pelvic thrust, the following procedure may be able to help alleviate lower back pain while making love: Before penetration, either on your own or in some way during foreplay, begin by softening the muscles of the lower back by physically activating the dai mai channel with very gentle circular and rotating pelvic movements. Your movements should be similar to playing with a Hula-Hoop, only smaller (even tiny) and less rigorous. Alternate the motions in both directions.

After penetration, with either partner on top, make very slow and tiny circular motions with your hips and back, both clockwise and counterclockwise. As you do these circular motions, dissolve and move your own and/or your partner's qi from the genitals to your lower tantien, to your dai mai and around this belt in the same direction as your pelvic rotation. Going round and round, transfer energy until you feel your own and/or your partner's weakened or damaged lower-back muscles soften.

Typically, lower-back pain that is primarily muscular in nature (rather than issues involving discs or other problems in the lumbar spine) will negatively affect the kidneys.

Allow the slow movements and circulating qi to work in these two areas of your body so they become very soft and liquid. Have as many internal orgasms as you need here. With your mind, dissolve this area around and around your waist until the muscles around the dai mai and the kidney area turn soft. Keep any gyrating and wiggling motions to a minimum and avoid rapid movements until and unless the muscles around your dai mai and kidneys have become soft. However if you are feeling exhausted, remember that you should avoid targeting internal orgasms in the area of your kidneys.

Cautionary Note: Once you have finished this exercise, only after the involuntary hardening in your muscles has released is it prudent to begin pelvic thrusting, and even then you should do so carefully and think about moving more slowly.

STRATEGY 1: SUBLUXATIONS IN THE VERTEBRAE

This is an intermediate level qigong technique that is not recommended for beginners or anyone with serious back problems. If in doubt, consult your healthcare practitioner before trying this exercise.

As mentioned earlier, it is not advised to attempt to have internal orgasms inside the spinal cord, or any of the structures between the spinal cord and the bones, unless specifically taught in person by a highly qualified master. There are too many important details that must be considered that are beyond the scope of this book.

However, to help resolve back problems associated with badly aligned vertebrae (subluxations) that are pinching nerves, there is a two-part process that can be used, though this is still best undertaken only under the guidance of a master. Spines are delicate things and the following general instructions, although sound, are never guaranteed to fit the needs of specific circumstances. If during your practice, you experience pain that is over and above your normal baseline, stop immediately and seek the advice of a healthcare professional.

Let's say your problem is with three contiguous vertebrae. First, with or without physically moving, circle your energy round and round the dai mai until the muscles influencing the pain near these three vertebrae feel soft. A release in the soft tissue in one area *can* extend to the vertebrae above or below the vertebrae at the specific site of the pain.

Next, build up and have internal orgasms in the painful vertebrae and in the same number above and below those vertebrae. To be specific: if only one vertebra is painful, also direct your internal orgasm only one vertebra above and below the painful one; if two or three vertebrae are in pain, also direct the internal orgasms to two or three vertebrae above and below the painful ones. When the author was in China, he observed that this procedure gave quite good results in relieving back pain.

By having internal orgasms above and below the offending vertebra or vertebrae, your back should progressively soften as the tension and pain starts releasing from the offending vertebrae in the middle. Once you can have internal orgasms in the vertebrae that are causing the pain, you are less likely in an ordinary orgasm to shake or flop like a fish and thereby strain back muscles, ligaments and vertebrae. The failure to address the situation and have sex while "pushing through the pain" is often what prevents people with back pain from getting better.

STRATEGY 2: PUMP YOUR KWA

This strategy is for intermediate and not beginning sexual qigong practitioners. If in doubt, consult your healthcare practitioner before trying this exercise.

While you are building up to an internal orgasm in the spine, continue pulsing your kwa internally, without moving your pelvis. Deliberately move energy from your genitals up and down your spine, from the top of your head to your tailbone, going gently back and forth. Continue moving the energy in your spinal vertebrae regardless of whether or not you have an orgasm. In most cases, this will be immensely helpful for your back.

PAIN MEANS STOP!

As mentioned several times earlier, if you have significant pain, it is best to just stop and not force the situation. Even receiving fellatio is questionable when you have severe back pain. When you combine severe pain with sex, you can cause your nerves to contract and initiate a cascade of negative events. In a worst-case scenario, your back muscles can go into spasm causing the vertebrae to misalign, which may squeeze the discs and compress the nerves in your spine. Searing pain can result.

Severe back pain coupled with sex can pattern your nerves to say, "No!" and set you up for more pain and diminished sexual pleasure downstream. For example, let's say your back is too tender to have intercourse at all, so you consent to letting your lover give you fellatio. There are anatomical connections from the penis to the lower back. Simply having fellatio on an erect penis can pull on and strain the anatomy of the lower back. This can result in pain or potential back destabilization soon thereafter. Many men seeking the pleasure of oral sex will often ignore or not mention this pain to their partners. The contracting nerves may very well leave a residual memory that signals your nerves to contract, which can continue to trigger back pain even after the oral sex is over, sometimes for a day or more.

HEADACHES

A headache can reduce your libido and take you out of the mood to make love. If you or your partner has a headache and you have a way of diminishing it, there's no doubt that lovemaking will become more enjoyable for both of you.

Dragon and Tiger and other forms of medical qigong use the methods described in Practice 28 and Figure 14-2 A–C to help relieve headaches. Both men and women can do this for their lovers. Out of the bedroom, this method can be used on friends and family to release the stresses of the day and to soothe cranky children. You can even do the technique on yourself. It works by pulling stagnant energy either out of your own body or another person and releasing that stagnant qi to the boundary of the etheric body.

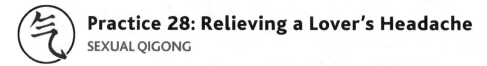

Practice 28: Relieving a Lover's Headache
SEXUAL QIGONG

If you do this technique on your lover, you can tell if it is working in several ways. At the very least you can see or feel the tension release somewhat from your partner's eyes and facial muscles. Then his or her mood may brighten and the headache may lessen in intensity or completely disappear.

1. Rub your palms together until your hands become soft and warm, so that when you touch your partner's head, the warmth of your hands will cause his or her nerves to relax rather than become more tense. You then gently place your palms on the back of your lover's head and forehead so your hands feel from front and back as if they are sinking into his or her head (Figure 14-2 A). You contact the tension within it so it feels like you are holding the headache's tension in your hands. Then you feel, mobilize, loosen and ideally dissolve the stagnant energy within your lover's head.

2. From your rear palm, you push the stagnant qi inside your lover's brain forward. Simultaneously you slightly cup the other hand at the front of his or her head and pull the stagnant qi out of the head into your palm, moving that energy away from your partner's head (Figure 14-2 B).

   An alternate way of doing this part of the technique is to pull the stagnant energy out of your partner's head and into your fingers. Some people find it easier to feel and grab qi with their fingers rather than their palms (Figure 14-2 B1).

3. You point your palms hands away from his or her head and push the stagnant energy out of your palm to the boundary of your lover's etheric body in order to release the stagnant qi as much as you can (Figure 14-2 C).

   A variation on this is to point your fingers away from your partner's head and push or project the stagnant energy out of your fingers to the boundary of his or her etheric body, thereby releasing as much of the stagnant qi as you can (Figure 14-2 C1).

You may need to repeat the entire process shown in Figure 14-2 A–C several times to obtain the maximum benefit. ●

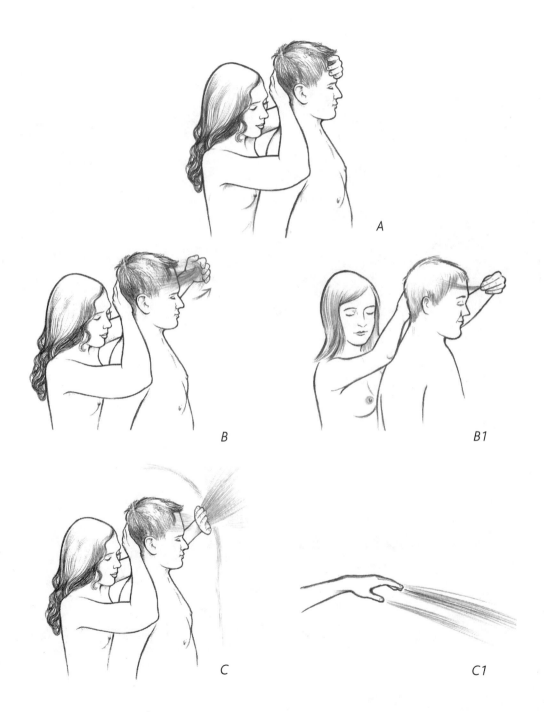

Figure 14-2 A–C: Using Qigong to Relieve a Lover's Headache

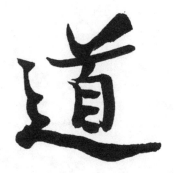

SECTION 5

TAOIST SEXUAL MEDITATION

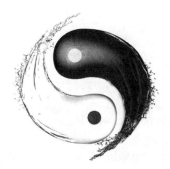

CHAPTER 15

The Inner Dissolving Meditation Method

The living traditions of Taoist meditation have sought from their inception to balance the realities of the human condition—namely, that a Being or soul lives in a temporary physical body and also at the same time has the potential to establish contact with a permanent, directly-experienced spiritual center.

This chapter expands on the Outer Dissolving meditation methods taught within sexual qigong and explains the Inner Dissolving meditation method, which is significantly more powerful. Taoist meditation is primarily concerned with uncovering Universal Consciousness. To that end, Inner Dissolving is applied to the deeper blockages primarily within the third through seventh energy bodies— emotional, mental, psychic, karmic, and essence—which upgrading the energetic system of the body alone cannot resolve.

Chapters 16 and 17 describe the methods through which a practitioner can arrive at the body of individuality, or essence, an advanced stage on the path of Taoist meditation. Chapter 18 describes the ultimate journey, where a Being's essence works towards arriving at the eighth energy body, or the body of the Tao.

A NEW MEDITATION PARADIGM

The words "meditation" and "sex" are not often used in the same sentence or the same context. While the majority of people associate meditation with solo practices, it can be done with a partner through sexual meditation. This book explores a possibility new to the West: using sexual meditation as an accelerated spiritual path.

The methods of spiritual development in sexual meditation empower a couple to embark on a unique journey, beginning with enhancing the physical, emotional, mental and spiritual parts of themselves so that they can be at home in their ever-changing physical body and circumstances. These ancient Taoist sexual meditation practices enable couples to energetically merge and, eventually, move outward together as one, past all corporeal limitations, to dissolve whatever blockages are encountered until either or both partners can realize and fully merge with the Tao.

Using the Inner Dissolving methods in this chapter, partners can learn to release deep blockages and inner "demons" in their energy bodies, until they can reach the level of awareness that brings them to the heart-mind (see Chapter 5, "Connecting to the Heart-Mind"). They gain access to new dimensions that may have never before been available.

Once the deeper blockages are released, energy flows more freely and dormant capacities within each of the partners' eight energy bodies activate and begin to come alive. Surprising new aptitudes and faculties emerge. This upgrades the essential energy anatomy of the body and is the outcome that dedicated practitioners of sexual meditation move toward.

During this meditation path, every aspect of your experience is enriched until you are brought fully present in the moment, connected to the earth and resting with an open heart.

SEXUAL ENERGY TO ACCELERATE MEDITATION

We all want to evolve and grow, and most would like to see this happen at a relatively fast pace. The truth is that most people simply lack sufficient excess energy reserves to resolve the deeper spiritual blockages in the higher energy bodies, or to even to resolve the blocks in the lower five bodies. If a person lacks sufficient energy to bring to the situation, they flirt with the inner blockages rather than work through them to full resolution.

A common pattern for those doing deeper spiritual work is to back off when the energy within a blockage hits a certain vibratory pitch or when they stand at a precipice that is uncomfortable or perceived as dangerous. When this happens, a person may approach the same block hundreds of times, without ever fully releasing and resolving the stuck energy within it, even though he or she may want it resolved. This is why people develop calcified personality structures, repeatedly struggling with the same unresolved issues. This can occur lifetime after lifetime until the person resolves the block, and during these lifetimes they often will have formed even more blocks that require resolution. Thus the cycle of conscious evolution unfolds very slowly. The Taoists found that by using the energy of sexual meditation and working with a partner, what initially might seem like an insurmountable blockage could be resolved much more quickly than in any other manner.

ACCESSING FOUR TIMES THE ENERGY FOR MEDITATION

The easiest way to understand the power of sexual meditation is by looking at the amount of energy that is available during lovemaking to apply to qigong and meditation practice. In all Taoist practices, the amount of energy a person can bring to bear on a blockage at any point ranges from one to four. During Taoist solo practices such as qigong or sitting meditation and even with moving practices such as tai chi as meditation or spiritual martial arts, a practitioner has just one unit of energy available to work with and direct toward his or her blockages.

But there is another possibility. Two practitioners who fully engage in Inner Dissolving sexual meditation practices can access to up to four units of energy each. In other words, one plus one does not equal two, but rather each partner can individually have up to four times the amount of energy to apply to blockages in the energy bodies. This can dramatically accelerate the path of meditation.

The following is an energetic progression in the context of solo and dual cultivation (partner) practices:

1 Unit of Energy: If one partner does sexual qigong within himself or herself, but the other does not, the practitioner will energize and develop his or her own subtle qi significantly more than with ordinary sex. This can result in a dramatically better experience for both, because sex will become more alive and satisfying.

1 to 2 Units of Energy: If both partners practice sexual qigong, the energies inside both their bodies will be activated and developed to a much greater extent. This can generate more qi than either partner could access by doing any sort of solo subtle energy practice

2 Units of Energy: If only one partner practices sexual meditation and is capable of Inner Dissolving on both his or her own body and that of a partner, then the practitioner can get twice the energy that is available from meditating alone. Again, the non-practitioner stands to benefit because the sex will become more alive and satisfying. As an added bonus, the non-practitioner can benefit from being relieved of blockages in the first four or five energy bodies (physical, qi, emotional, mental and possibly psychic), which can result in significant improvement in his or her quality of life.

4 Units of Energy: If both partners practice sexual meditation together and simultaneously use Inner Dissolving, each individual partner will have access to four times the energy they would be able to access meditating alone. (see Chapter 17, "The Magic Moment: Experiencing the Essence of Another").

Three Levels of Taoist Meditation

There are three primary ways that Taoist or any other form of meditation is normally practiced, especially in the West. Although this information may seem very basic, often people think they are doing meditation for spiritual growth, when in fact they are not. Each higher level of meditation requires a progressively greater commitment of time and energy:

1. For the purpose of stress relief. The covers the majority of meditation that is taught in West and is the most common reason why people begin and practice meditation. This requires practicing between five minutes and thirty minutes a day.

2. For the purpose of achieving inner peace. To accomplish this, real commitment, connection to a teacher from an authentic lineage and comprehensive teachings are needed to maximize anyone's chances of success. This will often require dedicating at least an hour a day to not just a practice but to a proven time-tested meditation system.

3. For the purpose of achieving enlightenment. This is quite often a multi-lifetime journey that becomes the primary aim for more advanced souls on the planet or those who live in spiritual communities. When this becomes the main directive in a person's life, practitioners will dedicate much of their day to doing meditation in its many forms. All the practices of advanced Taoist sexual meditation fall into this category.

PRELIMINARIES TO SEXUAL MEDITATION

All methods of Taoist practices exist along a seamless continuum. Each new stage of development on the path is built on energetic proficiencies acquired in earlier stages of practice. You can start at different places on the path—healing, martial arts, general health practices and sex—however you will eventually need to master certain fundamental skills to achieve the higher potentials of the Taoist path. No matter where you start, no stage on the path can be skipped, and the required abilities cannot be feigned. Before a serious practitioner can actually engage in the more advanced sexual meditation methods in a meaningful way, the following five foundations must be in place.

1. Practitioners must have a reasonable ability to perform the basic methods that Taoists prescribe for ordinary sex. Lack of skill, sensitivity and endurance on the physical level would make it impossible for the practices that sexual meditation

requires. Specifically, men in the early learning period must be able to maintain an erection for a bare minimum of fifteen to twenty minutes and preferably longer (see Chapter 8, "Classic Taoist Techniques for Prolonging Sex").

2. It is essential that both partners have arrived at a place where they have acquired emotional stability. It is not uncommon in meditation practices to lose the distinct boundaries between you and your partner. The primal bedrock of the ego structure—a sense of the self as a separate being, which provides a sense of psychological security and identity—can readily be shaken. When the inner structures that bind the ego begin to loosen, enormous eruptions and challenges can occur. This is why a significant amount of emotional stability is a prerequisite. In the long run, the ego's power to induce suffering and imbalance will lessen, but in the short run, eruptions can be disruptive, unsettling and at times have the potential to be completely overwhelming.

3. Practitioners must be competent at sexual qigong (or some parallel energy system) and be able to open up the body's internal energy structure to arrive at the launch point for sexual meditation. They must be able to:

   • Direct both partners' qi to anywhere in the energy bodies of either partner (including all relevant energy channels, points and centers, especially the lower, middle and upper tantiens) as well as being able to use this ability for a multitude of specific ends.

   • Recognize experientially if either partner has energetic blockages within the first four energy bodies (physical, qi, emotional and mental) and use Outer Dissolving to resolve those blockages.

   • Ascertain the effectiveness of their dissolving practice; that is, upon conclusion of Outer Dissolving they should be able to discern whether an energetic blockage has been fully resolved, partially resolved, or not affected at all.

4. Practitioners must be able to do the Inner Dissolving method described in this chapter. Generally a practitioner first learns Inner Dissolving while sitting. Then, in sexual meditation, the Inner Dissolving method becomes an engine to consciously and deliberately move qi within the first through sixth energy bodies (physical, qi, emotional, mental, psychic and karmic).

5. Practitioners must be able to recognize the energetic blockages that reside within their first six energy bodies, and can use either Outer or Inner Dissolving to resolve these blockages either partially or in full.

As practitioners move from one level to the next, they will often circle back to previous levels, continually making sure that their foundation remains solid.

LAOZI'S INNER DISSOLVING MEDITATION METHOD

The Inner Dissolving meditation method is the core practice within Laozi's Water branch of Taoist sexual meditation and is a yin rather than yang meditation approach. Inner Dissolving works on resolving all blockages, but is particularly useful in addressing the fifth up to the eighth energy body.

The Outer and Inner Dissolving methods are different in both aim and result.

The primary purpose of sexual qigong and Outer Dissolving is to develop physical health and strength and the mental capacities that derive from them. To achieve this, Outer Dissolving releases trapped energy externally away from the body. The result of this energetic healing is a better-functioning body as qi flows freely through areas that were previously restricted or blocked. As more qi flows, you work to develop dramatically more energetic sensitivity and the ability to direct qi much more accurately within yourself and your partner.

Sexual meditation, in contrast, is primarily concerned with helping you achieve Universal Consciousness. The Inner Dissolving meditation method uses the energy trapped within blockages as fuel for moving into unbound "inner space," ultimately imploding dissolved energy to the internal empty core of your Being where pure Consciousness resides.

Inner Dissolving uses energy trapped within blockages as fuel to move into unbound "inner space," ultimately imploding dissolved energy to the empty core of your Being where pure Consciousness resides.

THE PROCESS OF INNER DISSOLVING

For thousands of years, the Chinese have described the Inner Dissolving meditation process with the phrase "ice to water to inner space." Inner Dissolving is extremely effective for resolving the deeply buried, temporary and long-term emotional, mental and psychic stresses that can take the joy out of life. Through Inner Dissolving, your mind penetrates the defined clumps of frozen energies that make up your deepest blockages until they become relaxed, amorphous and flowing.

This part of the process is called "ice to water," just as it is in the first two stages of Outer Dissolving. The unbound energy can now go about its natural function, part of which is helping to heal whatever potential ailments the original blockage may have caused. Once the energy is flowing, you move your mind deeper and deeper inside your energy field and consciousness, dissolving through layer after layer, until you trace the energy back to its source.

You follow and let the dissolved energy open a door within a door within a door, leading you deeper and deeper into the inner space at the point where you began dissolving. You then implode each layer of energy inward into that point, however far the source extends within your higher energy bodies. In the final step, you reach a place where the blockage originates and its blocked energy fully releases into emptiness and naturally dissipates or comes to a stop.

This process may proceed very slowly—the amount of time it takes cannot be specified. Depending on your individual nature, you might experience this endpoint as a complete yin or yang energy. Yang may be experienced as a feeling or vision of light. Yin may be experienced as a sense of unbound fluidity, calmness, peace, mind expansion, infinite space or emptiness.

When you find yourself at that deep place, you then rest within that endpoint and, over time, develop the ability to return to that spot through all the layers of your energy at will, and especially in the midst of life's most stressful and difficult situations. Eventually, by dissolving deeply enough into any one spot, sooner or later, you will end up at emptiness, which is the doorway to Universal Consciousness.

YIN AND YANG QUALITIES OF INNER DISSOLVING

Taoism does not aim for a philosophical ideal of physical or psychological androgyny, whereby the yin and yang characteristics of each sex are blended beyond recognition. Rather, the aim is to liberate the full range of yin and yang that naturally occurs in a man and woman, through the practice of Inner Dissolving.

Regardless of how a blockage diminishes or is released through either Outer or Inner Dissolving, it always has a yin and a yang side. The originating energetic or external event that caused the blockage could be either yin or yang. Once you have a blockage, it can express itself in yin and yang ways as regards both your outward behavior and your innermost thoughts and feelings.

For example, in both men and women, some deep emotional hurt, with the same cause, could be expressed outwardly with raging anger or inwardly with extreme passivity, powerlessness or depression. Although, in general, men express yang emotions more easily and women yin emotions more easily, there are always exceptions. When a blockage resolves into emptiness through Inner Dissolving, often both men and women find they can express the less dominant yin or yang side of themselves more easily and effortlessly. Inner Dissolving practices helps people get in touch with both their dominant and non-dominant natures.

The yin-yang symbol always has yang within yin and yin within yang. When a blockage resolves, it allows a smoother flow between yin and yang in both directions. Further, it diminishes the pain and limitations of excessive polarization.

Men and women with different personality types mix yin and yang uniquely. There is no set way the mixing happens because each individual morphs, changes and evolves in stages on the way to becoming more spiritually awake. Women who resolve yin or yang within themselves could express it in a more yang feminine way, or just as easily, in an even more yin feminine manner. Likewise men could express resolved yin or yang in a more yin masculine way or in an even more direct yang masculine manner.

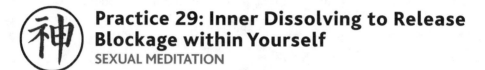 ## Practice 29: Inner Dissolving to Release Blockage within Yourself
SEXUAL MEDITATION

1. Scan your body to find a blockage to work with, such as one in your neck as shown in Figure 15-1 A.

2. Use the Inner Dissolving method of "ice to water to inner space" to move from the outside to the inside center of the blockage (Figure 15-1 B).

3. Go deeper and deeper into the inner space of the blockage (Figure 15-1 C).

4. If you can, continue until the blockage begins to resolve into emptiness. It may release inner light from the movement into emptiness (Figure 15-1 D).

5. If you reach a successful conclusion working with this blockage, it will fully release into emptiness. Among many potential experiences at this point is a complete release of silent vibration or inner light, which can fill your entire body from the inside (Figure 15-1 E). ●

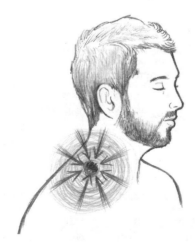

Figure 15-1 A: Visual Representation of the Inner Dissolving Process

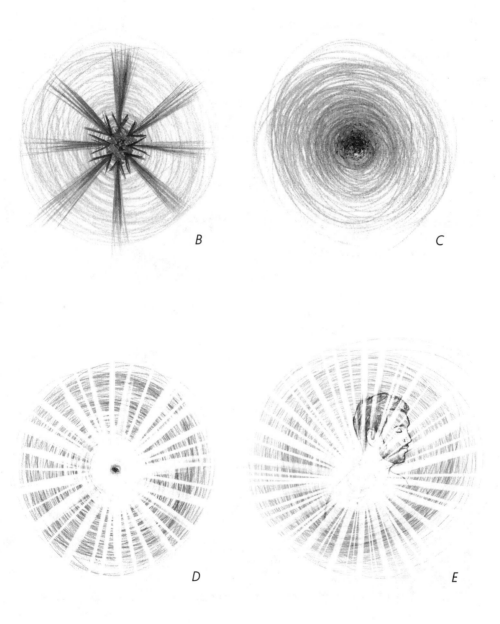

Figure 15-1 B–E: Visual Representation of the Inner Dissolving Process

Why There Are More Male Than Female Spiritual Adepts

Initiates in many (although not all) Taoist priesthood communities would receive instruction and guidance from elders of both genders. Even so, historically, there have been many more men among the elders than women. Taoists are not unusual in this respect; at higher levels of accomplishment, men outnumber women in virtually every major spiritual tradition. This doesn't mean that the option to awaken isn't equally available to women—it certainly is, if they are willing to take up the arduous discipline required.

Taoism has examples of women making the climb up the spiritual ladder. For instance, in Taoism, the Eight Spiritual Immortals have a prominent place. One of these was a woman, He Qiong, also known as He Xiangu. She took a vow to remain a virgin and never had a family.

A more recent female Taoist of note was Sun Bu-Er, a wealthy married woman who lived in the twelfth century C.E. After raising her children, she took up Taoism later in life and became a Taoist Immortal. Her poetry has become part of Taoist classical literature.

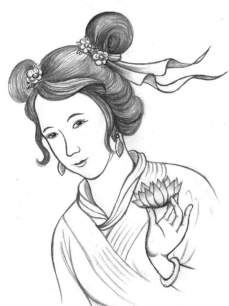

Figure 15-2: He Xiangu, one of the Eight Spiritual Immortals of Taoism.

In *Passionate Enlightenment: Women in Tantric Buddhism*, Miranda Shaw gives many examples of female adepts in the Tantric tradition. She writes, "Although parts of the historical record of women in Tantric Buddhism have been lost and erased, there is sufficient evidence to show that this was a movement in which women actively taught and freely introduced new practices, deities and insights that they discovered in their meditations."[1]

---

1. Shaw, Miranda, *Passionate Enlightenment: Women in Tantric Buddhism* (Princeton, NJ: Princeton University Press, 1994), 198.

In both ancient India and China it was a potentially dangerous undertaking for women to take on the role of a wandering seeker of spiritual knowledge as was commonly done by men. They could easily be assaulted, captured, sold into slavery or killed. To mitigate this problem, many wandering Taoist women became extremely skilled sword masters which relieved them of the need for male protection and afforded them freedom of movement.

On the spiritual journey, perseverance is mandated for accomplishment. Success requires prolonged work and an immense amount of personal drive derived from a specific aspect of yang energy. The doggedness and the sheer ability to keep going forward, no matter what, comes more naturally to men because of the preponderance of yang energy in their physical biology. A woman's biology, in contrast, tends to have a preponderance of yin energy, and her fierceness is more likely to be catalyzed by a threat to her children or tribe than by personal or spiritual aspirations. A man may forsake his wife and children to go meditate in a cave. A woman would be much less likely to give up her family to pursue her own spiritual development. Generally, yang is dramatically more goal-oriented than yin, which serves a man well on the steep, upward climb toward enlightenment. Nevertheless, the ordinary worldly drive for success is completely different from the often soul-wrenching work that is part of the rigorous spiritual-development process, where no one can validate you except yourself.

Often, the typical discussion about men and women having more yin or yang in their personality is conducted with minimal understanding of the universal energies involved. A direct encounter with these unmistakable forces within creation is in itself a rare attainment. In this context, whether a woman has a psychologically yin or yang personality is less important than whether or not she has a naturally arising and sustaining yang drive toward spiritual evolution.

This quality is normally present at birth and, according to the Taoists, related to karmic factors. Women who do possess the required staying power for the spiritual path are likely to have been born with an innate yang drive to begin with and then, from that higher baseline, have gone on to develop their tenacity and determination. These women often become leaders in a wide variety of worldly arenas, including business, politics, the arts and athletics. In the past it has been rare for them to take their talents into the spiritual field, especially when in their youth—however this too may change in the future.

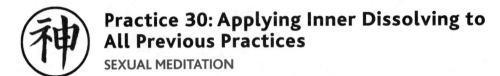

Practice 30: Applying Inner Dissolving to All Previous Practices
SEXUAL MEDITATION

When you first begin Inner Dissolving, it is recommended that you practice it within solo sitting meditation where it is easiest to learn. Once you have learned the process of Inner Dissolving meditation in solo practices, then you can revisit *all* the previous sexual qigong practices in this book that you did with Outer Dissolving and repeat them using Inner Dissolving. This will help you use Inner Dissolving with what you already know, so it will be easier to integrate the Inner Dissolving process into those practices. This is an important building block and should not be skipped. Only when you have completed all previous practices up to this point with Inner Dissolving, that is, through Practice 28, should you move on to the more advanced methods of using Inner Dissolving. ●

STAGES OF INNER DISSOLVING

Inner Dissolving meditation has many different variations that you can use, depending on your skill level, your partner and the specific practice. The method involves a number of specific abilities that are learned progressively over time, so that the partners can:

- Dissolve only themselves, only the other person, or each other simultaneously.

- Link to each other's energies, up to and culminating with their central channels. Dissolve until both lovers can effectively remove the blockages that prevent them from recognizing their essence in the seventh energy body.

- Create a combined neo-central channel between them.

- Pulse the neo-central channel equally in both directions (that is, going deeper inside into inner space and externally into outer space) until the pulsing of the neo-central channel creates a sphere of energy between and around both lovers, the boundary of which is the edge of the etheric body of the neo-central channel. This neo-central channel sphere can be much larger than the auras that the individual practitioners would normally have.

- Pulse the neo-central channel to move equally inward and outward toward the end of the universe, without regard to the billions of galaxies that lie in the middle. While this cosmic pulsing is done, everything that is contacted with Inner Dissolving is released into emptiness.

Once a practitioner reaches this point, he or she is approaching the culmination of all forms of meditation in the Taoist tradition. Having contacted, linked to and cleared all there is, from big to small and, simultaneously, recognized and merged with all there is, he or she achieves the body of the Tao. The rare practitioner who reaches this stage earns the title "Spiritual Immortal" alongside, for example, Laozi, Zuangzi, and the author's teacher, Liu Hung Chieh.

CONNECTING WITH THE MINDSTREAM

Many meditation traditions refer to a state of consciousness called "the witness," an aspect of awareness that simply observes whatever is arising with equanimity, free from judgment. This function allows the content of experience to come and go, while the awareness always maintains an unshakable observing quietude. To reach and maintain this state is a significant accomplishment for a meditation practitioner. However, in Taoism, the witnessing mind is only the beginning of developing higher states of consciousness.

As you become more familiar with the process of being aware of awareness itself, you may also begin to sense a deeper and even more subtle stream that pervades your awareness. This is the Mindstream, the contact point that eventually leads you to Universal Consciousness itself. According to most, if not all, the world's mystic traditions, the Mindstream is naturally present in all living creatures.

This Mindstream is quite distinct from the motion of mind that drives the familiar flow of constantly arising thoughts that jump from one to the next.

Unless explicitly sought and given full attention, the Mindstream usually remains hidden for the majority of human beings and even for most meditators. Ordinary awareness is so preoccupied with external events that this subtle but important connection to the water of life is lost.

Once discovered, however, you begin to discern incredibly subtle phenomena as you develop deeper levels of awareness, layer-by-layer and shade-by-shade, gradually uncovering and revealing all the previously hidden content within your first seven energy bodies. Part of the uncovering at the level of the Mindstream is to become directly present to the energy of all your karma. This can be both extremely liberating and terrifying.

As you apply the Outer and Inner Dissolving methods to your deepest physical, mental, emotional, psychic and karmic tensions, you will enter intermittent periods of stillness and emptiness during which your innermost tensions disappear for progressively longer periods. You then experience periods of peace and clarity that penetrate right to the core of your Being. It is at this point that most practitioners begin to consciously experience the Mindstream, which usually initially appears in vague or fuzzy ways.

Profoundly nourishing to the mind, body and soul, such fleeting episodes of the Mindstream will come and go, but each interlude will deliver you to a clearer, more relaxed inner place from which you subsequently fully engage in life. Each encounter with stillness leads to more awareness and new qualities of the Mindstream, as progressively clarity emerges with respect to the spiritual state of your various energy bodies. This is how the intricate developmental process of spiritual awakening unfolds.

Making Space for a Regular Sexual Meditation Practice

In our busy world, many find it difficult to set up a regular practice, yet this is one of the keys to becoming a successful meditator. This is critically important when you practice solo sitting meditation, just as it is central in sexual meditation with a partner. If setting up a fairly regular schedule seems impossible at first, redouble your efforts, compromise if you have to, and do whatever is necessary to pull it off.

If it still proves impossible to keep a regular schedule, get creative and find ways to make each sexual meditation encounter connect and build from the previous one. This continuity is important, as it reinforces the energetic bonding, allowing your practice to grow as strong as possible.

Adjusting to life's irregularities is a high art. In today's ever-accelerating world, adaptability is essential if you want to find and maintain any measure of internal stability and stillness. Find some way to set aside a regular practice time until you and your partner reach the point of being able to easily dissolve each other, anytime, anywhere, with or without sex.

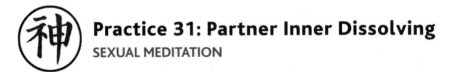

Practice 31: Partner Inner Dissolving
SEXUAL MEDITATION

A bare-bones sexual meditation practice would involve these three procedures after you dissolve any energies of third parties hanging around both of you (see Practice 33 and Figure 15-3 A–D):

1. Initially, while in bed, flesh to flesh, use the Inner Dissolving method to dissolve each other. As your experience in bed together grows, you can extend the experience of Inner Dissolving to include times when the two of you are alone and just hanging out, without being overtly sexual. Regardless of anything else that might be happening, continuously develop your ability to link at deeper and deeper energetic levels. Without touching, dissolve the blockages you encounter, both in yourself and your partner.

2. With stubborn blockages—those that arise with such strong energy that they take

many sessions of Inner Dissolving to resolve—work with the blocked energy in between your regular sexual practice periods, possibly using solo or moving meditation. The key to this procedure, either alone or with a partner, is to immediately work with and resolve the energy whenever it arises spontaneously in the flow of daily life.

3. When the energy of that blockage comes up, time allowing, sit across from each other without touching and attempt to dissolve the energetic glitches around the issue for either or both of you. This practice of sitting across from or next to each other in between regular sexual practice periods is especially useful for major blockages that otherwise might take weeks or months to resolve or might never be completely dissolved. ●

TEN WAYS TO USE INNER DISSOLVING

Laozi's Inner Dissolving meditation method can be used to work through many different types of blockages in relation to sex. It can also be used to release positive emotions that have lain dormant or been repressed in your life or over many lifetimes. Here are ten ways you can use Inner Dissolving meditation:

1. AN ANTIDOTE TO SPIRITUAL STRESS AND DEEP REPRESSIONS

The Inner Dissolving methods of sexual meditation have a great innate capacity to release deeply blocked energies and repressions in the higher energy bodies—psychic, karmic and essence—and to ultimately clear what lies between you and the Tao itself. Releasing repressed pleasure in the higher energy bodies can commonly create dramatically greater joy and bliss during sex.

Although overcoming blockages through Inner Dissolving meditation is extremely liberating, the middle ground between starting and full resolution can be quite difficult and disconcerting. The potential emotional and psychic pain encountered during Inner Dissolving can lead to a strong resistance to dealing with what has been repressed. Feeling this pain can often weaken the perseverance needed to successfully follow through and resolve blockages. Bliss derived from Inner Dissolving partner practices can counteract the drudgery and deep internal resistance needed to dissolve difficult blockages.

One major reason for the resistance that a person encounters on his or her spiritual path is the strong negative energy stored within the blockages that often contain energetic strands from many sources, such as childhood abuse, long-term negative conditioning, birth trauma and severe karmic issues. Encountering these difficult blockages during solo meditation can create insurmountable internal resistance that leads to a cascade of unsatisfactory resolutions and postponements that are perpetuated for much longer than they need be.

Using pleasure to overcome internal resistance is one of the reasons why doing either Outer Dissolving or Inner Dissolving with a sexual partner can be a less arduous meditation journey. Sexual partners can help each other overcome the grimness of dissolving difficult blockages. They will be able to use the highs of the joy and bliss to help them get through the lows of working through a blockage's difficult content. They can encourage and support each other to get to the source of a blockage and stay with it long enough to successfully resolve it.

In many Fire methods of Taoism and other traditions, joy is engineered by visualization methods and ramping up the qi of the energy channels, glands and emotions, however this can be short-lived. Water method practitioners progressively and increasingly gain these qualities by releasing their blockages through Inner Dissolving. As they stabilize, integrate and balance the growing feelings of joy inside themselves and each other, emptiness emerges as a joined and natural quality in their consciousness.

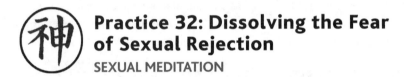

Practice 32: Dissolving the Fear of Sexual Rejection
SEXUAL MEDITATION

For many people, the fear of sexual rejection is a big blockage that has solidified within various energy bodies. This blockage makes a good starting practice after you have learned Inner Dissolving. This can be done alone in sitting meditation or with a partner during sexual meditation.

Rather than feed the fear of thinking about sexual rejection, follow the energy that fear generates back to its source inside you. While meditating, dissolve the roots of every sexual rejection you've ever experienced. Stay the course and you can eventually reach a relaxed point internally where it's genuinely okay that you were rejected. Dissolve through every present or past sexual rejection until you arrive at the emptiness space that has no beginning or end. This method of developing nonattachment through total immersion can be applied to many of life's most primal fears as well as other emotions. ●

2. ELIMINATE "GHOSTS" IN THE BEDROOM

After thousands of years of experimentation, the Taoists have concluded only the rare couple can withstand the complexities of a completely open relationship for any length of time. Intellectually, it may be a wonderful ideal, but, as a practical matter, the Taoists have found that it is not terribly wise. As the Taoist would say, "Don't bring any ghosts home with you." It is best to not bring the energy of other sexual involvements into the bed you share with your primary partner, or any other partner for that matter.

The main point and guiding rule of all practices in this book is to be fully present to each encounter, so that no secret part of you is with the ghost, memory, or fantasy of another lover. If you are pair-bonded with a spouse, or a steady boyfriend or girlfriend, and you choose to be sexual with someone outside that relationship, it is incumbent on you to clear the energy of that encounter out of your system upon completion. You want to make sure that there is no bonding residue with this third party at any level—physical, emotional or psychic—that can enter your primary relationship through your energy field or your mind.

To accomplish this, practitioners of sexual meditation intentionally, even habitually, use Inner and Outer Dissolving to totally and completely clear the energy of another lover after the sexual encounter. This is accomplished by dissolving inside yourself and, if you can, within the other as well. You want to avoid carrying the sexual energy forward into whatever comes next in the flow of your life. This is quite the opposite of what many typically do: savor a past sexual experience, using the memory and energy of an encounter to shore up sexual self-esteem or to stay somewhat turned on.

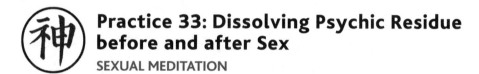

Practice 33: Dissolving Psychic Residue before and after Sex
SEXUAL MEDITATION

This practice is for both couples who are monogamous and for those who are non-monogamous. It involves clearing the psychic residue before sex and then using the time after to continue the dissolving process.

If monogamous, this practice can make every sexual encounter completely new. It relieves the all-too-common problem of sexual boredom and mitigates any tendency toward possessiveness or desperation. Moreover, releasing many—if not all—of the energetic blockages within either of you enables you to truly see one another, rather than look through the filters of habit. Rather than a stagnant energy field that limits the relationship, you effectively allow the waters of life to flow through both of you, keeping the relationship buoyant and happy.

If non-monogamous, this practice will help you develop discernment and recognize the difference between sexual curiosity and real sexual pleasure—two very different worlds. In time, it will enhance your ability to recognize and connect with the rare individuals with whom you can form a deep, ongoing relationship, whether or not you decide to have children together. Even in the sexually-free Western world, many enter into long-term relationships simply because they are lonely and find someone who will put up with them. Rare are the pairings in which two people genuinely connect and fit together on multiple levels.

Here are the four steps to do this Inner Dissolving practice:

1. If you are in a monogamous relationship, simply dissolve any psychic residue from any people or events in the day. If you are non-monogamous, you may need to focus on the energy of another lover that you need to fully release. If this is so, both partners dissolve them until they are gone and it's just the two of you (Figure 15-3 A).

2. The two of you, and only the two of you make love in all the ways you wish (Figure 15-3 B).

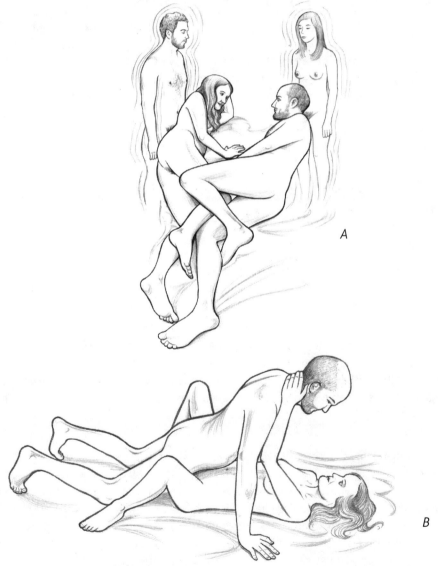

A

B

Figure 15-3 A–B: Dissolving Previous Lovers to Prevent Ghosts in the Bedroom

3. After you are done, the two of you dissolve each other and release the energy of the other and your attachment, so the next time you can sexually experience each other in a fresh, renewed way (Figure 15-3 C).

4. Lie, and cuddle and rest in each other. Enjoy your empathy together as you continue to meditate (Figure 15-3 D).

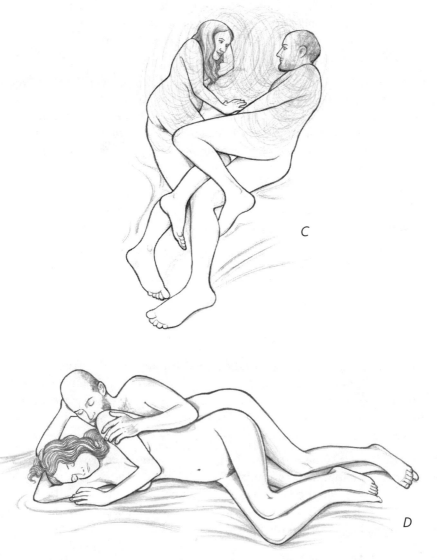

Figure 15-3 C–D: Dissolving Previous Lovers to Prevent Ghosts in the Bedroom

A critical part of this practice is that immediately after making love, you should sit or lie next to your partner and meditate. Start within yourself and dissolve all the physical energetic bindings of your first two energy bodies—physical and qi. These are the attachments that leave the physical body hungry for the other.

If the other person is a practitioner, he or she will do the same. If not, do your best to do this for both of you, even though the other may not be aware (or even need to know) this is occurring. It takes two to form an attachment. If the energy inside you is dissolved, it is significantly more difficult for the other person to form an attachment. The point is to remove any energetic residue that you may have left inside your partner as well as whatever energetic residue that person may have left in you. In effect, this brings you both back to the state that you were in prior to lovemaking.

Next, use the Inner Dissolving method on all the psychic residue and attachments in the higher bodies. Especially pay attention to releasing the karmic bonds between the two of you. Release and resolve every residual energetic connection to the best of your ability. Remember: intent goes a long way. Your aim is for everything that occurred during lovemaking to be converted back into energy, Spirit and emptiness. This has a number of beneficial effects from the Taoist point of view.

This isn't to say you shouldn't maintain a level of human caring and affection for a non-pair-bonded lover, you most definitely should if possible. It is very possible to be sexual friends with someone and genuinely share deep love without being "in love" with him or her.

In Taoist sexual meditation, this practice is highly recommended for married or committed couples, whether monogamous or not. After making love, one or both will dissolve the energy of what just happened. This makes it possible for the energy between you to be vibrant and fresh the next time you come together. ●

3. CONNECT TO THE SHEER JOY OF LIFE

Sexual meditation is designed to take a practitioner into the pure awareness and profound levels of consciousness that lie beyond ordinary dimensions. Such states have been given many names in spiritual literature, and the experience of them is magnificent. However, at the end of the day, they are simply what remain once blockages are resolved.

Our very nature is to be ecstatic and fully alive, connected with a profound inner wellspring of happiness and bliss. What's more, Taoist meditation practice nourishes an ability to be present with whatever arises. Once the internal burdens that energetically bind us are free, we can experience the sheer joy of life, independent of any external cause or circumstance.

4. UNDERSTAND THE KARMA OF RELATIONSHIPS

From the Taoist perspective, karma goes on a long time, and human beings are free to find out what relationships are all about. Different seasons bring different lessons. To become a free individual, each being has to work out and go beyond the yin-yang polarity—in this life or in another. When a relationship no longer suits you, it's best to break smoothly rather than with hatred and venom. Preserve any good human feelings that you had with the person rather than destroy them.

Taoists also emphasize the importance of noticing the qualities of your relationships as they develop rather than only after they have formed. Take note of the nature of any relationship and be aware of how it impacts your consciousness. Particularly pay attention to whether or not you can spiritually grow with a person. Always keep in mind that how you handle yourself with respect to another can result in your inner world either contracting or evolving.

To fully evolve and become free is an immense challenge, one the meditation tradition of Taoism holds is worth the effort and time it takes to see to the end.

5. RESOLVE THE FEAR OF DEATH AND THE FEAR OF LIFE

Relinquishing the attachment to sexuality as a primary feature of one's identity has benefits beyond daily life. Upon death, as the Spirit separates from the flesh, a Being can go through a rather disturbing period in which the mind and Spirit remain powerfully attached to the memory of the physical body. This is part of the natural process of moving from one incarnation to the next. During this transition a fixation on the desires of the now-deceased physical body can affect how and where you go next. Through Inner Dissolving you can develop a sense of peace about death, knowing that who you are is a soul or Being inhabiting a body.

The other side of being afraid to die is that many people are just as afraid to engage fully with life. Although not conscious of the fact, many in bed don't fully engage sexually, because the fear of death is always present in the background. Sexual meditation and Inner Dissolving can lead someone past the fear of death and bring him or her into a genuine appreciation and willingness to engage not just with sex but with life itself.

6. RESOLVE CURRENT AND PAST LIFE TRAUMA

The interconnected web that creates and sustains a blockage includes everything that effectively keeps us involuntarily separated from others, our essence and the Tao. Resolving energy blockages is a complex endeavor in which perceiving the fabric that weaves us all together is a major key. Unambiguously necessary to this endeavor is the ability to face old traumas and the impact they have on our human relations.

Trauma exists and solidifies as tangible energetic blockages within the human energy system, regardless of whether these are related to current or past life events. Such traumas occur in every form imaginable. Whether through a sexual, physical, mental, emotional or psychic injury or assault, traumas leave residual blockages in the first six energy bodies. These take away the joy of living, decrease our awareness, condition us and cloud our view of life. Traumatic events are always linked to a particular setting and circumstance, some more extreme than others.

Natural disasters (such as earthquakes, violent storms or tsunamis), famine, disease and war, as well as oppressive dictatorships and utterly inhumane governments—all can leave residual trauma in one or more of the subtle energy bodies. Throughout time humans have shown themselves to be capable of very nasty and evil actions—experiencing these in this lifetime or previous ones often creates major blockages in our energy bodies. Relational traumas such as overly prolonged anger, frustration, grief or depression, a ruptured bond with one's mother at birth, suicide of someone close, a breach of trust with a primary caregiver, or outright betrayal by a deeply entwined associate or lover can also leave a residue in the form of stuck, blocked and frozen energy.

Taoism, along with a number of Eastern spiritual traditions, recognizes that unresolved trauma—whether from a current life or from one or several past lives—can and does continue to play itself out in real time. These unresolved traumas can play havoc with a sexual relationship. Karmic replays of past patterns can be resolved during sexual meditation with Inner Dissolving.

7. EXPERIENCE TRUE PARTNER MERGING

Through Inner and Outer Dissolving, Taoists discovered they could directly merge with the consciousness of another person who was also a sexual meditation practitioner. The Taoist Inner Dissolving practices make it possible to experience what your "other half" is actually experiencing within his or her body, energy and Spirit. This goes way beyond the romantic idea of physical and emotional merging.

Imagine being able to actually directly feel what your lover is experiencing inside his or her body, energy and Spirit. You directly experience what your unconscious inner male (for a woman) or inner woman (for a man) is actually like, rather than having it be a hypothetical idea. This is not to be confused with practices of *imagining* or *visualizing* what the internal state of the opposite sex is like, as is commonly done by adepts of Buddhist and Hindu Tantra.

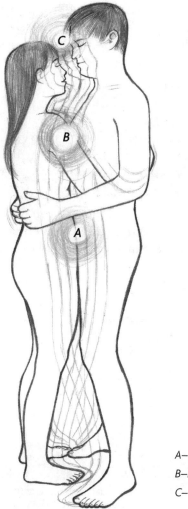

A—Lower tantien
B—Middle tantien
C—Upper tantien

Softly soak into your lover physically and energetically, including joining the three tantiens.

Figure 15-4: Partner Merging

In the Water tradition of sexual meditation, you directly experience your opposite polarity at its source—within the body and soul of the "other." The aim is to understand, balance and transcend the essential male-female (yin-yang) energies that compose all human beings and, in fact, all beings throughout the universe.

8. ACHIEVE NONPHYSICAL PSYCHIC LINKING

The ability to feel and activate not only your energy but also that of your partner becomes increasingly heightened and amplified when you begin sexual meditation. This includes psychic energy. When you find yourself attracted to someone or even having strong sexual desire, your new psychic abilities can help you sort through your feelings.

At this stage in your practice, you increasingly understand that visual appeal is a small part of being attracted to someone. What you want to know is whether you have the potential to be energetically compatible, whether for an evening or longer. Moreover, with a person who might not be a practitioner of Taoist internal arts, you might want to know if he or she has deeply blocked energies or emotional fixations that will impede your own progress and/or your future relationship with that person.

Taoist sexual meditation practices can teach you to "read" the energy of someone to whom you are attracted and answer those questions. You can unobtrusively enter and feel his or her energetic field without interfering, touching or manipulating his or her free will in any way, so when it's over, you leave them just as they originally were, without leaving any influence inside them. The motivation and way of doing it seeks to avoid any form of psychic influence or manipulation, as, for example, many proponents of Sex Magic are prone to do. It is important to understand that the "energy reading" of another person is a fairly advanced technique that must only be done in honorable ways unless you wish to incur heavy negative karmic debts.

This technique allows the following possibilities:

1. You could have the complete psychic experience of what it would probably be like to have sex or a short or long relationship with that person.

2. If you see that he or she is attracted to you, you can possibly release some or all of that person's curiosity about you, and, in so doing, you can have some choice in what happens next from a noninterference and neutral position.

3. You can dissolve and completely free the energy of your own desire until the attraction turns into a *wu so hui,* or "no big deal," situation.

4. If both partners are practitioners of sexual qigong or sexual meditation, both may be able to fulfill their sexual needs at a psychic level without getting physical.

5. If both are sufficiently developed, they can link, merge their energy fields and meditate together without even touching.

9. DISCOVER YOUR TRUE ESSENCE

From a spiritual view, after you clear enough of your karma, discovering and embodying your seventh energy body or essence enables a person to evolve and have a unified soul, or *ling*, (see Chapter 3, "Body of Individuality") capable of reincarnating whole. Otherwise, the Taoist view holds that when a person dies, he or she splits up and has to begin all over again, with much of what the person learned and accomplished in the previous life vanishing. Furthermore, until someone accomplishes the body of individuality, he or she is not equipped to begin the spiritual journey toward embodying and becoming one with the Tao.

Inner Dissolving is the method through which someone can release and resolve the blockages in their first through sixth energy bodies. These blockages must be mostly cleared before a person can arrive at his or her essence. The Inner Dissolving meditation method is the means and not the goal itself, which is in fact realizing the seventh and eighth energy bodies.

Even if one does not arrive fully at the body of individuality, doing Inner Dissolving is still beneficial. Releasing the earlier energy bodies makes your life more stress-free, smooth, relaxed and happy. Although you can arrive at the same place by doing solo practices—standing, sitting, moving and lying down—as mentioned before, your access to up to four times the energy through sexual practices makes the work go much faster.

The paths of sexual qigong and sexual meditation take courage. These practices can release repressed blockages within some people at a faster pace than they may be able to psychologically handle at that time. If these psychological issues arise and are too much, the advice is to step back, adhering to the seventy-percent rule or, even better, just take a break and return later if desired. When you take a break from sexual meditation you might consider returning to practicing only solo practices, and then, when you get a bit stronger you can try partner work again. Meanwhile, as you undergo a period of integration, you can still enjoy ordinary sex or sexual qigong without meditation before smoothly gliding back into it.

10. ENTER INTO UNIVERSAL CONSCIOUSNESS

Once you and your partner begin to work with the seventh and eighth energy bodies and your consciousness starts moving to the distant ends of the universe, you begin to connect with that which pervades everything—Source, God, the Divine, Tao or Spirit. Regardless of what you call this universal connection, joining and integrating with it in a totally relaxed way at every level is the ultimate goal of Taoist sexual meditation.

YIN, YANG, REINCARNATION AND THE HIGHER ENERGY BODIES

From the Taoist point of view, the earth is a dense training ground for spiritual evolution. Rather than taking an anthropocentric view (looking exclusively in terms of human values and experience), the larger perspective of Taoism is about what is true in all times and places in the universe. Through Inner Dissolving and sexual meditation you can begin to go beyond these limited earth views to have a higher context. As you move into more advanced stages of the Taoist path, everything starts to connect to everything else. Within this new understanding you begin to see the relationship between the energy bodies, qi, yin and yang, morality, incarnations and karma.

THE NATURE OF KARMA

Caught up in the swirl of red dust—in the transitory desires, attachments, illusions and fixations that consume our life force—most people never consider the mechanics of karma. Once a person starts to relate to life from the soul's perspective rather than a purely human point of view, two important distinctions come into view:

1. There is a wide array of energetic conditions and manifestations in which the soul or Being can reincarnate within the vast universe of localities and dimensions.
2. Each incarnation is unique in terms of how a soul or Being, corporeal or noncorporeal, experiences time.

With this broader lens we begin to see how qi and yin-yang affect us, not only on this earth and in this lifetime, but also in further incarnations as they impact the higher energy bodies: psychic, karmic, essence and Tao. Taking this into account changes the game entirely: the totality of life in the universe is now your reference point.

Now the practices you do not only improve your energy and life in the here and now but also train you for future incarnations. Getting clearer in this life (or, at the very least, not taking action that blocks your higher energy bodies) means you will be that much clearer in the next incarnation.

It is important to note that this transition from an anthropocentric, earthly viewpoint, to that of a citizen of the larger universe is fairly easy to adopt as a new belief at the conceptual or cognitive level. However, making the actual transition itself is exceedingly more difficult.

A key indication of this transition is the ability to recognize qi as qi and yin-yang energies as yin and yang, rather than only seeing the manifestations of these energies in physical or some other recognizable, definable form. Once this perceptual threshold is crossed, your soul will carry that knowledge beyond this incarnation into the next.

This is particularly relevant given the variants in other worlds, such as:

1. The experiential nature of widely divergent environmental contexts.
2. The infinite ways yin-yang energy can manifest in the ever-arising flux to appear in solid, not-so-solid and completely non-solid forms.
3. Radically different expressions of space and time that exist in other galaxies, dimensions or worlds.

In other words, when you land in your next incarnation, it is quite likely that all known markers, physical or otherwise, will have disappeared. How you experience and reference the first seven energy bodies may be entirely different in a new location and new incarnation.

For example, in terms of the first energy body, you may find yourself inhabiting a silicon-based body rather than a carbon-based body. You may even find yourself in a body that is only semisolid, amorphous, or totally noncorporeal (that is, without physical form). There are no guarantees that you'll have a solid body in any incarnation. Regardless of the substance that comprises the first energy body in each new incarnation, the yin-yang paradigm and principles are still operational in each of the seven bodies that lead up to the body of the Tao. The range of potential manifestations is far beyond what even the most fertile human imagination can conjure up.

This subject is presented not to frighten or intrigue the reader but simply to invite consideration of a much broader frame of reference for cultivating your spiritual evolution. The life of the average person typically only revolves around the first four energy bodies, although Westerners largely ignore the qi body, recognizing and validating only the physical, emotional and mental bodies. Most people rarely reflect on the higher energy bodies. They are even less likely to take them into account when deciding on a course of action.

Some people have access to the middle ground of highly developed intuition, which lies somewhere between the fourth and fifth energy body, but in general humans with a fully developed psychic body are quite rare. Those cognizant of and developed in their sixth (karmic) and seventh (essence) energy bodies are rarer still. From the limited frame of reference of the first four bodies, it is difficult to relate to qi or yin and yang directly or to comprehend one's existence beyond this earth except as an intellectual concept.

Karmic Propensities and Natural Ability

Many wonder about natural abilities—the type of innate talent that results in major breakthroughs in science, philosophy, art and music. A common reincarnation theory posits that such individuals developed the skill in a previous incarnation. This prior knowledge allows for instinctive recognition and adaptation to the energy in a new form. With minimal or no training, the natural talent shows itself.

According to Taoist philosophy, it is the understanding of yin and yang energy in the eight energy bodies that allows for any substantial transfer of knowledge between incarnations. Because of this, the motivation or perseverance to do meditation is a skill that one can "inherit" somewhat from a previous incarnation. This may also be the case for other abilities, such as scientific understanding and musical talent. These "inherited" reincarnation capacities account for why some are prodigies in certain areas including spirituality.

In Tibet, for example, a spiritual prodigy is called a *Tulku*. Many inaccurately think this means the "Tulku" was completely enlightened in a previous life. Although true for the rare few if the Tulku is genuine, most in fact were previously just highly spiritually advanced practitioners. If a specific Tulku is not genuine, then that title may have been given for political reasons.

Genuine prodigies may not necessarily be born with the knowledge consciously intact, although this does happen with a rare few. Instead, often what happens is that once a person with the karmic propensity from previous lifetimes is exposed to an aspect of spirituality or practice, he or she can immediately absorb, use and integrate the entire point viscerally, while others without an inheritance must go at a dramatically slower pace.

FUTURE REINCARNATIONS

Enlightenment can occur in any world or dimension, although it is far easier to succeed in a place with a heavy gravitational field such as the one we have here on earth. The density of our environment makes it easier to move between and resolve the various energy bodies and to recognize the qi of anything that manifests in them. Recognizing the underlying qi and yin-yang polarity in any manifestation is quite different from recognizing only the shape and form of its external appearance. It's important to recognize that qi is what's relevant, not the appearance of the manifestation.

The aim of all Taoist spiritual practice is a direct encounter and experiential recognition of the flux of qi—the essential yin and yang energy as it plays through each energy body. Secondary external forms through which combinations of qi reveal themselves and become obvious are always temporary. Qi relationships remain constant throughout various reincarnations and localities, although the way they manifest may be utterly unfamiliar. The energetic education you carry from one life to the next as regards your ability to instinctively recognize yin and yang can give you a leg up wherever you reincarnate.

Although sexuality is a powerful way to discern yin and yang on this earth, many other environments exist in other parts of the universe that do not feature this male-female polarity. The main point is not how yin-yang energies manifest in male and female bodies during sex. Instead the key is to develop a heightened capacity to adapt to changing circumstances and recognize the essential qualities of yin and yang itself, regardless of where or how you encounter them on the road to enlightenment.

TAOIST HIGHER MORALITY

Yin and yang can also be considered in terms of higher morality. First of all, for those whose ability to recognize qi is limited to the first four energy bodies, moral decisions are mostly made by relying on intelligence or by reacting to conditioning alone. By applying awareness to the Golden Rule, such individuals do their best to promote balance and compassion. This works quite well within the scope of this planet, but decisions made on this basis may or may not be relevant in other environments.

The emanating energy of what you do here may very well affect life forms billions of light years away. This may sound far-fetched until you can directly perceive the qi of the higher energy bodies, which connect to everything throughout space and time.

Secondly, in higher forms of Taoist morality you become progressively more aware of the immediate effect of any thought or action on your energy bodies, especially the fifth, sixth and seventh (psychic, karmic and essence) bodies. At this level of development, a practitioner begins to discern that the movement of qi through those bodies can be smooth or disturbed in various ways. Development in the psychic body gradually opens this gateway. You eventually begin to sense, see or in some way recognize which actions create energetic signatures of positive karma and which create negative karma. When this psychic door fully opens, as it does for some, you can, with training, gain the ability to keep your karmic body consciously smooth and even, at which point you neither create nor store karma.

From this refined perspective, any action that creates karma—either positive or negative—is immoral. This is because all karma, whether positive or negative, still needs to be released to attain enlightenment. Although positive karma creates effects that we normally call beneficial and this can smooth the road to enlightenment, karma is still karma. The unconscious desire for accruing the fruits of positive karma creates its own kind of weird blockages that prolong the spiritual path. The unconscious desire and attachment to positive karma never arise if you let go of any positive karma as it is being created.

To further understand this perspective, although ordinary moral thoughts or actions can potentially keep your normal emotional and psychic fields feeling smooth, normally it is almost impossible for this to happen if karma is being produced.

Although from an ordinary viewpoint, positive karma will benefit you in your life, and negative karma will ultimately cause you harm, from the perspective of the essence and the body of the Tao, both types of karma bind you and prevent you from achieving and embodying these final two energy bodies.

This stage continues until you can start to directly recognize and feel, on an ongoing bodily and energetic basis, the mechanics of how your karmic body gets activated and how it colors everything it contacts. Once this recognition dawns on you, the objective of the next stage emerges: to lessen the influence of any thought or action by either projecting less energy or absorbing less of the energy that accompanies the act. This reduces the karmic effects of that thought or action. For example, an emotional freak-out will definitely affect your energy and create karma. However, you can also have very strong emotions that move through you smoothly, creating no karma or long-term detrimental effects whatsoever.

In terms of eventually becoming fully spiritually awake, the motto at this stage could be stated as, "the greater the karmic effect, the less moral the act; the lesser the karmic effect, the more moral the act." The same process applies to your essence—the body of individuality. From this perspective, that which imprints your higher energetic bodies is of moral consequence or *you so hui*, while that which does not alter your authentic internal smoothness is of no moral consequence or *wu so hui*.

RELATIONSHIPS AND THE EIGHT ENERGY BODIES

For Taoists, the primary consideration in any relationship is its potential effect on the higher energy bodies (emotional to essence) of the individuals involved. If the interaction of sexual energy flowing between two people can be used to remove internal obstacles, blockages or stuck points in one or both, then everyone benefits from that forward spiritual movement. With Taoist sexual meditation practitioners, this mutual intention is assumed. Built into the free exchange of unattached sexual love between practitioners is the desire to help each other by dissolving each other's energetic blockages.

Included within this intention is the Taoist notion that it takes at least ten thousand lives to reach enlightenment. Thus, when Taoists engage in sexual meditation with somebody, for whatever reason, they aim to behave in such a way so as to avoid needing to apologize ten thousand lifetimes later. This takes into account that much of what people experience in their everyday states of mind and body is not what it seems.

Sexual meditation offers a golden opportunity to complete the unresolved karma of many lives. In any given pairing, you might be able to clear out your own karma, but not your partner's, or you might be able to clear out his or her karma, but not yours. Nevertheless, all practitioners should do their best to complete each other's karma as well as their own.

Above and beyond your personal karma with others, the essence that comprises the karma around relationships within you as an individual or with other partners must be resolved in order to reach enlightenment. In most of us, this core level remains denied or frozen. Only by accessing the body of individuality—your seventh energy body—can you enter this subtle environment of soul or Being. Both partners must be working toward accessing this energetic realm to do the practices described in Chapters 16, 17 and 18.

Taoist Sexual Meditation and Classical Tantra

Many inner meditation traditions actively, although often in a way that is hidden from public view, take the energetics within the human body and actualize its potentialities in Spirit and Consciousness.

Within the Taoist lineage to which I belong, it is considered quite appropriate to use sexual qigong not only for more satisfying sex but also to increase one's general reservoir of qi. Sexual meditation is different, however, as its aim is spiritual evolution and gradual awakening to the Tao. Although pleasure is part of the package, neither classical Taoist nor traditional tantric meditation traditions were focused on "spiritual entertainment." Rather, the primary emphasis was on developing a personal relationship with Consciousness itself. Sex was only a spiritual vehicle rather than the ultimate end in itself.

Similar to traditional Hindu and Buddhist tantric sexual practices, the Water Tradition of Taoist sexual meditation uses powerful positive or negative emotions in practices because they can be converted to Spirit and emptiness. This attitude and approach makes the whole sexual arena a lot more interesting and fun. Instead of shunning the darker animal sides of human nature, a practitioner converts his or her negative emotions into energetic fuel. Any powerful emotion, such as anger or fear, for example, is dissolved until the blocked energy within the anger or fear resolves into emptiness. The original destructive or frozen emotion is thereby erased at its source, which lies at or near the emotion's root. Left behind however, is not the downside of anger, fear or any other emotion but a greater degree of contacting emptiness.

Both the Fire and Water Taoist traditions can also be compared with other Eastern systems such as classical Buddhist Tantra (also known as Vajrayana) or Hindu Tantra. Vajrayana Buddhism normally does not openly teach sexual practices. In terms of both sexual and nonsexual overall practice methods and goals, the Taoist Fire tradition has many similarities to Vajrayana Buddhism, which influenced Taoist Fire method practices over a thousand years ago. Conversely, the core practice methods of Taoism's Water tradition are very different from Vajrayana Buddhism.

Tibet's Dzogchen tradition has similarities to the Water methods, both in terms of philosophy and key practice points, although the terminology, philosophical context and specific techniques are often quite different. Accomplished Dzogchen Master, Namkhai Norbu, echoes some of the language of the Taoist Inner Dissolving process when he describes the experience of dualism (that is, being separated from Universal Consciousness), "In the same way that flowing water freezes into solid ice, the free flow of primordial energy is solidified by the action of conditioned cause and effect, the functioning of the individual's karma, into a seemingly concrete material world."[2]

At the higher levels most authentic traditions were developed to arrive at a similar destination, although how they take a practitioner there varies greatly.

---

2. Norbu, Namkhai, *The Crystal and the Way of Light* (New York: Routledge and Kegan Paul, 1986), 111.

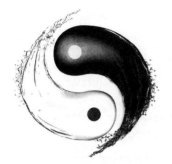

CHAPTER 16

Advanced Practices— Transmission, Sound and Vibration

Within Taoism there are powerful sound and vibration techniques, many of them advanced methods, which practitioners can use to access the flow of qi while making love. These advanced practices further refine inner awareness for healing and spiritual transformation. They can also help a practitioner move through particularly nasty blocks and can be used when a person is spiritually stuck.

An experienced Taoist teacher would traditionally prescribe one of hundreds of techniques and methods depending on the specific condition of the practitioner. Within Taoist groups, students practicing solo meditation, sexual qigong or sexual meditation would be watched closely for any signs of instability or imbalances in any of their energy bodies. New sound or vibrational practices would not be taught until the previous material had been fully mastered, assimilated and stabilized within the student. Unfortunately this type of attention and training is rare, as many attempt to learn from books or teachers whom they may see only intermittently.

Traditionally, over time, a Taoist practitioner's energetic system would gradually go through upgrading and refinement in order to be able to handle deeper and stronger practices. Through ongoing and consistent practice, what once was impossible to a student, would become possible and easy, as well as forming a new level of stability and awareness for the student to safely move to higher energetic levels.

This chapter explores some of the traditional Taoist sound and vibration techniques that were taught and how they can be used as intermediate and advanced spiritual methods within sexual meditation. The chapter ends with four case studies that highlight the importance of going slowly with intermediate and advanced qi techniques. There are many different kinds of qi practices that have different effects depending on the person. Some are easy, while others may be inherently more problematic, requiring that a practitioner proceed very carefully, ideally under the guidance of an experienced teacher.

SAFETY PRECAUTIONS

It is important to understand the risks inherent in sound and vibration practices. Meditation and qigong practices that give you a very rapid sense of increased physical or psychic power sometimes do so by overstraining the central nervous system. Practices that promote an even, steady progression of qi development are safer and usually more reliable for long-term progress. Short paths to spiritual awakening carry inherently more risk than longer, more conservative paths.

Sexual meditation combined with vibration techniques is a fast track that should be attempted only by those with great inner stability who have done the foundation practices. A very small percentage of those who engage in meditation techniques of any kind, in any tradition, can tip over into mental destabilization or worse. Specific case studies are included at the end of this chapter to give you an idea of what can happen when certain qi techniques are practiced incorrectly.

Some of the practices in this chapter go deep and may bring up many dark, repressed emotions and blockages that you never knew existed. **Do not take these techniques lightly.** They should not be practiced by anyone with mental health issues, especially those who have been diagnosed or treated for mental issues such as post-traumatic stress disorder, chronic depression, bipolar disorder and schizophrenia. Mental illness is relatively little understood. For example, it is estimated that one percent of the population will become schizophrenic by their late twenties, perhaps after stressful events, but often without discernible cause. These exercises are also not recommended for those with severe health problems.

Experimenting with the exercises in this chapter is unwise to do solely from reading the text. It is recommended to do them under the guidance of a trusted master. If someone gets in over his or her head, the master can make specific interventions to try to correct the situation, rather than leave the student in a bind. Bear in mind that in the West, qualified masters in this material will be hard to find. Practices in this chapter that *require* this supervision are marked as *advanced*. For reference, an intermediate practitioner would on average have approximately ten years of experience working with qi practices. This is also to remind the reader to stay away from even intermediate practices until sufficiently proficient in the preliminary Taoist meditation practices.

It is important that you do the foundational ordinary sex and sexual qigong work presented earlier in this book before even considering moving on to the more advanced practices such as those described in this chapter and beyond. The dividing line between having a deep release and stepping over into mental destabilization can be anything but transparent. Finally, if in any doubt at all, consult a health professional and do not attempt to do any of these exercises.

THE ART OF SPIRITUAL TRANSMISSION

Generally, in authentic Eastern spiritual and meditation traditions, a teacher's more profound knowledge in all forms is passed on to students through spiritual transmission. Traditionally, all sexual meditation methods were taught in this manner. The author was taught transmission as an entire area of study at the end of his Taoist priesthood training and during the years he spent with Liu Hung Chieh. It is rare to find teachers who can transmit and even rarer to find a teacher who can teach how to do so.

Transmission is a form of telepathy, distinctly different from mind reading or reaching into another's mind to seize control of that person's thoughts. Although telepathy is the closest word we have in English, it lacks precision. More accurately, transmission is a direct transfer, mind-to-mind and body-to-body, of the totality of a learning experience. The transmission of Taoist techniques and energetics, whether or not they involve sexual meditation, is as intimate a process for the teacher as is sexual intercourse. For the recipient it includes:

- Preparation for receiving the teaching
- What is to be learned
- All that is needed to integrate and stabilize the material.

Transmission gives the teaching to a student in a seed form. The teacher transmits by embedding information into outgoing energy emanations that meet and mix with the energy of the student's mind and energy bodies. This can be done through internal light, vibrations or sound that may or may not be audible. The transmission helps and empowers the student to learn and embody the fullness of the teaching over time. In this sense, transmissions give a student a template that is filled in and fleshed out through ongoing practice and by putting his or her awareness on the subject matter.

Recipients bring the knowledge to life through practice within their body, mind and Spirit. Although many who are receiving a transmission will feel an initial blast of energy, generally students will have to wait for the teaching to grow and come alive within them over time. Like the seed of a tree, a transmission must fall on fertile ground—the student's mind and energy bodies—and be given regular watering, or practice. Then the transmitted teachings can grow into experiential knowledge and, over time, into maturing wisdom.

Within Taoism there is also a more intricate form of transmission that occurs in some teacher-student relationships. This type of transmission depends on many factors, not the least of which is the balance between the teacher's skill and the capacity and willingness of the student to receive what has been given, as well as karmic influences. A dynamic can occur wherein the teacher psychically takes the student's energy and teaches him or her how to morph it over time.

This type of transfer goes beyond supplying raw information; it involves giving the student a boost in competence to attain the practice at hand. The teacher helps to fill in the knowledge gaps for the student, without the student actually being conscious or aware of the totality of the transfer. As the student practices, the information naturally pours out in such a way that the student thinks and feels as if he or she has made an original discovery of how to do the method. The transmission itself registers only at the unconscious level until practice allows the knowledge to emerge and consciously becomes the student's own.

If a skilled physics teacher could do transmission, he or she could actually silently transfer to students the essence of all they would need to know to develop quantum theories. However, this would not be a transfer of a formula or equation; instead, it would be the direct experience of the quantum event itself, as if the student were one with that event.

> *If a skilled physics teacher could do transmission, he or she could actually silently transfer to students the essence of all they would need to know to develop quantum theories.*

With transmission, talking the talk is insufficient; a teacher must also be able to walk the walk. Teachers can only transmit what they know both personally and experientially, what they can fully embody and demonstrate in their lives. At the higher levels, Taoist teachers learn the advanced energetic techniques of transferring subtle knowledge to another person through in-depth, one-on-one training.

Some spiritual teachers may know the words, and the words may even ring true, but they cannot do energetic transmissions. Yet in the bigger picture, even those teachers have an important place, because they make students aware of the inherent higher possibilities. However, when such teachers extend beyond their ability, a classic problem can emerge. When the blind lead the blind, both run the risk of falling off a cliff.

SOUNDS AND INTERNAL ORGASMS

Chapter 13 explored how to generate internal orgasms by directing your qi and intentions to specific locations in the body. Internal sounds provide another gateway to achieve an internal orgasm. To generate an internal orgasm during sex, the general process is to subtly focus your intention and bring your energy to the specific site where you desire an internal orgasm. Once the energy is located in a specific area, you learn to vibrate the area with fast oscillating vibrations or sounds, creating rapidly escalating openings and closings that will result in internal orgasm(s).

This technique can also be done while kissing or with mouths separated. With your lips fully engaged, you can generate an internal humming sound, usually centered in your spine (not to be attempted if you have a back injury). Advanced practitioners can generate the humming sound from specific internal organs or glands. If your mouths are separated, use any sounds or words you like. The important element is the vibratory frequency you choose, not the specific sounds, mantras or words.

FIVE STAGES OF LEARNING SOUND AND VIBRATION

Sexual meditation practitioners go through five stages of learning sound and vibratory techniques:

1. The sounds are clearly articulated, audible and fairly loud. Gradually the external, articulated sounds become softer as the strength of the vibrations proportionately increases inside your body.

2. Specific sounds, mantras or words will completely cease to be verbally articulated as, in tandem, the inside of your body vibrates with the sound; at the same time, other different frequencies and power may still be externally articulated and heard.

3. Once you have gained experience and can readily create vibrations inside your body (with or without articulating words), over time, as the audibility of the external vibrations emanating from inside your body decreases and becomes even quieter, there will be a commensurate increase in the qi produced when you internally vibrate.[1] The goal is to learn to modulate the qi power of your internal vibrations inside your body.

4. Once all external sound naturally ceases, it becomes possible to make any part of your body, or your entire awareness, silently vibrate at will.

5. At this stage you can direct specific frequencies or sounds with conscious intent alone and learn to regulate these inner vibrations to become lighter or stronger at specific bodily sites (for example, your wrist, elbow or erogenous zones), as well as to target specific energy bodies at the more subtle levels of your Being.

COMMUNICATION IS VITAL

Communication with your partner is vital when engaging in Taoist sexual sound and vibration practices. Ideally, you will be partnered with someone who shares your interest in Taoist sexual qigong and meditation and who is happy to fully participate. If that is not the case, you can handle the situation in any number of

---

1. India's Nada Yoga or Yoga of Sound focuses on this to an even greater degree. By creating internal vibrations, its yogis can make external, highly audible sounds emanate from the inside of their body that can be easily heard.

ways. With a casual, one-time, or occasional partner, rather than giving a complete explanation of the practice, you can simply say in a light-hearted manner, "I really like to make sounds while making love." Most will go along with the program as long as what you're doing doesn't seem dangerous, but just a bit weird.

Suppose you're with a regular partner who doesn't care to engage in sexual meditation practices, but is fine with you making sounds. Give him or her some context as to why you are making weird sounds during sex and make sure they willingly accept and align with your intention, without making them feel forced to participate. Explain that it might seem as if you're getting angry, sad or upset, but that letting the sounds out doesn't have to diminish the satisfaction you can derive from each other, and, in fact, it can add a new dimension of pleasure.

In any event, it is crucial to take the time beforehand to clarify what you are doing and let your partner know that you are being responsible and deliberate with whatever you are releasing. Be sure to make it clear that you are not aiming the intense energies of any release at your partner. Without this clarification, your partner could easily misinterpret the situation. This is understandably so, as the qi can be quite strong and can be felt or reacted to quite forcefully when you are sexually aroused. If your partner is not aligned and this freaks them out then you should avoid doing these practices with them.

POSSIBLE EFFECTS AND RELEASES

If both of you are practitioners, you may find that all sorts of blocked emotions begin to emerge with these practices, especially once you open your left and right energy channels. If your partner starts crying or laughing or howling, it is important to not judge or interpret it. Instead, take whatever energy arises in the moment and use it as best you can as part of your Outer or Inner Dissolving practices. This can be a little tricky at first, especially when powerful laughing and crying arises. This is because most readily experience strong emotions from others as a signal to blame themselves, thinking, "What have I done?" or "I must have done something wrong." However, if you know beforehand to expect the unexpected, you and your partner can have fun with the practice and use the energy generated without any unwarranted emotional reaction.

At the beginning of doing sound and vibration practices, the release of strong emotions can be a little unnerving, but over time the feeling that it's a big deal will usually give way to a "no harm, no foul" attitude. On the rare occasion when releases remain a a major issue or make your partner reproachful, it's best to discontinue the practice altogether with that partner rather than escalate the situation.

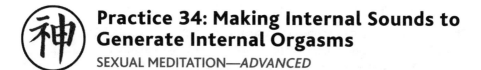

Practice 34: Making Internal Sounds to Generate Internal Orgasms

SEXUAL MEDITATION—*ADVANCED*

This is an advanced-level method to create internal orgasms with internal sounds. This technique is best combined with Inner Dissolving rather than Outer Dissolving, however it can be done with either. Practice this method generating an internal orgasm inside yourself first, and only then use this technique within your partner (if, and only if, they are willing). If either partner has any mental health issues, this exercise is not recommended.

1. Begin by putting your attention on your genitals for a few minutes. Then move the vibrational or other energies from your genitals up to your lower tantien, and stabilize your qi there.

2. Focus your conscious mind until it becomes very quiet and still.

3. Intuitively pick any part of your body that you can vibrate, regardless of location, for example, your genitals, fingers, knee, tongue or neck.

4. Feel for a sound that will help you do this. Don't try to rationally figure it out; just let whatever's inside you spontaneously pop up to the surface.

5. Start to vibrate the chosen part of your body as strongly as you can: hmmmmm.

6. Using your full intent and, as strongly as possible, move your qi from your lower tantien to wherever the vibration is located, hmmmmmmm.

7. As you vibrate into that spot, allow it to increasingly energetically pulse until it reaches a tipping point, and, in a relaxed way, you emerge into your internal orgasm.

8. After you can use internal vibrations to create orgasms inside yourself, you can use steps 1 to 7 to help create external or internal orgasms in your partner. If your partner is also a practitioner you both can project vibrational qi from your lower tantiens to mutually create or escalate orgasms within each other. ●

Taoist Esoteric Liturgies

Part of my training for the Taoist priesthood involved learning esoteric liturgies that used frequencies to balance and transform various energies.[2] Once a month, members of the community would gather in seclusion for an outdoor meditation ceremony under the full or new moon. These (often all-night) meditations involved deconstructing Taoism's liturgies—some three thousand of them.

---

2. The author has produced a CD set of guided meditation exercises utilizing these Taoist liturgies, *Ancient Songs of the Tao* (Energy Arts, 2008), that you can use in your personal practice.

The liturgies consisted of sounds from an ancient, prehistoric Chinese language now mostly lost to antiquity. Each liturgy was a teaching, and many of them involved the five elements and eight energy bodies.

Using these ancient sounds, each of the energy bodies would be activated. The purpose was not to make a pleasing sound, the way a choir might sing to praise or entertain. The aim was clear: to activate a specific energy body (or part of an energy body), first in yourself, then in others, then in trees and in the stars, so that one could eventually realize the vibratory quality of the entire universe.

Each of the eight energy bodies has a giant set of frequencies within it as well as shades of those frequencies—bottom, middle and upper, you could say, like tones in music or spectrums of light. Each energy body has a range of light, just as sound creates a light wave in an oscilloscope. Each energy body also includes and embodies traces of and connections to the other seven bodies.

During the liturgies, each individual energy body would be activated one at a time. The next step was the art of weaving the numerous minor frequencies into the major energy body being activated. For example, practitioners might fold the first energy body minor into the third energy body major, or incorporate the second minor into the seventh major, and so forth. At the end of each session, the first seven energy bodies would almost always interweave with each other in a carefully constructed, endless series of variations.

One of the goals was to eventually transcend the structures of the liturgies and be able to deliberately activate all aspects of the energy bodies without limitation. This is similar to a top jazz musician freely improvising after years of learning how to use virtually any musical structure fluidly and competently.

The liturgies were not using ordinary frequencies. In fact, they were exponentially stronger and more effective than audible sounds. These Taoist priests were trained to understand the intricate language of frequencies that coincided with the eight energy bodies. This was material that few outside the Taoist priesthood could perceive, much less understand.

The purpose of the liturgies was to allow one to connect with all and everything that is. Liturgies were also a key to learning the procedures of doing silent spiritual transmission in the initial phases. When teaching, the author sometimes uses these liturgies to help students learn the subject material.

ACCESSING AND RELEASING PRIMAL EMOTIONS

A basic principle of all Taoist meditation, especially sound and vibration techniques involves transmuting any strong emotion that comes from or toward you and using it as a fuel to help you dissolve the energy of those emotions. When the energy is liberated and a practitioner has a solid energetic foundation, the qi can flow unimpeded through your system and help you become a more balanced, compassionate and loving human being.

Taoists use sound and vibration as a powerful way to access deeply buried emotions that lie underneath the rational mind. These can be emotions and energetic impressions from our preverbal, early childhood years. In ancient times, the Taoists taught how to use sound and vibration to access such repressed emotions as fear, anger, frustration and jealousy so that they could be released in a relatively short amount of time. Contrast this to our modern times where for some it can take years or decades to approach such repressed emotions with psychotherapy.

The goal of these particular Taoist practices is for the qi of the emotion—be it anger, grief, sorrow, frustration, sadness, fear, loneliness—to fully emerge so you can dissolve and resolve it. Why? Whereas you might need twenty-five hours to dissolve a stuck blockage to its core by doing solo meditation practices, the same resolution might be accomplished in half an hour or so with sexual meditation, as the intensity is exponentially stronger. These sound meditations require you to stay present and neither disassociate, suppress nor censor emotional energy in any fashion.

For example, a woman who was abused as a child might be incapable of saying words that accurately reflect her repressed emotions without feeling like she is being choked. But she might be able to utter a string of sounds with emotional vigor that enables her to access and express the feelings that have never stopped bothering her. This may release some of that energy and set the stage for her to become more integrated and whole.

A fully trained Taoist adept whose subtle perceptions are highly developed can, at times, actually "hear" the vibrational qi sound keys that lock down a person's energetic system and keep emotions repressed. If the adept can communicates this knowledge and the student can understand and consciously replicate it, then those keys can help him or her unlock or unravel the blocked energies at a significantly more rapidly rate than otherwise possible. The ability of a student to do this will greatly depend on his or her foundation and level of inner development.

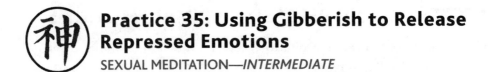

Practice 35: Using Gibberish to Release Repressed Emotions

SEXUAL MEDITATION—*INTERMEDIATE*

One method used in Taoist sexual meditation for releasing energies of repressed emotions involves speaking gibberish. Commonly known as speaking in tongues, or (less commonly) "glossolalia," this practice involves the fluid vocalization of sounds that resemble speech but are nonsensical. Allowing your tongue to fly freely in this way can greatly enhance the movement of sexual energy and allow repressed emotions to be expressed. This intermediate-level exercise is not recommended if either partner has any mental health issues.

These emotions may include a full spectrum of feelings. Vocalizing the shock and horror of traumatic events are at one end of the spectrum, while the natural emergence of ecstasy and bliss are on the other. Taoists don't view ecstasy and bliss as "special" emotions; they're just energies that unfortunately tend to get repressed in people.

The sounds themselves have no rational meaning and may range from screams to groans, from whimpering to intermittent explosions, from incoherent verbal diarrhea to what may sound like a highly articulate language from somewhere beyond this galaxy. Using gibberish combined with spontaneous sound vibrations (high- and low-pitched frequencies) can be very effective in releasing and resolving blocked emotional energy. That is, as long as you can handle it!

These emotional sound release practices can open people to deeper parts of their Being than they have previously encountered. It is especially helpful for individuals who are ready to open up but can't express emotions in any meaningful fashion. Many quiet people sometimes reveal their inward beauty when relieved of the pressure to put how they feel into the limited structure of words.

Sometimes when this practice is done while having sex, either or both partners may go so far as to begin screaming and making loud, visceral noises that do not map onto any recognizable human language. When done in the container of a safe relationship, this can allow a person's primal, innermost feelings to rise to the surface without any of the normal pressure to explain what's going on. We could even say that this level of feeling is quintessentially personal and therefore affords a person the type of privacy that ordinary language automatically circumvents. When that is the case, a person might choose to share the perceived experience with his or her lover afterward, or not. It is best, however, to avoid breaking the flow while in full flush. Having permission *not* to speak in understandable words is what gives this method its innate transformative release power. ●

DON'T BELIEVE EVERYTHING YOU HEAR

One note of caution is to be aware of the tendency to assign meaning to any of the sounds that come out of you. What your conscious mind comes up with as an explanation for what happens may have little to do with the real significance of the sounds. Don't make the mistake of overanalyzing the feelings that emerge during Taoist sound practices and turning those analyses into "facts" about some situation that happened long ago. Keep in mind that recovered memories may be real, imagined, a mixture of both or entirely irrelevant.

Be especially careful to avoid the temptation to make a big drama out of recovered memories, as the potential for emotional or mental distortion is considerable. In fact, memories are inherently unreliable and fraught with distortion. They may be merely a jumble of images mixed with the general energy of what was happening around that period of time. Whatever was actually bothering you that got locked in the recesses of your mind is somewhere in the mix, but you can't assume your interpretation is true. What you perceive as a shocking flashback may be a composite sensory feeling that is one-quarter true and three-quarters created.

What is important is that you release the blocked, unconscious energy and become free of it, rather than perpetuating it with a new storyline. Focus on the release, not on creating another story or drama. Sometimes silent dissolving techniques alone are insufficient to release deep emotional or psychic traumas. When this is the case, Taoist sound practices can play an important role to access, loosen and release these blockages.

AFTEREFFECTS OF ENERGETIC RELEASES

There are many different ways people react to the energetic releases that can occur during sexual qigong and sexual meditation. If your body has a massive release, three aftereffects are likely:

1. Your body may become hyper-energized. If so, just give yourself some time for the qi to reabsorb inside you and to become smooth before continuing to make love or going on to the next activity.

2. Your nerves may feel shattered. If so, take a pause or break. If you want to talk or be silent, do so. You may or may not want to be touched or hugged, depending on what is transpiring inside you. You could be just fine, or you could be completely physically, energetically or emotionally overwhelmed. If your partner verbally or nonverbally communicates that he or she needs space, be considerate and provide it. When your partner has chilled out, only go with what he or she comfortably wants to do, and don't push it.

3. If you are a Taoist meditation practitioner, you may need to fully process the powerful state of emptiness this practice can induce. If so, before going back to making love, you may need to rest and reintegrate. Take the needed time to reabsorb and smooth your energy into a calm and fluid state. You or your partner may even want to engage in a solo meditation to integrate the experience. Honor whatever comes up and relax into the experience so it can have a full integration.

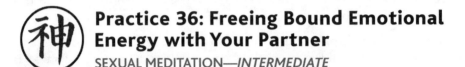 ## Practice 36: Freeing Bound Emotional Energy with Your Partner
SEXUAL MEDITATION—*INTERMEDIATE*

This is an intermediate-level practice method to augment your dissolving practice during foreplay or lovemaking when a stubborn energetic blockage won't release. Again, if you or your partner has any mental health issues, this exercise should not be attempted. It's also best to do this specific practice in an isolated area where you will not disturb others. It's not appropriate to do it near neighbors or sleeping children unless you are certain that you can modulate your voice to avoid waking them up.

Make sure you let your partner know beforehand that you are going to do this practice using gibberish and that strong emotions may be released in the process.

1. Both partners should begin by letting their minds become very quiet. Let go of any agendas about what may or may not happen.

2. Continue to feel the energies of yourself and your partner as you wait to see if any sounds emerge, regardless of whether they make sense. Remember that however odd or unnerving the sounds may be, they could be the key-in-the-lock of a storehouse of lifelong repression within the body-mind.

3. If your partner begins to make sounds, you can join him or her in making the same intense nonsense sounds, offering a strong, nonverbal sense of support that communicates, "I am with you."

4. With conscious intent, feel and locate where the emotional energy is bound and trapped inside one or both of your bodies. After you hone in on any single or multiple locations where blockages reside, you may find that you can't express your feelings. Focus all your sexual energy on the body part that is energetically constricted. Start making gibberish sounds or vibrate the blocked area. If you can, activate an energy channel between the blockage all the way through your body to inside your throat notch and out your mouth.

5. Once you have achieved a resolution of the blockage, pull the energy of your entire body into your lower tantien and concentrate it there before you finally let it release and spread throughout your entire body. If the internal orgasm is strong enough and

truly a full-body experience, this method can generate a release at the core of emotional or psychic tensions that have been frozen in your lower tantien. This type of release is unlikely to happen within the logical construct of ordinary communication between a sender and a receiver.

6. After the releases run their full course, they may circulate energy in your body, causing one or multiple internal orgasms to occur.

Important points to remember with this practice:

- Do not censor what you are compelled to express.

- Allow the sounds to change volume and/or emotional content, moving with whatever seems to want to arise spontaneously from inside you.

Sometimes the sounds will be normal in volume, at other times, harsh and deafening. Sounds can also come out very softly, as low groans or whimpers. Be reasonable and bear in mind that you don't have to scream at the top of your lungs; you only need to verbalize enough to let the energy come out fully and uncensored.

With practice, you can raise the energy higher and higher by using vibratory frequencies. This can propel one or both of you into an internal orgasm and even into emptiness. If you can't seem to "go all the way," don't worry. It will develop over time.

This method takes courage and stamina. It is not a practice for the meek. If you have any doubts as to if you can handle it, whether before, during or after doing the practice, back off immediately. When this sound process really starts to activate, an incredible amount of energy can pour out of both of you as you ride the energetic wave and let nature take its course.

In the event of a major release, it is important to note that the aftereffects can be substantial. Vibratory methods can serve as a catalyst for one or both of you and may lead to a seemingly unrelated major spiritual awakening within a short period of time. ●

Is Your Partner Willing to Play?

During an extended stay in India in my twenties I contracted a highly virulent form of amoebic hepatitis that killed two of my friends and severely damaged my liver. For the next few years, while I was very involved in Taoist sexual practices in Taiwan, my liver would unpredictably overheat. On several occasions, it got so hot that I passed out completely while having sex. Overstimulated liver qi can easily create the energetic condition for anger, and during that period I was feeling it with a vengeance.

My teacher instructed me to use vibration and sound during sex to convert that angry energy into incredible physical strength and healthy qi, which I could then use to heal my liver. Knowing how to appropriately work with the energy of anger is a worthwhile skill to develop, especially when it carries no malice.

A fairly insensitive young man at that time, I still had a lot to learn and at first didn't bother to explain to my partners what I was doing. After a few complaints, I decided to let the women I was sleeping with know that I was doing this odd practice for medical reasons. I told them (in Chinese, of course), "I might appear to be angry, but it's just energy that we can use to have more fun and help you get more orgasms," which is exactly what happened.

Now, every woman responds to strong male energy in her own way. Some women got really turned on, although most needed a short adjustment period before they could fully let go into the experience and enjoy it. Some women could never get into it, and wanting to do the right thing, I either ceased the practice or stopped seeing them. Either with or without conscious awareness, the women sometimes became angry themselves or moved toward depression. Fortunately, many women did not take what I was doing personally and agreed to participate, seeing it as an enjoyable lovers' game we could play together.

The goal of the practice at the time for me was to resolve the energetic root of the mechanism that turned anger inward, and to release it so that the problem eventually would resolve itself and go away permanently. Over time, I learned to gauge how my Taoist sexual meditation work was affecting the other person, and I would stop doing any technique with that partner if I sensed that it was not working for her.

Just as some of the women in Taiwan couldn't deal with my anger, similarly, female Taoist practitioners in the group I belonged to reported that there were many men who had trouble handling strong female penetrating emotions, such as rage, that the woman might be working through.

The bottom line is to let the other person know up front what might happen. Let people opt out if they do not want to engage and don't judge them for it. Turn the practice into a game with all the rules on the table, so your lover will never be completely uncertain of what might come next. Be prepared, however, that even when women or men initially agree, they might, after a while, find they don't like it after all. If you see any signs of this reversal in your partner, be prepared to check in with them immediately and to stop doing the practice if they so wish.

CAUTIONARY TALES

Editor's note: The examples in this section have been adapted from the author's book, *Opening the Energy Gates of Your Body,* Appendix C, "Importance of Correct Qigong Practice." Although specifically relating to qigong practices, the point is equally relevant to some of the stronger and/or more advanced meditation methods, especially those involving vibration and sound.

To be forewarned is to be prepared. That which can be immensely beneficial, if done incorrectly may carry risks. In rare instances, qigong and meditation done improperly has the potential to make a person ill or worsen his or her mental and physical health. The Chinese term for this is *dzuo huo lu mo* which translates as "fire goes to the devil."

If your body, mind, emotions, or psychic perceptions are getting weird or painful, simply stop practicing whatever you are doing until you find out clearly what is going on. Whatever your strength or capacity, your qigong and meditation practices must be internally comfortable. Forcing yourself radically beyond your individual limitations may cause harm to your nerves, glands, internal organs and brain. Overdoing any internal energy practice, including sexual qigong and sexual meditation, can be compared to the overtraining that leads to physical damage in athletes in every kind of sport.

Be aware that it takes much less time to do damage to your qi and energetic system than to fix it, and that the chance of finding genuine experts in the West capable of treating these kinds of energetic problems are slim indeed.

CASE STUDY: VIBRATING QI TECHNIQUES CAN HAVE UNPLEASANT EFFECTS

A student of tai chi in San Diego had learned a form that involved vibrating the mind, body and breath. He was in his teens at the time, with no martial arts background, and mistakenly thought this was traditional tai chi chuan. His first year felt good and relaxed, but then his teacher wanted to increase the pace. More breathing practices were added to increase the vibration. About two-and-a-half years into his training, the student developed the ability to discharge energy in martial arts on a crude level, and he felt he was really coming along.

Unfortunately, he also began to notice some side effects. These included:

1. Frightening hallucinations of his consciousness leaving his body and drifting uncontrollably away.
2. A feeling that things were moving much faster than they actually were—especially dangerous when he was driving.

3. Feeling his body become increasingly stiff internally.

4. Developing a thirst for power.

5. Feeling constantly hyper and unable to calm down.

6. Experiencing involuntary body spasms.

By the time this young man came to see me, he had not been practicing for three years, yet most of his symptoms had not abated. He literally feared for his mental and physical health. I found that he had condensed the qi in his body in the wrong way. Through various techniques, including Outer Dissolving, I re-patterned his energy and taught him how to continue this process at home. I also taught him techniques for removing the damaging qi from his body. Two years later, his problems had pretty much resolved.

CASE STUDY:
MIXING QI TECHNIQUES AND OVERTRAINING CAN BE HARMFUL

Bai Hua (Liu Hung Chieh's only other disciple aside from the author), taught a student the basic hsing-i neigong practice of sinking the qi to the lower tantien and after about two years of practice this student began to get very powerful. Around this time, Bai Hua left for another city and his student began to visit a number of hsing-i masters, looking for secret techniques from each. What he learned he practiced diligently, knowing that his first technique had worked so well.

Unfortunately his perseverance backfired. After a year practicing these other techniques, though none individually were inherently bad, the combination of various techniques from different systems resulted in all sorts of problems. In his effort to build energy in his lower tantien he ended up forcing his qi below his tantien and into his genitals. He effectively emptied the qi from his middle burner (the area from the diaphragm to the lower tantien, including the internal organs therein) into his lower burner (the area of the body between the lower tantien and feet). The breaking of the natural energetic seal between the middle and lower burners left his middle burner qi in total disarray. This resulted in mental and physical problems, including involuntary semen emissions and hallucinations. He lost his job, and his impending marriage had to be postponed indefinitely. It took Bai Hua and an herbal master three years to bring him back to near normal.

CASE STUDY:
FORCEFUL SEXUAL QIGONG CAN CAUSE PROBLEMS

While in Taiwan, I came across a system that includes techniques such as forcibly sucking energy up the anus and spine and hanging weights of ever-increasing amounts from the testicles and penis to develop sexual power. Around 1970, Wang

Shu Jin, my first teacher and a man known for his Taoist sexual abilities, warned me against this technique. Then, when I mentioned it to my next teacher in Taiwan, Hung I Hsiang, he gave me a one-hour lecture to caution me about practicing ridiculous forms of esoteric sexual qigong.

For example, in *Bonk: The Curious Coupling of Science and Sex*,[3] Mary Roach reports an interview with Dr. Geng-Long Hsu, a urological surgeon in Taiwan. The doctor tells her that, earlier in the year, he had "repaired a penis that had ruptured during a performance of jui yang shengong," an art that has been described as penis qigong. Dr Hsu exclaimed that the man had "tried to lift one hundred kilograms with his penis!"

Lesser problems are even more common. I have met many people who have practiced sexual control techniques and damaged their sexual apparatus. It is easy to overstrain the system, especially if the sexual organs are genetically weak to begin with. Some common problems include swollen testicles and internal bleeding. While these practices may lead to the ability to maintain erections for a longer time, the increased pressure can damage the underlying tissues. Women, too, can be damaged by inappropriate sexual qigong practices, resulting in problems such as false pregnancies and erratic periods.

For men, another sexual qigong and martial arts practice that can cause problems involves sucking the testicles up into the body. In martial arts this technique is used to protect oneself from groin kicks. Wang Shu Jin advised me not to practice this technique because I was traveling too often, and he couldn't monitor me closely enough. He also said that even with close monitoring, a certain percentage of people are damaged by the practice if it is begun after puberty.

CASE STUDY:
THE DOWNSIDE OF PACKING QI

One of my teachers, Hung I Hsiang, had a brother who was a practitioner of White Crane Qigong. One of the common techniques of White Crane Qigong is to force, or "pack," energy into the body, much like forcing clothes into a suitcase. This involves forceful breathing, body contractions, and a sense of physical and energetic strength. By overdoing it, Hung I Hsiang's brother actually caused one of his lungs to hemorrhage, and died.

In the West, I have seen people practicing all sorts of qi packing exercises, and these techniques are all potentially dangerous if not carefully supervised over time by a master. Forceful packing can potentially cause internal hemorrhaging, imbalances in the overall body energy, damage to lung tissue and susceptibility to respiratory diseases.

---

3. Roach, Mary, *Bonk: The Curious Coupling of Science and Sex* (New York: W. W. Norton, 2008), 131–32.

One man, an assistant instructor of a well-known East Coast martial arts master, was told to practice working with the Small Heavenly (Microcosmic) Orbit in a forceful way, using reverse breathing to generate heat in the lower tantien, which was then circulated. This person was also told to squeeze his anus and forcibly lift energy up his spine with his breathing.

The more he did this, the stronger and more powerful his energy felt. As in other qigong techniques, often the greater the force used, the stronger the experience generated. Unfortunately, he was burning himself up, especially his kidney and heart energy. When he began to experience symptoms such as cold, clammy sweats, involuntary tremors, extreme sensitivity to cold, and loss of vitality he was told to keep practicing, to "burn through the blockage."

Once he stopped these practices, it took more than five years of working on the problem to get rid of the symptoms. The fact that these symptoms arose is not in itself dire, since they could have been corrected at an early stage. His teacher had failed to pay attention to the warning signals and, instead, made the student feel that there was something wrong with him!

If your body or mind experiences great difficulties when you practice any qigong or meditation technique, sexual or not, simply stop. You either may not have a strong enough foundation in the necessary preparatory material, or the trouble may not reside in you, but rather in faulty teaching or your misunderstanding of the instructions.

The Taoist Fire tradition includes some forceful techniques that have the potential to create a variety of problems. This is one of the reasons why the author chooses instead to teach Water method practices that focus on letting go, balance and natural movement. The key is to use full effort without force, always being careful to observe the seventy-percent rule.

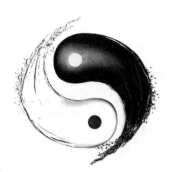

CHAPTER 17

Two Become One

In this chapter, the dance of intimacy expands into truly extraordinary realms. This is not about two-become-one in the "let's get married and join our lives" sense; rather it is two-become-one meaning joining as a holographic, multi-dimensional Being. The Inner Dissolving sexual meditation practices lead to directly experiencing the transcendental essence of each of you and merging your essences so that two become one.

What has been presented in this book up to this point will work, more or less, even if you are dissolving yourself and your lover but you are with a partner who does not know how to do Outer or Inner Dissolving. However, the material in these last two chapters can only be done if both lovers are sexual meditation practitioners. All exercises should be done with Inner Dissolving unless specifically stated otherwise. With both partners practicing, sexual meditation has the potential to really take off and achieve its ultimate spiritual goals.

ONE CONTINUOUS DANCE: FOREPLAY AND INTERCOURSE

At this stage in the practices, the distinction between foreplay and intercourse begins to blur. Optimally, all will be flowing in a beautiful, energetic dance between you and your partner. The ability for total energetic merging between lovers is a necessary prerequisite to continue into the more advanced practices of sexual meditation.

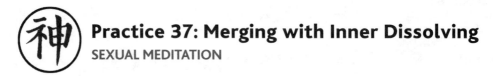

Practice 37: Merging with Inner Dissolving
SEXUAL MEDITATION

This practice looks at the bigger picture of how Taoist sexual meditation progresses from foreplay to intercourse to merging. Keep in mind during each stage of this practice, each lover can both send and receive energy at the same time.

Part 1: Merging and Orgasm

The process of merging during foreplay begins when you dissolve the energies bound in all of the different parts of your lover's body. You might start dissolving your lover's foot while you simultaneously dissolve your own. At a certain point, both of your feet will energetically merge as you experience them both as one foot.

The boundaries between his and hers, yours and mine, gradually disappear. You repeat this dissolving and merging process with other corresponding body parts: knees, eyes, genitals, and so on. Eventually, you reach a point where he dissolves and pulses her energy and, simultaneously, she reciprocates. You take as much time as you need to allow for this full merging to occur.

A couple can work on corresponding body parts (each focusing on the other's left knee, for example) or he can pulse her knee while she pulses his chest. As you progress and merge and dissolve more parts of your bodies, it becomes a wild dance between the two bodies. While you each bring plenty of attention to the process, you simply follow the movements and feelings of energies as they ebb and flow rather than have anyone "leading" the dance. The net effect is that as his energy enters hers and as hers enters his, the boundaries between what's his and hers disappears.

As you feel the foreplay heating up, rather than going for a big orgasmic release and climax, you want to slow down to shift your focus to the opening and closing of your kwas instead. This will enable you to fully circulate energy between your left

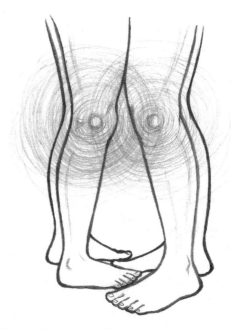

Figure 17-1: Dissolving Each Other's Knees

and right channels and thereby flood all the energy channels in both your bodies. This sets the stage for an ever-escalating ability to generate internal orgasms.

Eventually, you will naturally move on to intercourse and orgasm. Once penetration occurs, you can choose to use the spinal pump method of Bend the Bow Qigong (see Figure 17-5 A–C and Figure 17-6 A–C later in this chapter) and pump the spine before and during orgasm (whether internal or external, and regardless of whether one or both of you are coming). Then release the qi from the local orgasmic site to spread throughout the body.

Part 2: Transferring Energy after an Orgasm

Immediately after the release or orgasm, draw into the center of your awareness. Apply the solo channel work you learned in Chapter 12, using your hands and genitals to transfer energy to your spine. From the point of contact with your partner at the genital connection, dissolve and penetrate inside your lover's body, using your consciousness to go either down or up his or her channels.

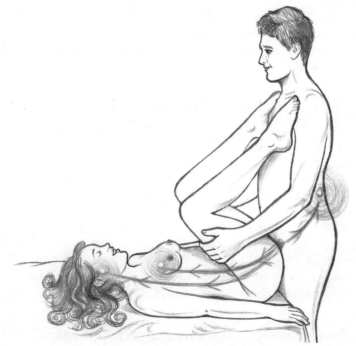

1. *His energy goes from his erection to dissolve blockages both in her breast and in her head. Through these points, after the blocked energy is resolved, he could activate her Microcosmic Orbit or left, right or central channel.*

2. *Her vagina projects energy through his pelvis to his lower tantien and then to his spine to dissolve a blockage there. From these points, after the blocked energy is resolved, she could activate his Microcosmic Orbit or left, right or central channel.*

Figure 17-2: Woman on Her Back with Feet on the Man's Shoulders Connecting Energy

You can both be directing energy into each other or you can both focus on just one partner's body, reversing which of you is doing this energy penetration, as required. The ideal situation, whether she is on top, on the bottom or on her side, is that the man should hold her legs or feet with his hands, if possible. This allows the energetic circulation between their bodies to maximize the yin-yang relationships flowing between her lower limbs, feet and vagina and his upper limbs, hands and penis. Figure 17-2 doubles this connection by having his arms on her legs, and her feet on his shoulders.

Projecting energy to specific points and through different channels of the body is more difficult in some positions than others. Your aim is to place your physical bodies at the best angles that allow you to most easily project energy into your lover's body along whatever channels seem blocked while at the same time maximizing energetic circulation and pleasure. Continue to play around, intuitively sensing what needs dissolving and resolving, until whatever is blocked gives way.

At a certain point, you will transition into the all-important moment in Taoist sexual meditation, in which there's no longer a sense of your body and your partner's body, your energy and your partner's energy, your Spirit and your partner's Spirit. Now only one mechanism is doing the actions—the subtle consciousness that transcends and pervades all manifest existence. ●

THE MAGIC MOMENT: EXPERIENCING THE ESSENCE OF ANOTHER

In *Finding God through Sex,* David Deida[1] writes, "Sex affords us the opportunity for letting go of ourselves without reservation and merging with our woman in pleasure and love. This feeling of two merging into one is the epitome of sacred and secular pleasure." At the advanced levels of Taoist sexual meditation, this unification goes beyond just feeling to becoming a concrete known reality.

At the core of the central channel, in the deepest transcendental essence of a person's soul or Being, there is no difference between male and female. Before you attain this depth of focus, there truly is a difference. As the merging process progresses, a magical moment can occur: an instant jump of consciousness wherein man and woman spontaneously merge.

> *As the merging process progresses, a magical moment can occur: an instant jump of consciousness wherein man and woman spontaneously merge.*

---

1. Deida, David, *Finding God through Sex* (Boulder, Colorado: Sounds True, 2002, 2005), 115.

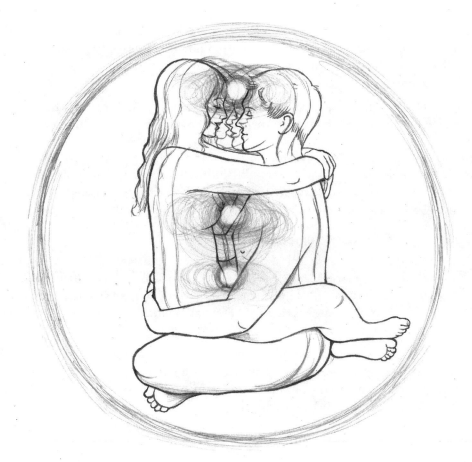

Figure 17-3: Complete Merging of Bodies and Energy Fields

Now two become one body, one qi, one undivided psychic space, one inseparable unit without distinct boundaries between self and other. Now you begin to actually feel the specifics of what it is like to be the other person's body, qi and emotions.

This means not only to be inside the other person's body, qi, emotions and ordinary mind but to actually become your lover. This is the point of real merging. It cannot be said when or even if this magical moment will occur, but when it does it creates a significant inner spiritual shift.

Encountering this world within can make a human being significantly more universally-oriented than a person who remains sexually polarized. On a purely personal level, perhaps the true cure for that part of spiritual malaise often referred to as "the battle between the sexes" is the moment when two people truly merge to become one.

Upon reaching this point of transcendence, a man or woman can directly experience what the opposite sex is feeling. They come to know one another fully—not through intellect, not through empathic pathways, not even through compassion or unconditional love, but through direct experience.

The net effect of this on a man is that he starts to experientially realize what the yin is inside his nature. For a woman, she starts to realize her yang. This gives each a whole new expanded perspective. Aspects of the opposite sex you may have previously disliked or simply didn't understand, will no longer carry the same charge. Your lover's deepest secrets and hidden recesses suddenly feel familiar because you have become them. What was once foreign and separate—the unknown territory of "other"—can now become normal familiar ground.

Doubling and Re-doubling of Energy

The first significant advance in sexual meditation comes after you have gained access to your own energy, developed the ability to dissolve blockages and learned to have internal orgasms. When you reach this point you have essentially doubled the amount of energy that you can use in sexual meditation: yours added to your lover's. It's the simple arithmetic of one plus one equals two.

By order of magnitude, the second advance in Taoist sexual meditation is far more expansive. It isn't just the next new advance in awareness—it's a jumping-off point. You're about to leap into the unknown. As the merging between you and your lover stabilizes, you not only access each other's energy, you each double the other's energy. Now each of you has four times the energy to work with than you would have on your own. When this energy is channeled in sexual meditation you are afforded the potential to dramatically accelerate your spiritual growth. You truly begin to move into the realm of that which is "larger than yourself." Knowledge of this merging between lovers, whether direct or implied, is why many of the world's ancient traditions view sexuality as a direct bridge to the Divine.

Opening of the Spirit

This merging and experiencing the essence of another occurs spontaneously. You cannot engineer it, nor should you try. When you start pulsing and the qi releases—when both of you are dissolving body parts—there will come a sudden "Boom! Wow!" Experientially, everything opens and all of sudden the two of you are one.

The "boom" may be experienced in many unpredictable and indescribable ways. Words can't begin to approximate this opening of the Spirit. Often accompanied by an explosion of light, this *interdimensional shift* has a magical flavor. It arrives with a sudden "Poof!" like when a magician pulls a rabbit out of a hat, or—to make an even more accurate metaphor—when something as huge as an elephant appears out of nowhere.

This rarely occurs without long-time practice. All you can do is simply be available for it to happen. It really depends on your karma. Once you've thoroughly dissolved the left and right channels, and you've reached a point where the shift happens, the sense of him and her existing as a separate entity drops away. Now you are working with only one body and energy.

Merging the Right and Left Channels

At this point you can extend the merging even further to make your partner's left channel join with your right channel and vice versa. This allows you to transfer qi across your systems. Now you start experiencing what it's like to be a woman's yin in a man's body or a man's yang in a woman's body. The process of moving past your personality as your identity has begun.

Your heart becomes hers and hers becomes yours. In the presence of this fusion, you don't experience yourself as either completely male or female because, psychically, you begin to experience everything going on within the other. Who and what your lover is, through progressively deeper and deeper layers, becomes apparent. You find out who and what a man or a woman is, beyond cultural conditioning. You are really stepping into the other person's shoes, energetically speaking. Only at a biological level do the two of you remain separate.

By repetitively immersing yourself into this commingled energetic space, even the most macho male can actually start to directly experience the female essence. And the most feminine female can come to know male essence within her own body and Being.

This is what makes sexual meditation so much more powerful than meditating by oneself. Only the dynamic interplay and dual cultivation practices of two can allow for the universal yin and yang within each of the sexes to genuinely begin to comprehend and experience each other.

MAINTAIN YOUR INTRINSIC NATURE

You should continuously be integrating your experiences without endangering your intrinsic nature. If a man brings out a tremendous amount of female energy inside him and fails to incorporate it properly, he can damage and even totally destroy his masculinity. Likewise for a woman, if she brings out tremendous yang energy without integrating it properly, she can do serious damage to or destroy her femininity. It is a tricky balancing act. It is helpful to know that you need to carefully integrate your experiences, because then you can shift your focus and intention to do just that.

This integration is unlikely to occur purely through intellectual thinking or referencing philosophical ideas of what men and women could be or should be.

The Taoists approach at this point is to go beyond intellectual musings, right into the center of how the universal energy matrix works, regardless of all variations within time, dimensions and space.

With each bend and bump on the road of integrating the newfound energies, you develop the internal discernment to know if it allows the smooth engagement and movement within and between the personal sense of your yin and yang essence. If it does not, your ability to integrate your experiences in sexual meditation can only be partial and at worst damaging to your intrinsic yin and yang masculine and feminine natures.

This consideration of how to integrate these advanced experiences only arises after a person can directly recognize and understand his or her own yin and yang natures, after two partners have become one. Before this happens it is best to focus on preparing the way for the event to occur.

Once you become aware of the yin and yang sides of your inner self, you need to be artful about how you express your opposite side so that no harm or damage occurs. You'll want both sides of your nature to grow in a spiritually healthy way. Understand your opposite-gender nature, but don't deny or twist your own earthly biological yin or yang genetics in the process.

THE EMERGING INNER SPACE OF TWO BECOMING ONE

As you continue joining and dissolving over time, a spiritual space will begin to open up. Energy dissolves and moves, internal orgasms occur, emotions release and resolve and the space of two becoming one begins to open. This space makes direct emotional and psychic communication possible. Now you have direct access into the depths of each other—not secondary inference or a vague, intuitive sense of the other, but direct access to spiritual intimacy.

In this space, you can move energy within your channels in any combination you like. Choosing either the left or right channels, you can dissolve up and down one channel, dissolve up and down the other channel, dissolve both of them together, or cross over from one to the other. Follow your intuition and do every up and down permutation possible until the left and right channels in both of you are fully open. Stay with the basic principle: "do what's easy first and what's difficult later."

As long as this incredible space between you continues to naturally open bit by bit, allow it to do so. Merge into an expanded space of emptiness with total communication with your lover. Let the gift of this space keep losing its boundaries as far as it can.

REST TO ALLOW TRUE SPIRITUAL FRIENDSHIP

When doing this practice, be sure to notice if the space inside of you ceases to naturally open or begins to contract. At this point in sexual meditation you may want to stop making love and simply relax. You have successfully arrived at the meditation launch point—don't abandon it purely to satisfy animal needs.

Do not continue sexual play simply because you can. Instead, stop and relax even more. Relaxation opens the space, whereas any kind of tension will close the space down, and it will start to diminish. If you recognize any tension, just relax for a few moments and let your lower tantien and kwas gently pulse.

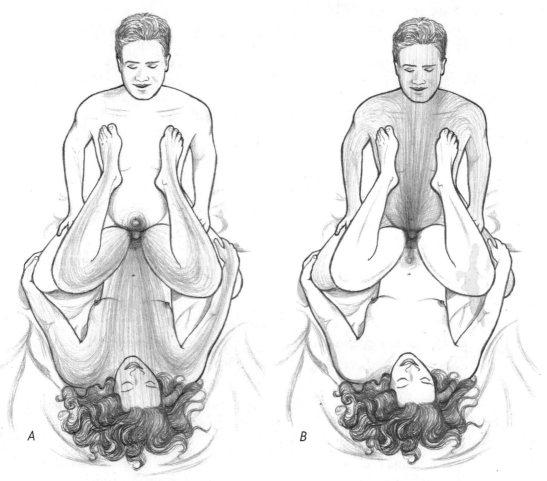

A) He withdraws the whole of his energy from her entire body back into his lower tantien.

B) She does likewise, withdrawing the whole of her energy from his entire body back into her lower tantien.

Figure 17-4 A–B: Partners Pull Energy Back into Their Bodies

Allow whatever energies that remain in both your own and your partner's genitals and tantiens spread throughout your bodies (both your entire energetic and physical nervous systems) until both of you are internally calm and balanced.

When it's time to withdraw, each partner pulls his or her energy from the other's body back into his or her own lower tantien. Then you just hang out, cuddling or lying separately. Sit up if it seems appropriate. Grow into and share the meditation space together. Taoists view this type of sharing as the beginning of true spiritual friendship.

THE MICROCOSMIC ORBIT: PREPARING TO ACTIVATE THE CENTRAL CHANNEL

Special warning: Before attempting to activate the central channel, you must have experience and skill with the Taoist sexual meditation methods in the previous chapters—directing internal orgasms, dissolving internal blockages (especially emotional and psychic) and activating the left and right channels effectively—otherwise you are likely to be wasting your time with these more advanced practices.

Assuming that you can do the practices in this chapter and your sexual teapot has begun to boil, it is time to activate your left, right and central energy channels during intercourse. Once the whistle on the teapot blows with your qi hot and moving, the main point is to actively convert your sexual energy and/or orgasms into Spirit and, later, into emptiness. Once you are capable of working with the ever more refined levels of emptiness, this conversion of your sexual energy into emptiness allows you to jump beyond your body, beyond the limitations of time and space and even beyond the limitations of life and death.

> *The conversion of your sexual energy into emptiness allows you to jump beyond your body, beyond the limitations of time and space and even beyond the limitations of life and death.*

This is the ultimate objective of sexual meditation—to gain access to these limitless spaces using the three energy channels (left, right and central), with the central channel playing an especially important role.

Your central channel contains the psychic and karmic content you can carry from one life into the next. By freeing yourself of all bound energies within the central channel, you can free your Spirit from the deepest, most subtle tensions we experience in this life. Even more remarkably, once you move past karma into essence, you can potentially eliminate the need to involuntarily reincarnate.

The central channel begins in the center of perineum, located at the center of the underside of the pelvis. It continues through the center of the torso, neck and brain and finishes at the bai hui point on the crown of the head. Keep in mind that the central channel and the spine are *not* one and the same, even though various traditions confuse their functions.

There are many ways to activate the central channel. The following is a description of one method to do so in progressive stages. It is not presented in the form of detailed instructions because this advanced material must be learned directly from a qualified master.

PREPARATION PHASE 1: SMALL HEAVENLY OR MICROCOSMIC ORBIT

Before approaching the central channel, you can use the Taoist Bend the Bow Qigong[2] spinal pumping and pulsing techniques to open up the small heavenly circulation of energy (also known as the Microcosmic Orbit—see Chapter 11, Figure 11-6).

Bend the Bow consists of two parts: bending the bow (literally your spine) and shooting the arrow (the energy). When doing the Bend the Bow technique, the neck and spine slightly curve forward on the close (bending the bow) then straighten on the open (shooting the arrow).

To ensure safety when you do the Bend the Bow method, it must be accurately learned from a qualified teacher and then mastered as a solo practice before it is used sexually. This technique involves small and extremely important details that are essential to protect your spine which are beyond the scope of this book. The stages of learning and working with Taoist Bend the Bow methods are in some ways parallel to how you work with the energy of what in India is called Kundalini.

If you are already familiar with Bend the Bow as a solo practice, Figures 17-5 and 17-6 are examples of how this technique can be incorporated into sexual practices. This is not recommended for any beginners. When doing Bend the Bow during sex, stay connected with your lover at the genitals until both your Microcosmic circulations come into synch.

---

2. Bend the Bow Qigong is one of the core programs within the Frantzis Energy Arts System. This qigong set must be learned directly from an advanced instructor to ensure that safety protocols are observed and the spine is adequately protected.

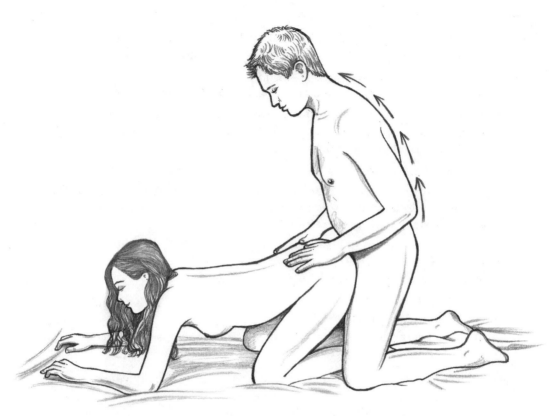

A) As the man withdraws, he bends the bow, curving his spine and pulling the energy within his penis and her vagina up his spine or central channel to the crown of his head.

Figure 17-5 A: Bending the Bow upon Withdrawal

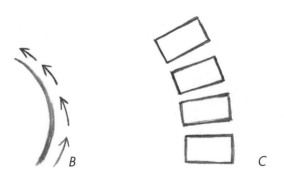

B) Motion of the spine while bending the bow. C) Bending of vertebrae.

Figure 17-5 B–C: Curving Motion of the Spine and Vertebrae for the Bend the Bow Technique

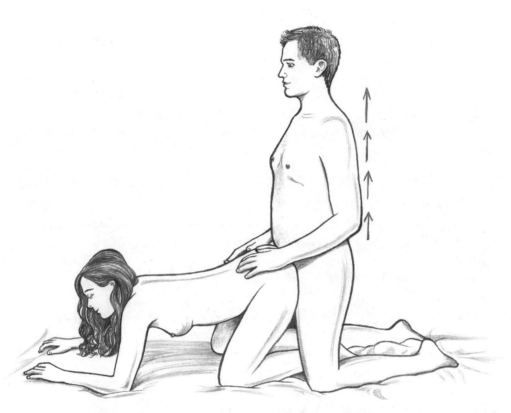

A) Entering her, the man shoots the arrow, straightening his spine while he sends his qi downward via the front of his body (not shown in figure) or central channel to his perineum and penis, and from there into her energy system (not shown).

Figure 17-6 A: Shooting the Arrow upon Insertion

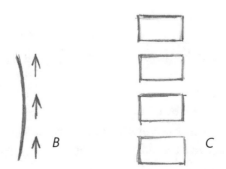

B) Motion of the spine while shooting the arrow. C) Straightening of vertebrae.

Figure 17-6 B–C: Straightening Motion of the Spine and Vertebrae for the Shooting the Arrow Technique

TEN PHASES OF USING THE MICROCOSMIC ORBIT TO AWAKEN THE CENTRAL CHANNEL

The Small Heavenly, or Microcosmic Orbit is presented in many books as just one flow of energy. However, in reality, it has a series of distinct phases that culminate upon arriving inside the central channel. In each phase, on the centerline of the torso, neck and head, the orbit begins at the perineum, goes up the torso to the crown of the head and from there descends to return to the perineum where you began. Certain variations reverse the up-and-down directional flow of energy, but the specifics of how these energetic reversals are done, under what conditions and for what specific purposes are beyond the scope of this book.

The ten main energetic techniques are related to ten primary phases of activating the Microcosmic Orbit. In the Taoist Water tradition, each of these energetic techniques is normally taught progressively, one by one, until a practitioner is equally skilled in all of them. The following is an overview of the ten Microcosmic Orbit phases:

1. Beginning at the perineum, upwards from the upper part of the buttocks, then the entire back of the torso, to the entire back of the neck and skull to the crown of the head. Then down the entire forehead, face, neck, chest, belly, pubic area and returning to the perineum.

2. From the perineum, to the tailbone, up the back (posterior) of the spine, neck and centerline of the skull (the bai hui point). Then down the body's centerline from the crown of the head, face and throat on the front of the torso and returning to the perineum (referred to in Chinese medicine as the "governing and conception vessel").

3. Up the front (anterior) part of the spine and down the centerline on the front of the torso.

4. Up the spinal cord through its various layers, then down the centerline on the front of the torso.

5. Up the central channel and down the centerline on the front of the torso to the perineum.

6. Up the anterior part of the spine and down torso's centerline, midway between the spine and the central channel.

7. Up the anterior part of the spine and down torso's centerline, midway between the central channel and the skin of the torso.

8. Up the anterior part of the spine and down the central channel.

9. Up the spinal cord through its various layers and then down the central channel.

10. Up and down within the central channel.

When you do the later stages of the Taoist Bend the Bow spinal-pumping methods, it is ideal to close your vertebrae and bring your qi from your perineum through the spinal cord rather than only along the vertebrae or through the cerebrospinal fluid. Then, when you open your vertebrae, you dissolve and move the qi from the crown of your head, down your body's centerline to your perineum as best you can.

For most, in the beginning stages, moving energy through the cerebrospinal fluid is relatively easier than moving energy through the spinal cord. This assumes a practitioner has a clear conscious distinction of the differences and can direct his or her qi with intent.

The strong unwinding movement of cerebrospinal fluid and related anatomical structures is what often causes people to writhe or undulate during sexual meditation practices. Within some Eastern traditions, these same phenomena are considered Kundalini experiences. After the cerebrospinal fluid is sufficiently activated, it may take a while before your consciousness is able to directly focus into the spinal cord itself. Let the unwinding takes its natural course. Notice if you enter into a calm, clear space—that is often the point at which it becomes easier to bring qi through the spinal cord.

PREPARATION PHASE 2: LINK MICROCOSMIC ORBITS

Until now, both of you have been focusing independently on getting the energy moving through your Microcosmic Orbit. Staying connected at the genitals, you will now progress to the next stage: simultaneously increasing your lover's circulation as well as your own until both Microcosmic Circulations synch with each other. This often happens naturally, with minimal effort. At this point you should be able to feel what the other person is doing and feeling. Continue this linking, pumping your spine and bringing energy up and down the spinal cord and along the centerline of the front of your torso.

Linking with Nature, Natural Forces and Planets

Within the Taoist tradition there are two great subdivisions. The lower, or initial stage, is the path of Taoist shamanism and the higher, or later stage, is the path of Taoist meditation, including sexual meditation.

Shamanism is about truly understanding what power is. When you understand what it is, you can let it go. This allows you to go beyond power and not have the power control you. The prime purpose of Taoist shamanic practices is for a human to pragmatically encounter, gather and become comfortable with his or her own personal power. Through unambiguously knowing power, a person can drop the all-consuming drive to acquire power in its millions of forms. You must attain power before you can give it up. When this is done, an individual can release and resolve what is false inside him or her. This opens the door to meditation, which in time leads to what is true within a person's seventh and eighth energy bodies.

As a part of the Taoist shamanic path, one learns to energetically link with the forces of the environment for a wide variety of purposes. This is first done with living things in this world, starting with trees, all living plants and then moving to linking directly with animals. Many people can do this quite naturally with their dog, cat, horse and other pets. Linking with animals and other elemental forces leads to a better understanding of the subtle energy flows that nurture compassion and love for all living beings.

Near the end of the Taoist shamanic path, one engages with the bigger bodies of this world. Taoists do this on a case-by-case basis, including what they consider to be living beings, such as mountains and large bodies of water, including the ocean. The Taoists view the earth as a living being whose blood is the ocean. The earth and the ocean also have eight energy bodies. A Taoist shamanic practitioner might link with one or more of the eight energy bodies of the ocean to use and borrow its power to aid in dissolving energy blockages. Practitioners can amplify his or her individual ability to release and resolve the blockages within themselves by linking to larger energetic forces in this way. Much as a practitioner would ask for permission from a human partner, the protocol for linking with other beings would be to ask for permission to do so.

One can also link to and use the power of the earth, as well as that of the sun, moon and planets in our solar system and even beyond, to that of the stars, all for a variety of purposes. Within Taoism, the North Star, or polestar, is a particularly popular body to link to. The same can be done with important nonphysical entities that inhabit the universe for a variety of purposes.

Truly understanding power and linking to the subtle energy bodies in our natural world gives the Taoist shamanic practitioner the ability to discover and sustain what many strive for in vain, a direct experience of power that is grounded in the world around us. That being said, the main purpose is to see the nature of power and then release the need for it so you can next move forward onto the deeper path of Taoist meditation.

AWAKENING THE CENTRAL CHANNEL

After you have done the preparation phases for activating the central channel, you are now ready to fully awaken it. There are three primary methods which will be briefly described. The full instructions for these are beyond the scope of this book. It is important to learn this material from a qualified master who can incorporate all the necessary safety protocols.

METHOD 1: THE THREE TANTIENS LINK TO THE SPINE

Once you've got the energy moving up and down the spinal cord, start to focus on where your qi is located at any given moment. Notice when the energy of the spine is parallel to your lower, middle or upper tantien (see Figure 17-7). These three tantiens, like chakras of the Hindu and Buddhist traditions, are located on the central channel. Practice until you can deliberately hang out and stabilize your energy at each individual tantien for as long as you choose. Over time, you should be able to experience the qi building and accumulating in one or more of your tantiens.

When enough energy has built up in any of the three corresponding tantiens, it is time to link the energy of your spine to the energies of the three tantiens along and within the central channel. Specifically, you want to link the lower tantien to the spine, the heart center to the spine, and spine to the upper tantien in the center of the brain either from the brain stem or, ideally once you are able, from the third eye, the area above the middle of the eyebrows (see Figure 17-7). After you can first accomplish this within yourself and stabilize the connection, the next stage is to do the same between you and your partner, initially linking each tantien and spine connection as one.

Once you can activate all three tantiens simultaneously, you move into another realm, where they truly become vibrantly alive in your awareness. This is the first stage of joining to the central channel. Most likely, at first you will only be vaguely aware of your central channel. Just as night gradually turns into the newly arriving dawn, this linkage to your central channel will become more and more obvious. Over time and as you persist with the practice, eventually you will become aware of your partner's central channel as well.

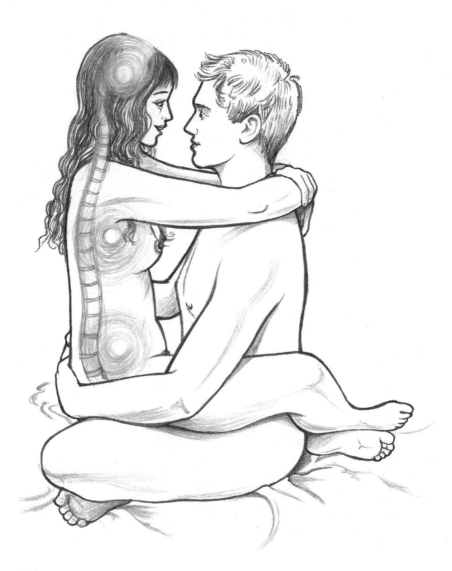

She is awakening her three tantiens and linking them to her spine as he will do next with his own tantiens. This step must be achieved before the partners can mutually attempt to link to each other's individual tantiens.

Figure 17-7: Connecting the Spine and Three Tantiens Energetically

Regular and Instantaneous Jump Method of Linking Energy

All energetic linking or transfer of energy in Taoism's Water tradition is accomplished in two distinct ways. The first is by gradually dissolving and moving energy on some kind of direct line. This has been the technique employed up to this point for all sexual qigong and sexual meditation methods.

The second method is by focusing your mind on the two places you wish to connect, dissolve, jump and thereby link them instantly. The nature of this jump-link method is not a gradual moving of energy along a line, but rather an instantaneous jump that immediately links energetic consciousness. This happens outside our normal sense of time and sequential events, with no sense of gradual transition.

The actual "how to" of jump-linking is learned in one of three ways:

• Through copious effort, experimentation and rigorous self-analysis of what is more and less successful until you finally figure it out on your own. This is the most difficult method to accomplish.

• By being with someone who can jump-link, so through him or her you experience how to do it.

• By mind-to-mind transmission from an adept, who directly patterns and teaches a student at the psychic level.

After you can jump-link relatively effortlessly on your own, you can progress to doing it with your partner. Using this instantaneous jump method with genital and bodily contact, jump between your heart center at the middle tantien and that of your partner, back and forth, until this happens readily without much effort. Then do the same for the lower and upper tantiens. Finally do all three centers simultaneously. Most likely you will need to practice this for many months, or longer, until it becomes fairly effortless.

METHOD 2: TRANSFER OF ENERGY FROM THE SIDE CHANNELS INTO CENTRAL CHANNEL

In this method of awakening the central channel, during penetration you will be moving energy through the three channels (left, right and central). It is important that you avoid simply visualizing the energy moving through your three channels. If you do this you risk turning pleasurable body sensations into a dissociated head-trip or an exercise in mental gymnastics.

To increase your ability to move energy through your three channels, gently squeeze and concretely feel your left and right kwas open and close. The energy from the genitals joins the left and right channels at the kwa region on each side, so this method is highly effective. The energy from the genitals can join the central channel both at the perineum and pubic mound or mons pubis area (where your abdominal muscles insert into the center of your pelvis) which is between the left and right kwa.

Although this central area is technically not a kwa, it functions like one in terms of how it opens and closes to move energy through the central channel. As such, it can be considered the central kwa, as opposed to those on the left or right.

The three external sections of the kwa are located just within the muscles of the pelvis above its energetic center either left, right or in the middle (Figure 17-8). Energetically the actual kwa is located deep within the center of the body half way between the skin on the front of the torso and the back of the spine.

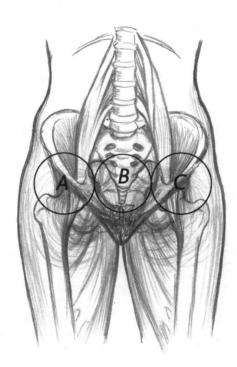

A–Right channel and right kwa

B–Central channel and central area between the kwas

C–Left channel and left kwa

Figure 17-8: Anatomical Structures Connected to the Kwa

With practice, a woman can easily link the contractions of her vagina and perineum to pulsing within any part of her kwa, and a man can link the pulsing within any part of his kwa to corresponding movements in his perineum, prostate, anus and penis.

When closing your kwa, pull energy from your partner's genitals into your genitals. Then, when opening your kwa, project energy from your genitals into your partner's genitals.

In the center of your pelvis, between the left and right kwa, is the primary central channel energetic junction box that is not located on the surface of your skin, but deep within your body.

There are three clear sections: the left kwa, which governs the left energy channel; the right kwa, which governs the right energy channel; and the central region in the pubic mound just above the genitals, between the top of the pubic bone and the lower tantien, which governs the central energy channel (Figure 17-9).

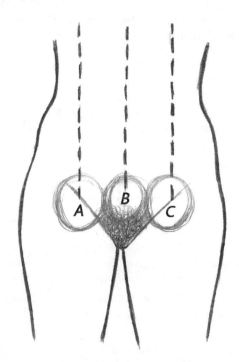

A—Right channel and right kwa
B—Central channel and central area between the kwas
C—Left channel and left kwa

Figure 17-9: Three Sections of the Kwa

You can move these three areas in five ways:

1. To move energy only in the left channel: open and close the left kwa only, **not** the right kwa and center section.

2. To move energy only in the right channel: Open and close the right kwa only, **not** the left kwa and central section.

3. Alternate the opening and closing of two of the areas while leaving the third still, in order to transfer and join the energies of two channels together, or to completely withdraw the energy of one channel into the other, while not affecting the third (for example, left into right, or either right or left into or away from the central channel).

4. To move energy solely in the central channel: Open and close the center area only and keep the right and left kwas closed. This closing of the left and right sides will bring the energy of the left and right channels continuously into the central channel.

5. Opening and closing all three sections of the kwa simultaneously in order to strongly circulate qi evenly throughout the entire body.

Next, to fully activate and work with the energy of the central channel, a practitioner must move energy from the right and left channels into the central channel. To do this, you close the left and right sides of the kwa to draw their energy into the central channel. To maintain and ensure the energy of the left and right channels are being absorbed into the central channel, you continue to keep the left and right sides of the kwa ever so slightly closed with a comfortable pressure. When you do this your energy should now be in the central channel.

Now that the energies of the left and right channels are stably inside the central channel, open the center pelvic section very gradually to systematically move energy through the central channel upward, or you can close the center pelvic section gradually to bring energy down the central channel.

You can reverse the flow even more strongly to bring energy from the lower tantien or entire central channel into either or both of the left and right energy channels. The methods of opening and closing the left and right kwa and the central area in between them is especially helpful to either move energy into or away from the central channel.

After you have done this effectively, the next stage is to slowly and steadily bring the newly arrived energy from your lower tantien up and down the central channel. This should be done in tiny enough stages so that you can move energy in this way without strain in a very stable and relaxed manner. Practice until you can smoothly stabilize the energy entering the central channel and move it to your heart level. In this way you can then energetically link your lower tantien to your middle tantien.

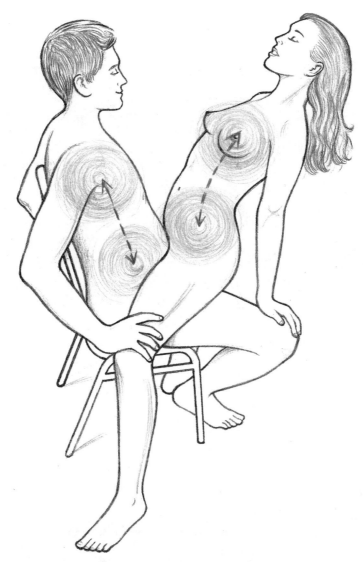

Figure 17-10 A: Linking the Lower Tantien to the Middle Tantien

After you have linked your lower and middle tantiens you move onto the next stage where you link to your partners tantiens from the central channel. Continue to practice this method until both you and your partner can either pull or project energy between your lower tantiens (Figure 17-10 B). When this link is established between your lower tantiens, you will feel a laser beam of energy between these energy centers that connects your physical bodies.

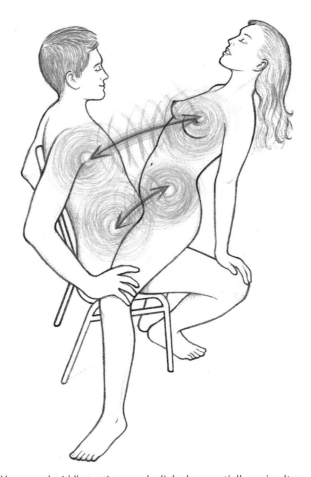

The partners' lower and middle tantiens can be linked sequentially or simultaneously.

Figure 17-10 B: Partners Push and Pull Energy between Their Lower and Middle Tantiens

After you link just your tantiens, you go deeper to now link your central channels together from your lower tantiens until each person's consciousness joins together as one in the central channel.

Then repeat this same process using the middle tantien in both partners. Once you have established energy moving both up and down the central channel and between the lower and middle tantiens, link the entire section between both your central channels, that is, between the perineum and middle tantien, which is your heart center (Figure 17-10 B).

Be aware that linking heart centers can invoke very strong emotional and psychic reactions. If this occurs, take it easy until the initial flush or reaction passes.

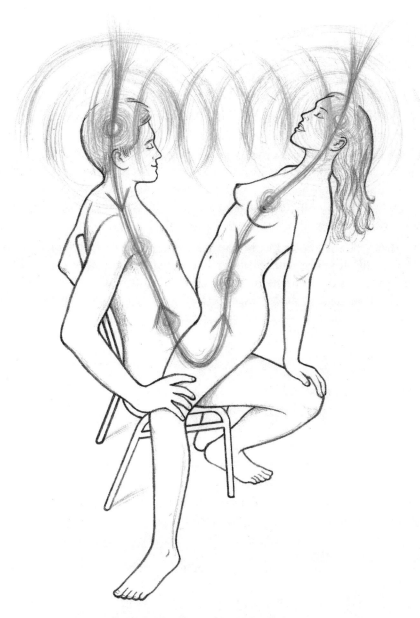

Figure 17-10 C: Lovers Link Their Central Channels

The next step is for you and your partner to link energy completely up, down and through each other's central channels. Energy is pushed and pulled through the lower, middle and upper tantiens inside both central channels (Figure 17-10 C).

METHOD 3: SPINAL PUMPING TO MOVE ENERGY IN THE CENTRAL CHANNEL

In addition to using the central pubic area of your kwa, you can also move energy up and down or in and out of the central channel using Bend the Bow Spinal Qigong energy pumps (see Figures 17-6 and 17-7). When you do this pumping technique, you are going for a balance between maximum strength and evenness to get the best effect. Observe the seventy-percent rule.

By opening and closing the spine in a pumping fashion, you not only bring qi up and down the spine, you can also control the movement of energy within the central channel. When opening your spine (penetrating), you project energy into your partner's genitals and central channel, and when closing your spine (pull out), you pull energy from your partner's genitals and central channel.

Due to the different yin and yang natures of men and women's physical bodies, they often initially experience moving energy with a yin or yang quality quite differently. This is true whether a person works with solo practices or with energy flows between themselves and a partner. The following is a partial list of the various energy flows you can play with in sexual meditation.

Close the spine and pull energy:

- From above the crown of your head down the spine into the genitals.
- From the fingertips (or from beyond, in your etheric body) to the spine and down to the genitals.
- Up from (or from below) the feet and legs into the genitals.
- Simultaneously from (or from above) the crown of the head and fingertips down the body and to the feet (or below).
- Simultaneously toward any of your three tantiens from above or below it, with the top being the crown of the head and fingertips (or beyond) and the bottom the toes (or below).

 Open the spine and project energy from your genitals, spine or central channel:

- Up the spine and/or to the crown of the head (or above) and the fingertips (and beyond).
- Down the legs to the feet (or beyond).
- From (or from below) the feet up the body to (or past) the crown of the head and the fingertips and the boundaries of their etheric body.
- Simultaneously away from any of your three tantiens, or any other point on the central channel, from either above or below that point.

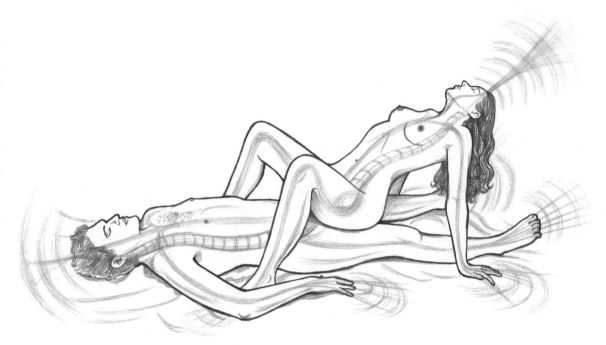

Each partner moves energy through his or her body, emitting qi from the crown of the head, spine, fingers and toes out to the etheric body.

Figure 17-11: Opening and Closing the Central Kwa Area to Move Energy through the Entire Body

By using the energetic pumps of both the spine and the three parts of the kwa separately, an individual can consciously move energy:

- From the center (genitals) to the periphery (head, fingers and toes)
- Up and down the body from head to feet and vice versa
- Simultaneously up one channel and down another by having one of the three sections of the kwa open, as another part closes.

As you master these methods with your partner, you are no longer two separate energy systems. By linking these procedures with your partner you can blend and combine to form a single harmonic energy system. What comes next is truly out of this world.

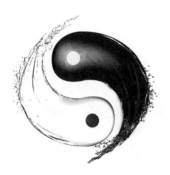

CHAPTER 18

Two Become More than One

Once the central channel has been awakened, using the methods described in the previous chapter, the next step is to continue linking and joining your central channels. You now are presented with a unique opportunity to make an exponential jump to higher levels of nonordinary consciousness.

The advanced Taoist spiritual meditation practices described in this chapter provide partners with the potential to go beyond the physical body into expanded places within themselves and to the most distant reaches of the universe.

LINKING THE CENTRAL CHANNELS OF BOTH LOVERS

The entirety of both your central channels will now become linked through each of the three tantiens. Once discovered and fully embodied, this joining of central channels can be accomplished with or without genital contact, in any juxtaposition of your bodies that naturally interests you. Skilled practitioners can even link their central channels while sitting across from each other with no body contact.

Now that your mind is beginning to enter the central channel, the time has come to pulse, or open and close, the energies within the central channel. When you close your central channel, pull energy from your partner's central channel into yours. Then, when you open, project energy from your central channel into that of your partner. Your central channels will link at the groin and at the boundary of your etheric bodies (see Figure 18-1).

At this stage you link only at the three tantiens. Later you can do it at any point along the central channels. With internal sensitivity and inner stillness, after some weeks or months, you can gain the ability to bring energy up and down the central channel, initially moving through all the points between the lower and middle tantiens. Ultimately, the process should become effortless.

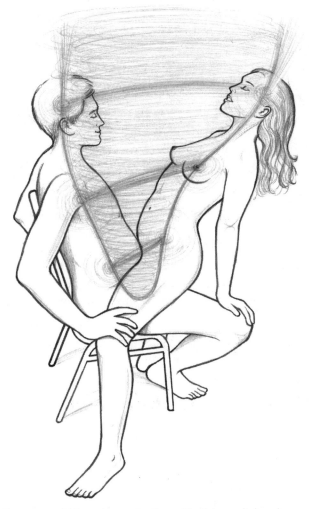

The upper, middle and lower tantiens of both lovers link and merge.

Figure 18-1: *Lovers Link Their Central Channels and Tantiens*

Next, use the previous procedure of linking the lower and middle tantiens to join both central channels at all the points between the middle tantien (heart center) and the upper tantien (brain center), all the way to the crown of the head (Figure 18-1). Particularly when linking at the throat energy gate (see Chapter 12, Figure 12-9), you may want to use the sound and vibration methods discussed in Chapter 16, as these are very effective for expanding consciousness.

Once your energetic linkages become stable at all points as you go up or down between the middle and upper tantiens, then go back and again focus on connecting with your lover at the heart center.

Doing this often with your lover creates a tremendous tenderness and warmth that allows the two of you to forge a profound loving bond—human being to human being—that goes beyond what is normally available, simply because heart-center energy is the essential "connective tissue" in relationships of many kinds, especially emotional.

Linking both lovers' heart centers is important. Doing so allows you to go past seeing the other as an object to connect with the other person's soul or Being. This heart connection method is of tremendous value and holds true regardless of the nature of the relationship, whether you're in a romantic, "I will love you forever" mode or making love with someone you've only just met and may never see again.

UPPER TANTIEN AND BEYOND

Let's recap for a moment. You've moved through early stages of lovemaking. Now you can continuously maintain having your qi move up and down between your own genitals and upper tantien along the central channel as it links with your partner's central channel. What's next?

Beyond just moving and linking energies, you now have the opportunity to dissolve every energetic binding, constriction, blockage or uncomfortable spot in any of your own or your partner's first seven energy bodies. Allow your inner perception to make you aware of any part of this subtle world that is not completely free and open and, if you find any blockages, dissolve them. Keep in mind that these blockages and constrictions are what stop your conscious mind from making the jump into higher levels of non-ordinary consciousness.

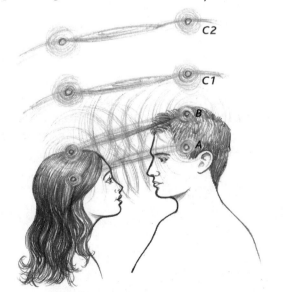

The three distinct locations of the upper tantien:

A—The third eye in the middle of the brain.

B—Just below the crown of the head.

C—The etheric body above the head. This has two potential locations:

C1—The eighth chakra of yoga.

C2— The ninth chakra of yoga.

Figure 18-2: **Lovers Link Their Upper Tantien Centers**

To more fully activate the central channel and move higher up the body will require you to progressively link with the upper tantien, which includes thirty mini-centers inside the brain as well as the centers shown in Figure 18-2. Initially, the upper tantien is most easily linked to at three distinct locations:

1. The center of the brain, behind the space just above the center of the eyebrows, commonly known as the third eye.

2. Just below the crown of the head, the bai hui.

3. Within the etheric field above the crown of your head (according to classical Indian yoga and Tantra, this is where the eighth and ninth chakras are located).

LINKING WITHIN THE ETHERIC FIELD ABOVE THE HEAD

When the crown linkage becomes strong, this is when the upper tantiens of both partners can truly connect. *At this point, it is important to stabilize everything you have previously learned before moving ahead.* This may require that you repeat the previous process until you are sure there are no gaps along the central channel.

Once you are confident your foundation is stable, you want to extend above your head into your etheric field and link at the upper tantien center located there. Within your central channel, start by moving the qi from your middle tantien to the crown of your head.

Then continue piercing the top of your head and extending above it energetically to the naturally felt boundary at the end of your etheric body. The end of the etheric body's energy field can fluctuate moment by moment, extending or shrinking anywhere from a few inches to a few feet above your head. How far the field extends depends on the strength of your individual or combined fields.

Once both partners can naturally extend the energy of the combined central channels to the tantiens above their heads, proximity alone usually causes the two channels to link naturally. This occurs with almost no effort. When this exquisite link occurs, your energies will tend to keep merging into each other's emotional bodies, as well as the other energetic bodies. This yields a tremendous sense of truly satisfying emotional and psychic unity with your partner.

Having successfully moved the energy of both partners' central channels above your heads, you can now start dissolving down the central channel. Repeat the dissolving and linking procedures you just completed going upward, only now do them all going downward.

Each practitioner links and dissolves the other simultaneously, helping each other through difficult or blocked areas. Many find it easier to give rather than receive, or vice versa. This limitation must be consciously worked through until you can dissolve your lover, or have your lover dissolve you, with equal comfort.

Begin above your heads and simultaneously dissolve down both bodies until you get to the bottom of your feet. Then keep going to the end of your etheric bodies, where the human energy anatomy joins the energy of the earth, and link there. Once you make this link, it easily stabilizes and usually stays in place without much effort. Once this stabilization is complete, your whole-body energy linkage happens effortlessly. Then simply dissolve whatever comes up and enjoy each other's presence.

INTER-DIMENSIONAL JUMP-GATES

Only for those with sufficient psychic potential and capacities, the part of the upper tantien above the head is an energetic gateway that allows a person to consciously leap between dimensions. It is no exaggeration to call the upper tantien an inter-dimensional jump-gate.

Upon activating one of these jump-gates, suddenly you might somehow find your consciousness nonphysically outside your body, and end up somewhere far away in space or time. In the West, some refer to this as astral travel. The greater the energetic and sexual turn-on, the easier it is to initially access these inter-dimensional jump-gates.

However, you should heed two warnings. First, do not try this experiment on your own. As a practice method, jumping between dimensions is best learned under the supervision of an adept versed in a multitude of complex and sometimes tricky details beyond the scope of this text. Second, such jumps may occur naturally at the most unpredictable moments. Fear not, for they are neither dangerous nor worthy of obsessing about, as they usually only happen to a small minority of practitioners. Should you happen to be among that minority, you can, over time, hone this jumping ability and control where you end up within all the potential realms of existence. This may sound far out, but this conscious jumping is in the range of what is possible with Taoist sitting meditation, sexual qigong and sexual meditation.

Cautionary note: If you should find this happening to you, it is especially important that you maintain a strong awareness of your physical body, regardless of where your energetic and psychic perceptions or visions lead you. Not staying fully connected to the body while experiencing realities beyond it can result in extreme psychic dissociation. According to some Taoist mediums, jumping out to another dimension without staying connected to your body can open the door for another entity to enter, kick your consciousness out, and, for varying periods of time, leave you floating out there without a clear way to return to your body.

Surreal, Out-of-this-World Experiences

Far-out experiences quite beyond conventional expectations are known to happen in this work, whether you've had an education in the paranormal or not. Taoist training can prepare you for this. Nearly every religion has branches which recognize that the paranormal exists, and Taoism is no exception.

As emphasized earlier, should you have a paranormal encounter, it is of utmost importance that your mind remains fully present in your physical body, no matter how far you move into inner or outer space. You could suddenly find yourself in a distant star system, for example, or inhabiting the infinite space between your cells. These surreal experiences can produce very odd sensations. Stay connected to the sense of your entire physical body no matter what.

Every encounter with Spirit takes you past the thinking, rational mind and further into the outer space of galaxies beyond planet earth while, simultaneously, you come to an incredible awareness inside of you. Whenever you encounter an energetically blocked sensation or your consciousness seems frozen (computer people would call it a "glitch"), pulse it. The glitch you're pulsing could be a phenomenon that is far from local. It might very well have its origins someplace way beyond your personality—some fifty thousand or five hundred thousand or billions of galaxies from your physical body, for example, or in the space between blood cells, or even in the space between organelles within your cells. Some glitches originate somewhere so deep inside that you will never know the exact location or what it might be called.

You may even find yourself stumbling into the theater of the absurd. Suppose a blockage is actually an entity, and you don't dissolve it strongly enough to clear it. Then just go for it again the next time. You might also find yourself having sex with numerous noncorporeal beings simultaneously! When you start going out into psychic territory, you can easily encounter other sentient energies that don't belong to either of the two people in your bed. These energies may be perfectly happy to have sex with you for any number of reasons.

Taoists have observed situations where energies enter a human being to tempt that person to play with them. Practitioners are generally warned against succumbing to this, because they can get distracted at that psychic level and spend years wandering in a psychic playground. Do not get seduced or overly absorbed with these energetic entities flying around on the edges of your consciousness. Fun or not, these distractions are clear and present obstacles to your progress in Taoist meditation. Keep dissolving. Always have the sense of two lovers becoming one.

SOUL MERGING:
CREATING A COMBINED NEO-CENTRAL CHANNEL

Special note: Only two practitioners who can skillfully amplify each other and cooperate intimately in the psychic realm will be able to effectively attempt, let alone have any chance of successfully completing, the methods offered from this point forward.

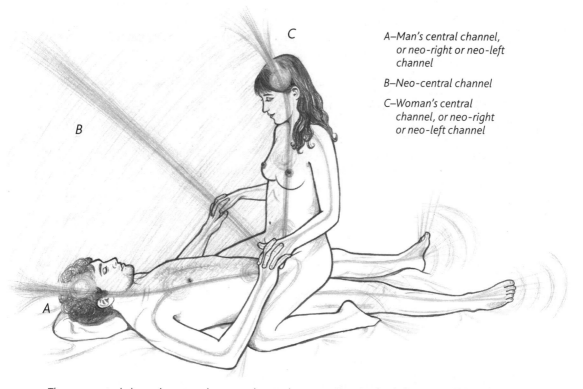

A—Man's central channel, or neo-right or neo-left channel

B—Neo-central channel

C—Woman's central channel, or neo-right or neo-left channel

The neo-central channel emerges between the two lovers, connecting both their central channels.

Figure 18-3: Neo-central Channel Linking

By linking your three tantiens and central channels together from bottom to top and then top to bottom, you and your partner have naturally created the conditions to link the circulation of your central channels. Instead of two energetic entities, you have now become one energetic entity. The two of you are no longer separate—you have become one dynamic energetic system.

Now, in the center space between your individual central channels (that is, between your physical bodies), partners can begin to create a third entity, the combined neo-central channel.

With this soul merging, the entire physical body and central channel of each individual partner will, in effect, become either the neo-left or neo-right channel of your combined neo-central channel. Either of you at any moment can freely switch from being the neo-left or neo-right channel. A couple can play with infinite variations on this consciousness-expanding magic-carpet ride.

Now you can strengthen, ameliorate, transform or awaken certain yin or yang aspects of your consciousness, experiencing the inner man or woman in a myriad of forms. You may also tap into the universal essences of yin and yang energy. This is a much larger frame of reference than the one we humans ordinarily experience while living in an earthly body.

Experiencing Super-bliss States

Many experiences simply can't be described in words. One of my paranormal, earth-shattering experiences during sexual meditation occurred with a lovely woman who was not an initiate in the Taoist priesthood. It took me into a far different place than any intense emotional experience I had previously felt.

Afterward, my brain and my eyes felt like they were lit like sparkling diamonds. She felt the power of my experience and wanted some affirmation about her part in getting me there. "Did I make you happy?" she asked. "You look so happy."

I was having a difficult time reentering the normal world of words. I was rendered incapable of telling this wonderful woman about the sheer power of the bliss that had occurred. All I could do was mumble and waffle. Yes, I was beyond happy. I just wasn't capable of answering her. It seemed as though saying anything would diminish the pure magic of the experience. I have been sad ever since that I couldn't and didn't answer her.

During sexual meditation, I had connected with a paranormal level of bliss that permeated my entire system. I took a magic-carpet ride through the many dimensions of the universe, experiences that I would eventually take many times, nonsexually, during solo meditation with my teacher Liu Hung Chieh. Tibetan Tantra has a parallel method to sexual meditation, which is called the "Four Blisses." For a thousand years, masters diligently tried to describe it. At the end it more or less came down to this naming convention: bliss *(ananda),* extreme bliss *(paramananda),* superb bliss *(viramananda)* and innate bliss *(sahajananda).*[1] If that's the best that a millennium of fully enlightened masters could do, it says a lot about how these paranormal, meditative states lie beyond the possibility of words.

---

1. Snellgrove, David, *The Hevajra Tantra: A Critical Study* (London: Oxford University Press, 1959), 38.

OPENING, CLOSING AND DISSOLVING THE NEO-CENTRAL CHANNEL

Once the neo-central channel emerges between you, each of you can begin to open and close your kwa with ever-increasing fluid strength. This is the ideal precursor to pulsing the newly created combined neo-central channel. Then you can initially pulse it in the following four ways:

1. From the central channels of both partners, pulse into the neo-central channel. Then from there pulse all the way to the ends of your combined etheric bodies or beyond.

2. In and out of your skin and physical body, pulse and dissolve into the pure energetic awareness within the neo-central channel, the neo-left and neo-right channels—that is, the original central channels of both lovers.

3. Each of you pulse and dissolve from your body into the center of your neo-central channel, and then back to your body or individual central channels (which have become neo-left and neo-right channels of the neo-central channel).

4. Pulse from your central channels, center to periphery, periphery to center, ad infinitum, to and from the neo-central channel, using the opening and closing principles of neigong at increasingly sophisticated and powerful levels.

A NEW PULSING ENERGY BALL ARISES

Once you have joined and unified your bodies, having established a comfortable, stable sense of these four opening and closing techniques, a fifth pulsation will eventually start within the combined neo-central channel. This typically begins at the level of the middle tantien, or heart center, although it may occur at the level of the lower or upper tantiens.

First Phase of the Pulsing Energy Ball

In the first phase, this spontaneously arising pulsing will get stronger and stronger. Soon it will spread outward, filling your entire etheric field to its spherical boundaries in all directions. This will unify all the physical and etheric energetic fields around until everything within both of you becomes one big, pulsing energy ball.

Allow the energy to circulate unencumbered within this pulsing ball, dissolving into emptiness any blockages that naturally emerge within the sphere. Then, at a certain point, a psychic moment will occur; you will both get a signal or nudge from within. At this juncture, you want to consciously direct all sensations within both of you to move into the center of the neo-central channel. You and your lover will do this simultaneously, as both continuously dissolve the neo-central channel.

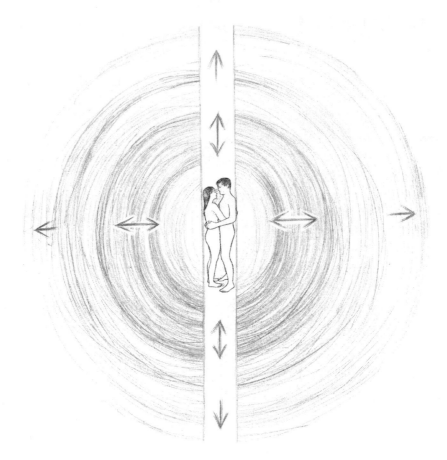

A-neo-central channel pulsing spherically in all directions.

Figure 18-4: Pulsing Energy Ball

Continue moving strongly into the neo-central channel. Naturally, and of its own accord, the pulsation will start to liberate whatever is coming out of or arising within both of you. This is the process of getting energetically unbound, or "working out your stuff," at the level of your higher energy bodies, where it can truly be resolved.

While continuously dissolving, pulse between the neo-central channel and your physical bodies, the central channels of which are now the neo-left and neo-right channels. As you close, dissolve inward as far into the neo-central channel as possible. As you open, dissolve as you expand outward until the size of this neo-central channel begins to grow large enough to encompass both your bodies all the way out to the edge of your skins.

Through this dynamic energy dance you will be commingling the psychic content that is within both of you, as he dissolves her, and she dissolves him. At a certain point, you will feel a sensation of energetic fusion. This happens instantaneously. Now each of you will know what the other is experiencing, and both of you can dissolve whatever comes up that needs resolving.

Second Phase of the Pulsing Energy Ball

In the second phase of working with the energy ball, you will not be able to separate your "stuff" from your lover's "stuff." It all becomes one pulsing ball of stuff with no separate identity of what belongs to whom. You simply want to move the energy of all of it, blocked or not, into the combined neo-central channel where it can be dissolved.

HOW THE COMBINED NEO-CENTRAL CHANNEL PULSES

The neo-central channel has a universal opening and closing rhythm which, in progressive stages, can eventually carry you to an awareness of the Tao via your eight energy bodies. The pulsing occurs in several ways:

- Vertically to the end of your energy bodies above your head and below your feet, in all directions simultaneously.

- From the periphery of your etheric body to the center and from the center of the neo-central channel to the periphery, thereby creating a pulsing energy sphere out of your two bodies.

- As the clearing strength of the pulsing continues, you can find yourself going further and further into the outer space beyond your body. Your third to eighth energy bodies extend exponentially to billions and possibly trillions of galaxies in all directions. As this occurs, you clear how the energies in the extending spaces of the third to eighth influence each lover and also how each lover has influenced them. This continues until the influences are freed and you realize the body of the Tao.

- As the pulsing becomes completely stable, a type of stillness with an undifferentiated center arises and the entire central channel loses all sense of location. This happens as you become present to an infinite number of openings and closings. This type of pulsing is difficult, if not impossible to describe. It exists at the outer edge of esoteric practice.

Ultimately, Consciousness itself is in charge of the pulsing, so you need not be concerned about "getting it right." By this point, your mind will be sufficiently open to accept that all flows can happen at once simultaneously. Don't be concerned about actively doing anything. By simply becoming aware of the flows, they begin to happen automatically. Once the neo-central channel and energetic sphere are pulsing, the intrinsic nature of the pulse will manifest and start to guide or create the lovemaking. You'll find yourself merging with and following the pulse, rather than leading it.

GOING INTO THE CORE OF YOUR BEING

Sooner or later, if you continue to open to the pulsation, it will expand beyond your bodies in all directions simultaneously. Then, when the expansion reverses and awareness returns to your neo-central channel, Inner Dissolving will go dramatically deeper within than before. With each expansion outward and subsequent return, you will go deeper into your cells, deeper into the inner space of consciousness and deeper into the core of your Being.

The pulsing of the neo-central channel is to be encouraged or allowed, rather than visualized and willed into existence or forced. As your linking capacity grows, this pulsing energy sphere emerges naturally. It is a form of intelligence—a direct manifestation of the universal qualities of yin and yang. Allow this energy sphere to give you a profound demonstration of how yin and yang naturally come together and separate in never-ending cycles. If you remain open and humble, this pulse can show you—in vivid, experiential detail—how all manifestation fluctuates from yin to yang and yang to yin. Words cannot begin to approximate the profundity of such an encounter with the fundamental workings of the universe.

GOING BEYOND THE PHYSICAL BODY: INNER AND OUTER SPACE

Here is a simple truth about the nature of consciousness and Spirit: things aren't always what they seem. Our basic ways of perceiving our own consciousness and the external world are often quite limited. Taoism addresses this conundrum with a spiritual maxim, "There is as much external space outside you as there is internal space or consciousness inside you." When Inner and Outer Dissolving are coordinated, the reality behind this statement becomes evident. This is where esoterica, quantum physics, string theory, enlightenment and God are likely, sooner or later, to meet.

There is as much external space outside you as there is internal space or consciousness inside you. When Inner and Outer Dissolving are coordinated, esoterica, quantum physics, string theory, enlightenment and God are likely, sooner or later, to meet.

Ultimately, as you meditate, your Inner Dissolving will go as far inward into inner space as your Outer Dissolving goes outward into the most distant reaches of the ever-expanding universe. This rhythm of going in, into inner space, and out, to outer space, is the crux of all intermediate and advanced Taoist sexual meditation practice. It is the dance of the universe manifesting within your body and higher Being. This is not an ordinary task. All the Taoist techniques practiced before have been to prepare you for this.

Once the inner and outer pulsation has been activated, foreplay, intercourse or simply lying in each other's arms will begin to follow this universal throbbing without effort on your part. All there is for you to do is deepen your relaxation. Resistance has never been more futile! If you hold any part of your body or mind stiff, you will inhibit or stop the pulsation.

Eventually, every single body part will begin to pulse. Everything you feel will go into the neo-central channel in between your physical forms. At times, one part of your body will become extremely sensitive, and that place will—by necessity—become the nexus of your pulsing ball. The pulsing will build to a crescendo right at the nexus point. Allow the rhythm to become very, very strong until an internal orgasm either explodes outwardly or implodes, carrying you deeper into inner space.

SPACE OF PURE CONSCIOUSNESS AND SPIRIT

Once you move beyond your skin and etheric boundary, you may reach a certain point where the opening and closing pulsations lose all sense of solidity. You may even find yourself being blown into the space of Spirit and afforded a direct encounter with pure Consciousness itself.

The space of Spirit doesn't have any clearly distinguishable characteristics. Prior to your arrival in this place, you will have experienced all sorts of energy moving. Cerebrospinal fluid operates within three distinct sets of frequencies, corresponding to *jing* (the energy of the physical and etheric body), *qi* (emotional, mental and psychic energy) and *shen* (karmic and essence energy). Many characteristics of sexual energy are commonly caused by the physical waves of cerebrospinal fluid moving up and down your spine. We experience these waves as the highs of sex: spinal undulations and explosive sensations in the penis and vagina. This level of energy is governed by the lowest set of energetic frequencies within your cerebrospinal fluid. These influence your physical and etheric energy bodies as well as the lower emotions.

Typically, when you dip your toe in the waters of Spirit, you are working with the second set of frequencies of your cerebrospinal fluid. After you jump to this higher set of frequencies, all of a sudden something altogether different opens up. The nature of your sexual sensations goes from enjoyable to extremely satisfying, albeit undeniably nonphysical. That's how you know you have jumped into the psychic arena. Now, with each orgasm, your conscious awareness will go further out into inner and outer space. You may or may not have concurrent orgasms in your physical body.

The awareness being generated by your neo-central channel now progressively moves outward into your eight energetic bodies. Over time, you can move past the level of your mundane emotional body to the higher emotions and beyond. Ultimately, you will start moving into what Taoism sometimes refers to as Pure Spirit or Buddhism calls Mind.

Universal Morality and the Body of the Tao

In this big universe, when a soul reincarnates into one of the many different times, dimensions and situations that can arise, most of these incarnations occur in ways that could seem to have no relationship to anything on this earth. If a human being is reincarnated into a totally different kind of existence, the yin-yang of karma and the Taoist view of morality or *Tao Te* continues.

However, the context, content and events transpiring may be unimaginable to an earthling at that moment. The universal morality of Taoism is expansive, including all the implications of energy interactions that may or may not become solid and material. After all, if someone ends up as a charged particle, most Mind of Man moral systems might not work terribly well.

And yet what happens on this planet is not different, in essence, from what happens elsewhere. It's just that in each different time period (today or trillions of years from now) or potential place or dimension, life has its current events that challenge a person regarding any or all of his or her eight energy bodies.

Taoists view each incarnation as having several basic possibilities. The highest possibility is that anyone could fully wake up to the body of the Tao and become enlightened. Likewise, anyone has the opportunity, moment by moment, to either engage with whatever will bring them closer to or take them farther away from the body of the Tao.

Although many of the principles of Taoist morality can seem perplexing, or even an affront to one's self-image or beliefs, Taoists simply view this as part of the learning process. Reincarnation has many unknown futures and each in turn will need to be dealt with. For all these reasons, inner Taoism is not particularly human-centric. What Taoists perceive as essential is karma and the continuum of all that is possible on the path toward the Tao.

EMPTINESS: YOUR ULTIMATE DESTINATION

Once the mutual energy ball dissolves past your emotional body, consciousness just continues to expand, going further into the external universe and into the depths of internal space. The more you go in, the more you go out; both practitioners just keep moving progressively more strongly between inner and outer space.

Then the next jump in consciousness occurs. Now your awareness becomes permeated by a space where the going in and out cease to be differentiated. Paradoxically, in and out somehow include each other. A third quality can emerge, a place where both in and out have dissolved into emptiness. At this point, you go past ordinary Spirit and move into emptiness, where indescribable light and vibration floods your entire Being.

This space of emptiness is supremely intelligent; it has a tendency to grow exponentially in a way that cannot be put into words. As this space increases, you will experience a totally different kind of orgasm, a stillness orgasm. Whether imploding inward or exploding outward, these orgasms leave no residue.

A stillness orgasm is like a deposit in a permanent bank account that's stored in your Being. You pulse in and out, in and out, and all of a sudden this *other space* emerges that fills your Being and doesn't go away after sex. The experience is like a hologram—what happens simultaneously connects to and influences all parts of your Being. This is a significant threshold in consciousness.

As you progress, you become truly comfortable with the core of your Being where Universal Consciousness resides. You fully embody your essence. You are now well on your way to the ultimate destination: to achieve the body of the Tao.

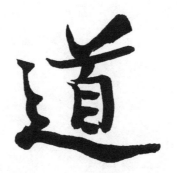

SECTION 6

APPENDICES

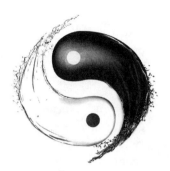

APPENDIX A

The Politics of Sex

Since ancient times, the Chinese have discussed the "Rules of Heaven" within the context of the universal laws of yin and yang; the issue of a God does not enter the conversation. The Chinese are not so much atheists as animists—the material world is organized and animated by a higher, unseen order. As such, every situation must move with the Rules of Heaven.

According to the *I Ching*, both heaven and earth give power to people. Heaven gives people invisible capacity, while earth gives us what is visible in the form of substantive elements. Everything under heaven and earth has its unique way of coming into existence and changing. Men and women are no exception. They come into existence so as to produce children and replicate themselves.

What is good or natural according to the Rules of Heaven? Men are yang, and women are yin. Therefore, for human males and females, it is better if yin and yang come together and have sexual relations than if they don't. What is unnatural, and therefore not good, is to be a celibate monk or to have chaotic excessive sex. For example, a man who ejaculates several times daily on a regular basis would be viewed as unnatural.

Of course, not everyone's lifestyle is conducive to sexual meditation, nor is the practice suited to everyone's disposition. In this segment, we will explore the various ways the Taoists approached the "politics" of sex in broad terms. These reflections are offered in the spirit of discovery to help you explore how you might integrate Taoist practices into your life.

CELIBACY

The Taoist view on celibacy is informed by their overarching attitude toward sex as a completely natural and healthy activity.

413

Sex is given to us by heaven, and yet everything under heaven is susceptible to instability. Just as an excess of water will cause a river to overflow its banks or explode in a flash flood, the human body can metaphorically explode from excessive pressure if sex is renounced in an unnatural way.

According to *Huang Di Nei Jing Su Wen (Basic Questions from the Yellow Emperor's Inner Canon):* "Just as heaven and earth open and close, yin and yang have changes. People must take yin and yang in measured proportions without excess. Without sex, yin and yang won't be in balance and your body can't produce its needs, which shortens the human lifespan."

According to the *Beiji Qian Jin Yao Fang,* also known as *Qian Jin Yao Fang,*[1] it is not permissible for men or women to abstain from sex. Purportedly, if a man has no sex, his mind's intent can waver and become anxious, while his spirit can become exhausted, resulting in an early death.

According to the Taoists, nature's law is that a celibate person can have an exceptionally long life *if* the lack of sex does not influence the individual's body or mind. Approximately twenty percent of any population will be dominated by the Metal element; these people are natural celibates. Abstaining from sex involves little or no effort on their part. Some Metal people actually prefer to entirely abstain from sex, or keep it at a bare minimum, as they are quite content that way and would be unhappy if required to have sex. Beyond that, the only exception to the natural law of celibates is the man who can genuinely calm his mind and have no anxiety regarding sex. Only one in ten thousand can do this with the energy of their body, regardless of their psychological willpower.

The Taoists say that men and women who unnaturally force themselves not to have sex will shorten their lives, the exception being women after menopause where the situation could go either way. According to ancient texts, for example, a man is likely to succumb to involuntary emissions and may have bad dreams of sex with unnatural women or ghosts; this can push his body in the direction of ill health. Thus it is best to be natural with sex.

As Stephen Chang writes, in *The Tao of Sexology,*[2] "From the Taoist viewpoint, practicing celibacy is about the most harmful thing you can do to your body. Denying attention or the right to function to any part of your body is foolish, as foolish as rejecting the use of your eyes and ears. Not using any portion of your body for its natural purpose will create a harmful imbalance which can affect every other part of your body, since all bodily functions are interconnected."

---

1. *Qian Jin Yao Fang* (Qian=one thousand, Jin=golden, Yao=important or want, Fang=prescription) means *One Thousand Golden Important Prescriptions;* the text was written during the Sung Dynasty (960–1279).

2. Chang, Stephen, *The Tao of Sexology* (San Francisco: Tao Publishing, 1986), 191.

People choose celibacy for many reasons—personal, intellectual and spiritual. The Taoists position remains the same. You don't renounce the world; the world renounces you. If celibacy comes about through natural circumstances or proclivities, so be it. When people become celibate for intellectual reasons or on the basis of some misguided belief that abstaining from sex accelerates their spiritual development, they risk running into problems.

If the sexual energy is not resolved in some way it is likely to cause churning in the mental, emotional and psychic body, which in turn produces bodily upheavals. People can mistake these upheavals for spiritual acceleration, when in reality their celibate state is like a car trying to pull a large bus at high speeds. Most people simply don't have the internal strength to do it. Even if a person has a strong will, unnatural or imposed celibacy still can tear him or her apart. Some may carry the belief that celibacy makes them pure or somehow superior, but it disrupts their primary energetic signature.

People often think that becoming celibate will allow them to conserve and build their energy. Or, after taking stock of destructive emotions and attitudes, they decide that becoming a celibate will take the sexual fuel out of the fire and ameliorate the situation. Some just decide that they are fed up with the messiness that can surround sex and don't want to play anymore.

Taoists have observed that celibacy usually doesn't work well if it doesn't come about naturally but instead derives from intellectual reasons. If celibacy creates a level of internal restlessness or agitation that can't be softened, it's counterproductive. With an intellectual decision to become celibate, the cure is generally worse than the disease, because pressures build inside your physical body and energy channels. People's minds can go to strange, messed up places—pedophilia, for example—if they don't have a natural outlet for their sexual needs and desires. Celibacy can twist their energy in perverse and unpredictable ways. What's more, if celibacy is unnatural, it can give a restless mind a real power boost by giving that restlessness a focal point. For a serious student of meditation, unnatural celibacy is particularly counterproductive.

On occasion, an individual who was sexual earlier in life will transition smoothly into celibacy as a natural, choice-less decision. For example, the author met an elderly man in Hawaii who had two former wives and fifteen grandchildren. He declared, "By age sixty, I just didn't want to have to deal with the whole 'woman thing' anymore. I'd rather just cook and take care of myself than live with a woman. I don't care about sex anymore. It was okay when I was younger, but it wasn't that great as time passed. I'm actually dramatically more at peace just being by myself." This man did not renounce the world of sex; the world of sex renounced him.

However, if people are facing celibacy for health reasons or some other unavoidable situation, it benefits them to learn how to open their channels and arrive at natural breath. Regular solo practices of Taoism—standing, sitting and lying-down qigong or meditation practices—can allow anyone to arrive at natural breath. This can relieve the natural burden of celibacy by making the qi inside a celibate's channels flow smoothly.

Taoist celibates do many of the internal energetic processes described in this book. However, rather than having a sexual partner, they work directly with the five elements to transmute their sexual energy into pure Spirit. This allows them to maintain a calm mind and a body that is not burdened by the natural force sexual hormones exert on the human condition. Moreover, these Taoists typically do this by withdrawing and ceasing to interact with this world—not because they decide to leave the world, but because the red dust of the world, with its desires and motivations, leaves them.

MARRIAGE

Humans are naturally inclined to seek companionship and make a life together with another in order to fulfill their physical, sexual, emotional, mental and psychic needs. Historically speaking, this has had little or nothing to do with romantic love or the notion of "the one." Romance did not come into vogue until the Renaissance, when the troubadours began to sing of the joys and sorrows of love.

As always, Taoists are eminently practical. Marriage is valuable insofar as it is the most cohesive social unit for raising children. Regardless of whether the parents are monogamous or not, the primary purpose of marriage is to produce offspring rather than ensure regular sexual contact.

The Chinese have traditionally been powerfully family-centered. If a marriage didn't work, and the parents grew to hate each other, the children would usually be given to the grandparents.

In general, the Taoists treat every glitch or blockage within the family system as an opportunity for meditation. With such high value placed on what is good for the children, problems in the family system will motivate the parents to evolve spiritually. Meditation—with its emphasis on clearing personal energetic, emotional, psychic and karmic glitches—can help men and women become better parents in the interests of the next generation.

MONOGAMY

Monogamy (from the Greek words *monos,*"singular" or "only," and *gamos,* "marriage") is held as the gold standard of relationship in many societies, and yet the failure to live up to this presupposed requirement causes tremendous pain and suffering between men and women. Expectations are changing, of course, as evidenced in common terms such as "serial monogamy," "semi-monogamy" and the fairly recent innovation known as "polyamory," the practice of openly maintaining more than one intimate relationship (not to be confused with polygamy, the practice of having more than one spouse, with or without the knowledge of all parties).

Historically, Taoists have accepted any and all of these approaches. They do not hold one model of relationship as better or more desirable than others. To the Taoists (and most traditional Chinese), any trend that lasts less than two hundred years is considered a fad. The attitudes and opinions about sex and monogamy a society holds in any given period is subject to change, and especially in modern times they can change in the space of ten or fifteen years. From one generation to the next, very different attitudes about what is or is not acceptable can prevail.

Not so very long ago, if a woman slept with someone "inappropriately," she was automatically viewed in a negative light. Now Western women can exercise a full range of choices, if they have the courage to claim that freedom. A similar loosening of social mores has occurred for men: not so long ago, a man who slept with many women was automatically viewed with disdain (at least by women) whereas today his behavior can be seen as quite honorable within a certain framework. No longer a tyrant or seducer, he might even be a skillful lover who is celebrated for spreading joy. Of course, how he's viewed will depend on where he lives and how he handles himself, but, overall, we have far less "fire and brimstone" and far more "live and let live"—at least among the more educated sectors of Western society.

What is natural for any specific individual? Biologically speaking, some seem to be geared more toward monogamy, while others are more inclined toward the opposite. In recent years, the notion that some of us have a "variety gene" (a specific genetic predisposition toward sexual variety) has been used to justify and normalize nonmonogamous behavior.

Sex at Dawn: How We Mate, Why We Stray, and What It Means for Modern Relationships, by Christopher Ryan and Cacilda Jetha[3] goes further, positing that monogamy is a fairly recent phenomenon, resulting from the rise of agriculture and individually-owned property, which made paternity an important matter. According to this book, for most of the few million years of human history, in hunter-gatherer

---

3. Ryan, Christopher, and Jetha, Cacilda, *Sex at Dawn: How We Mate, Why We Stray, and What It Means for Modern Relationships* (New York: Harper Perennial, 2010), 2, 12.

societies, "most adults would have several sexual relationships at any given time... and an open sexuality unencumbered by guilt or shame." The book claims that the truth about human sexuality was "so subversive and threatening that for centuries it has been silenced by religious authorities, pathologized by physicians, studiously ignored by scientists, and covered up by moralizing therapists." However, using the same sources as Ryan and Jetha, Lynn Saxon comes to very different conclusions in her book, *Sex at Dusk*,[4] in particular regarding monogamy.

Practically speaking, having more than one lover is a complicated matter. Some pull it off with great panache, while others get bogged down in never-ending negotiations for time, space and affections. Most people choose to keep their extramarital activities a secret, conducted outside the purview of their supposedly monogamous pairing. For many of these men and women, this choice may be more a matter of loving care and diplomacy than harmful deception. In fact, the Taoists have specific techniques for a practitioner to use to prevent bringing the energy of one sexual partner into the bed of another (see Chapter 15, Practice 33).

This brings up the issue of pride or honor, or what the Chinese call "saving face." A vital part of Taoist sexuality involves respecting your partner by doing what you can to spare him or her the feelings that "losing face" can generate. Even if a relationship is officially open, it's important to be protective of your partner's feelings.

Taoists take the viewpoint that there is no guarantee that you or those you love will be alive tomorrow, or even a few hours from now. Whatever a man and a woman share during a sexual encounter, long- or short-term, has the potential to be an extremely intimate and beneficial connection.

SAME-SEX RELATIONSHIPS

Throughout history, homosexuality has existed in China just as it has in other nations. The traditional Taoist position on same-sex relationships is not based on cultural ideas and prejudices common in the West, but on the energy dynamics and potential dangers involved. In *The Tao of Health, Sex and Longevity*,[5] Daniel Reid summarizes the Taoist view:

> [Homosexual relations] are harmless for women but highly detrimental to men, both physiologically and psychologically. Nature has made Yin passive and yielding, and two passive forces do not conflict. The Chinese refer to sapphic love as 'polishing mirrors', a term that reflects the fact that female homosexual practices are largely limited to the rubbing together of similar parts, rather than

---

4. Saxon, Lynn, *Sex at Dusk* (2012).
5. Reid, Daniel, *The Tao of Health, Sex and Longevity* (London: Simon & Schuster, 1989), 262.

actual penetration of the body. And even when the body is penetrated with a surrogate phallus, it is done through the orifice intended for that purpose. Like masturbation, sapphism was a common practice in the household harems of wealthy Chinese families, where up to a dozen women might find themselves completely cut off from male company for months at a time when the man of the house was off on official business.

Taoist physicians regarded homosexuality among men, on the other hand, as a dangerous practice—for several reasons. First of all, Yang is by nature an active, aggressive force, and, when two aggressive forces meet, a fundamental conflict of energies and intentions results.

From the energetic view of anal sex, a male-to-male encounter is yang meeting yang. According to the Taoist perspective, when yang energy meets yang energy during homosexual anal sex, the charges that this releases can have a negative impact on the central channel in either or both partners and disturb the natural flow of energy moving up the spinal cord into the brain. Taoists found that these effects tended to be exacerbated by sexual qigong and meditation practices. The energetic input would be too much for an already strained central channel to handle, which could result in severe consequences, such as physical, psychological, psychic and karmic damage to the practitioners and others.

The ultimate purpose of Taoist spiritual sexuality involves two partners creating a combined third central channel. This can only be achieved by a man and a woman, just as a man and a woman are necessary to make a physical baby. The Taoist system of sexual meditation was designed to specifically utilize the combination of yin and yang to create an alchemy that enabled deep spiritual growth to manifest. Outside this tradition, there may be esoteric sexual energetic practices that are deemed quite suitable for same-sex partners; however, these are outside the scope of this book.

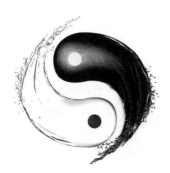

APPENDIX B

Man-Woman Concerns

CONTRACEPTION

Today, men and women can take advantage of a wide array of Western medical approaches for birth control. In ancient times, the Chinese relied on two primary methods: semen retention and intentionally-induced miscarriages using acupuncture and herbs. In addition, the Taoists developed a specific practice that works at the level of the karmic (sixth) body, which is also known as the body of manifestation. Because this method requires a fairly high level of attainment to be effective, it is rarely taught. An advanced practitioner can essentially close the door that allows another being to obtain a body (that is, reincarnate) through his or her sexual activities. At a later time, should the person genuinely desire to have a child, the door can be reopened to allow for conception, at which point it typically happens fairly quickly.

CONDOMS

Even people with very little energetic sensitivity can tell that condoms block what naturally moves between the naked penis and vagina. This fact must be judiciously balanced against the dangers of sexually transmitted disease and unwanted pregnancy. That said, in sexual meditation, condoms do limit the qi flow that would otherwise be available. Physical contact with the entirety of a partner's body maximizes the psychic energy two people can generate and use to penetrate and receive from one another.

MENSTRUATION

As a general rule if the woman or the man is uncomfortable having sex while she is menstruating, they should not do it. It is purely a matter of personal preference.

Some women particularly enjoy sex during their menses; intercourse and orgasms have even been known to relieve menstrual cramps. Taoists do caution that ideally, a man should not perform cunnilingus while a woman has her period. Also, if the man enjoys sex while his woman is menstruating, it is wise to make sure his body does not overheat during this time, as this can be an indication that his kidney fire is getting burned out. This is a condition that happens to some men if they have sex with a woman during her menses. If his body doesn't heat up, there's no problem about having intercourse at this time.

AGING AND MENOPAUSE

The glandular changes occurring in a woman's body during menopause parallel what many men undergo in their fifties, sixties and seventies. The author was familiar with Taoist methods of rejuvenation to retune, strengthen and balance the entire glandular system of older men, and most likely the same methods are just as effective for women.

HETEROSEXUAL ANAL SEX

The vagina is exquisitely well designed to have a penis thrusting away inside it. The anus is not. From an energy perspective, a woman's anus is very different from her vagina. Within her vaginal walls, a woman has energy gates that pulse and activate her vagina, literally pulling the yin energy from her entire body into her genital area. The vagina is clearly the most yin part of a woman's entire anatomy. This yin energy is absent in the anus.

In general, Taoists recommend moderation as regards male-female anal sex. They discourage excessive anal sex for these reasons:

- A woman's yin energy, which balances the male's yang, does not collect in her anus.
- The qi that collects in a woman's anus is more yang, as it is meant for pushing out to aid elimination. This prevents the man's qi from fully entering her.
- Many women (both in ancient China and the West) tend to have little enthusiasm for anal sex.
- Anal sex can irritate the rectal and sphincter tissues, which can be easily damaged. This activity can be painful and has the potential to cause problems such as hemorrhoids and anal fissures.
- Hygienic issues, including the transmission of parasites, were and are still very real concerns. If a man and woman choose to engage in anal sex, both should wash very carefully before and after.

Rimming is another way to increase sensation and sexual excitement for both men and women, although, again, this is a matter of personal preference. Rimming involves stimulating the anus or "rosebud" with fingers or tongue to a depth of one half to one inch, where the nerves are most sensitive. If you go much deeper than an inch, you will activate the energy gate of the anus. This can activate a channel that goes up the anterior (front) of the spine, which *may* be irritating or cause negative effects in some women.

For both men and women, moving energy through this channel may be very exciting. However, this channel doesn't link to other bodily systems in a beneficial manner. Some people may enjoy anal sex for the sheer pleasure of it. However from a Taoist view, in terms of balancing the lovers' yin and yang qi, anal sex is nowhere near as profitable—energetically speaking—as vaginal sex.

PORNOGRAPHY AND GETTING REAL

From a Taoist perspective, pornographic images are neither good nor bad; they simply lack the key element that gives sex its life-affirming qualities, and they therefore deplete rather than build your qi. The missing element is the energetic transfer that occurs between two human beings. Images without substance are not the real thing.

The same principle applies to your fantasy life. From the Taoist perspective, the only reason people have fantasies while making love is an inability to be completely present and involved with what is actually going on. In *Slow Sex: The Art and Craft of the Female Orgasm,* Nicole Daedone reports,[1] "Many women I meet create elaborate fantasy worlds where they retreat during sex. Many men, for their part, spend a lot of time with porn. Role playing, sexy lingerie, there are a hundred ways we bring fantasy into our sex...The problem is that fantasy is a way we step out of our experience with sex, rather than stepping further into it."

Being completely present is not a simple matter, of course. Conditioned patterns of dissociation and avoidance are fairly deeply entrenched, which is precisely why people need an effective method, such as dissolving, to break free.

If you need a fantasy to get you in the mood, go for it. However, after the initial titillation, come back to the real live human being lying next to you and drop the fantasy or visualization in your head. This is especially important when engaged in sexual qigong and sexual meditation, as these practices require your full presence. In fact, you could say that Taoist meditation is a highly effective mind-body-spirit training for entering fully into the now.

---

1. Daedone, Nicole, *Slow Sex: The Art and Craft of the Female Orgasm* (New York: Grand Central Life and Style, 2011), 47.

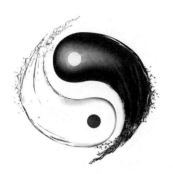

APPENDIX C

Ancient Texts on Sex

Editor's note: The author neither endorses nor disagrees with the advice given in the ancient texts cited in this book. He is merely passing on information that was popular in ancient China and continues to influence Chinese thought today.

Prior to the Communist Revolution, Chinese people enjoyed a very positive attitude toward sex. This was largely due to the influence of the Taoists, who authored nononsense sex manuals such as *Classic of the Plain Girl (Su Nu Jing)* and *Secrets of the Jade Bedchamber (Yu Fang Mi Jue)*. Along with erotic novels such as *The Carnal Prayer Mat (Jou Pu Tuan),* these texts afforded every literate Chinese household a basic education in Taoist methods for enhancing ordinary sex.

Liu Hung Chieh's only other disciple aside from the author, Bai Hua, who lived in Hong Kong, was the source of much of the information from ancient Chinese sex manuals that is quoted in this book. It is presented here for the sake of intellectual curiosity and cultural context, not to advise the reader on a specific course of action.

In all cultures in every period of human history, from cave dwellers to the most technologically-advanced societies the world has ever seen, people have engaged in sex. Times and conditions change, of course, but our basic needs and animal instincts are hard-wired. Although the ancient Chinese inhabited a world that was far less technologically advanced, they were still sophisticated in many ways.

Michel Foucault in *The History of Sexuality*[1] describes China, unlike the West, as a society endowed with erotic arts, where sex "is experienced as pleasure, evaluated in terms of its intensity, its specific quality, its duration, its reverberations in the body and the soul."

---

1. Foucault, Michel, *The History of Sexuality, Vol. 1: An Introduction* (New York: Vintage Books, 1978), 57.

The following are perspectives from ancient texts, with which you may or may not agree. They will give you an idea of some of the considerations of traditional, educated Chinese society at that time.

PROCREATION AND RELATED HEALTH ISSUES

Popular Chinese thought has been influenced by three ancient texts, all of which offer similar views on how the heart and mind of both sexes can be expanded and fulfilled through ordinary sexual technique and marriage.

These three texts were:

1. The *Tao Te Ching* by Laozi
2. *Huang Di Nei Jing Su Wen (Basic Questions from the Yellow Emperor's Inner Canon)*, a classic in Chinese medicine
3. The *San Qing (Three Pure Ones)*

All three texts advance the idea that, after birth, as a person's spirit begins to increase in size, his or her bodily elements also grow steadily in strength. When sufficiently grown, a man produces sperm and ejaculates, while a woman produces blood and menstruates, thus setting the conditions that enable them to produce children. At that point, an essential concern of sexual relations is to find out how the hearts of both sexes merge and cooperate.

In terms of sexual maturity, men are considered fully grown at twenty-five years of age, women at twenty. The five years after reaching sexual maturity (from twenty-five to thirty for a man, from twenty to twenty-five for a woman) is considered the ideal window for producing strong, healthy children. It is believed that the strength of the body begins to decline at that point and is therefore suboptimal for bearing offspring. If she bears a child beyond her prime, the baby will not be as strong as possible.

SEX AND FOOD ARE NATURAL NEEDS

The *Li Ji (Classic of Rites),* was one of the five classics of the Confucian canon. This text states that, along with the need for food, we have natural yin and yang needs. Similarly, Meng Tse (also known as Mencius, Meng Tzu or Mengzi), who was an important disciple of Confucius, said, "As decreed by heaven, eating and sex are the most natural events in people's lives." All life exists within this universal constant. No matter the environment or unique variations, all must follow this path.

AGE-APPROPRIATE SEX

The ancients believed that there were optimal times to relinquish one's virginity: between ages sixteen and thirty for a man, and between ages fourteen and twenty for a woman. Bear in mind that during ancient times, young girls were considered marriageable once they reached puberty. Specific age differentials were also established on the basis of yin-yang and acupuncture channel theory.

Three sets (young, middle-aged and older) of age-appropriate relationships were recommended. These were based on a complex numerical formula that was developed to determine the optimal ages of sexual partners. Ideally, both men and women would interact with the opposite sex in a manner that allowed the acupuncture meridians of each party to benefit energetically as much as possible from the other. However, this was not always the case, particularly, for example, when an old patriarch would marry a young virgin. His aim was to gain qi from a sexual encounter, rather than lose it to his partner. The underlying assumption was that the younger person had more qi, and the power of youthful qi would flow toward the older individual who had less. These suppositions were for average people rather than, for example, a case where the older person had significantly more qi than the younger, in which case the energetic advantage would move toward the younger and not vice-versa.

Using this formula, the best scenarios were as follows:

- Young female with an older male (*xiao yin* to *tai yang*)
- Middle-aged female with a young male (*jue yin* and *xiao yang*)
- Older female and a middle-aged male (*tai yang* and *jue yang*)

According to this age calculus, if both were depleted of qi, a sexual encounter between a very old woman and a very old man would harm (deplete) both partners.

GOOD AND BAD WAYS TO HAVE SEX

The Taoist *Huang Di Nei Jing Su Wen* and the *Ma Wang Dui* series both mention seven bad things you should not do and seven things that are good to do as regards sexual activity:

Seven bad actions:

1. Using willpower to forcefully stop sperm emission.

2. Premature ejaculation.

3. Excessive sperm emission.

4. When having difficulty obtaining an erection, trying excessive approaches in an attempt to get hard.

5. Having sex when the mind is anxious or disturbed.

6. Having sex when very tired or exhausted.

7. Using force and ejaculating quickly.

Seven good actions:

1. Generally paying attention to boosting your kidneys, which produces copious sperm.

2. Producing copious amounts of saliva (both lovers at the same time).

3. Having emotional feeling toward your partner, the ideal being genuine affection and love, before making love rather than just doing it for the physical sensation.

4. Letting the sensation of sperm build inside before you come, rather than ejaculating too quickly.

5. Making sure kidneys are warm and avoiding cold wind getting to them.

6. Waiting to begin until your erection has a lot of feeling and qi in it.

7. Resting after sex rather than engaging in daily affairs or work.

CHINESE AND WESTERN SEXUAL LANGUAGE COMPARED

Ancient Chinese texts about sex reveal a tendency towards flowery metaphors for various sexual activities and sexual anatomy. This, in a sense, elevates China's sexual literature to graceful poetry.

Daniel Reid, in *The Tao of Health, Sex and Longevity,* contrasts "coldly clinical" Western words such as penis and vagina and the crude slang of cock and cunt with the Chinese versions of these terms, Jade Stem and Jade Gate being the most commonly used. Reid cites eleven different Chinese metaphors for the vagina alone, and six for the clitoris, all of which would sound perfectly decent in polite company, unlike the Western words.[2]

The great detail to which the ancient Taoists analyzed sexual functioning is reflected in the fact that, for instance, specific parts of a woman's genitalia have their own enticing names in Chinese that either do not even exist at all as separate terms in English or are only found in medical textbooks.

---

2. Reid, Daniel, *The Tao of Health, Sex and Longevity* (London: Simon & Schuster, 1989), 313–15.

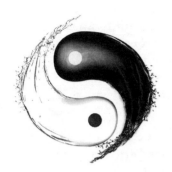

APPENDIX D

The Spelling of Chinese Words in English

N ote: This section is adapted from Appendix F of the author's book, *Opening the Energy Gates of Your Body*.

Any attempt to transliterate the sounds of Chinese words into English with any accuracy will fall far short. This is because Chinese not only has sounds that English does not have, but also uses a system of vocal "tones," which do not exist in English. Furthermore, English has sounds that are not present in Chinese. English speakers attempting to pronounce Chinese words will invariably add sounds from their own language, which will distort the pronunciation of Chinese.

None of the major systems for transliterating Chinese words is very accurate. Written Chinese is composed of ideogram pictures, each of which may convey one idea or several combined ideas. These ideograms, when spoken, are pronounced differently in the various different dialects of Chinese. For example, the word for family is *jia* in the "National Language" (Mandarin, or common-people speech), but it is *gar* in Cantonese, a regional Chinese sublanguage, or dialect, spoken in the province of Guangdong (Canton) and Hong Kong. There are yet more regional languages, each with different sounds for the same character.

Over time, the language of Beijing became the common medium of communication throughout China for the educated, which, in English, is known as Mandarin Chinese (from the days of the Emperors). Mandarin, as the official national language of all of China, is now what truly can be called Chinese, which every single person in China learns to speak. Throughout this book, all Chinese terms are in Mandarin and not in regional dialects.

There are three main systems of spelling Chinese words in English: Pinyin, Wade-Giles and Yale. In both the Wade-Giles system (invented by German monks, used in the old days by translators who mostly could only read Chinese but not speak it, and now used by the Nationalists in Taiwan), and the Pinyin system (developed for use inside China by the Chinese when the Communist government was trying to raise the literacy rate in China), many of the written English transliterations when pronounced phonetically do not sound anything like the Chinese sounds. The only system that was created to mimic the Chinese language as closely as possible using the English phonetic system was the Yale system, created at Yale University specifically to teach English speakers how to speak Chinese. At the present time, Pinyin is the most commonly used transliteration system.

For example, the Pinyin term qigong (or qi gong) in Wade-Giles is chi kung and in Yale is chi gung. In fact the way this word is said in Chinese is closest to chee gung. The qi of the Pinyin and the kung of the Wade-Giles are not accurate in terms of how this spelling would normally be pronounced in English. The internal martial arts written as taijiquan, xingyiquan and baguazhang in Pinyin are spelled t'ai chi ch'uan, hsing-i ch'uan and pakua chang in Wade-Giles. Wade-Giles gives us Tao, *Tao Te Ching* and *I Ching*. In Pinyin these terms are spelled Dao, *Dao De Jing* and *Yi Jing*. The ancient Taoist sages that in Pinyin appear as Laozi and Zhuangzi are written as Lao Tse and Chuang Tse in the Yale system, and Lao Tzu and Chuang Tzu in Wade-Giles.

This book, rather than adhering strictly to any one formal system of spelling Chinese words, uses a mix of transliterations that are either the ones most commonly used or that allow the English speaker to best mimic what the Chinese actually sounds like.

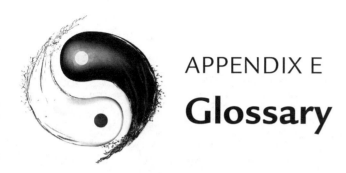

APPENDIX E

Glossary

A

Acupuncture: A form of traditional Chinese medicine that works with the qi of the body by inserting needles at specific points to treat various health conditions.

Alchemy: The process of changing one substance into another. In the esoteric field, alchemy has two main branches—external and internal. External alchemy occurs in a laboratory in order to focus human spiritual energies to transform ordinary herbs and minerals into super-medicines, to change base metals into gold, to create the Philosopher's Stone (which alchemists believed conferred physical immortality), and to gain direct knowledge of God. Internal alchemy (known in Chinese as *nei dan*) seeks through meditation and certain mind-body-spirit exercises to: 1) Work with the consciousness of an individual in order to become aware of the cellular vibratory energetic level of the body to heal disease; 2) Raise, bring out, and transform normally hidden capacities of the body-mind; and 3) Elevate ordinary consciousness to higher and more refined levels of superconsciousness until the mind expands to encompass the whole of the universe. All this is done inside an individual's mind-body-Spirit without the use of any external laboratory equipment.

Astral travel: Move one's consciousness outside the body to travel in space and/or time.

Aura: The energetic or bioelectric field that surrounds the living human body. See also Etheric body.

B

Bagua, bagua zhang (bagua jang, pakua chang): Literally, "eight trigram palm." Ba gua is one of China's three main internal martial arts. It is a Taoist practice based on the *I Ching*, which is simultaneously a longevity practice, a martial art, a healing modality and a spiritual meditation practice.

Bai hui: The exact center of the crown of the head that is known in Chinese as the "meeting of a hundred energy points."

Being: The word "being" means a person or sentient entity whether corporeal or non-corporeal. A "Being" with an initial capital refers to the essence or soul of a being.

Body of individuality: See Essence.

Body of the Tao: The eighth energy body, which entails joining one's human consciousness to the entire universe. To fully realize the eighth body is to achieve complete unity with the Tao, the ultimate aim of Taoist energy practices.

C

Causal energy body: See Karmic energy body.

Central channel (zhong mai, chung mai, jung mai): The main energy channel located in the exact center of the human body between the perineum and the crown of the head and extending through the bone marrow of the arms and legs.

Cerebrospinal fluid: A clear liquid surrounding the brain and spinal cord that protects these areas, as well as circulating nutrients and removing waste products within the central nervous system. According to classic Taoist energetic anatomy, human cerebrospinal fluid operates within three distinct frequencies. Western Craniosacral therapists are familiar with the first but generally not the other two. The three frequencies are: 1) Between 15 and 20 beats per minute, 2) Approximately 1,000 beats per minute, and 3) 10,000 beats per minute.

Cervix: Narrow passageway between a woman's uterus and vagina.

Chakra: A Sanskrit word meaning "wheel." According to Hindu and Buddhist traditions, the seven chakras are major energy centers of the body that play an important role in yoga and Tantra practices. The eighth and ninth chakras are located, one above the other, beyond the crown of the head within the etheric field.

Clitoris: Small erectile erogenous tissue at the front end of a woman's vulva.

Confucius (kong zi, k'ong tzu, kongfuzi, k'ong futzu)**:** The ancient philosopher upon whose thoughts the foundation of China's traditional secular culture is built. His concepts strongly influenced social interactions, etiquette, customs, and the hierarchical nature of most of the martial arts of China and Japan (see Confucianism).

Confucianism: Philosophy based upon the beliefs of Confucius, as described in his three texts: the *Analects, The Doctrine of the Mean* and *The Great Learning*, written 2,500 years ago (see Confucius).

Crazy wisdom teachers: Taoist teachers such as Zhuangzi (Chuang Tse, Chuang Tzu) to whom conventional norms and values don't apply. Such teachers aim to enable those they interact with to advance spiritually at the greatest possible speed. They achieve this with what may appear to others as unexpected and radical behavior in order to expose and explode hidden karma, so it can be resolved in the fastest manner possible.

D

Dai mai: Also known as the "great meridian," this is one of acupuncture's eight extraordinary meridians, a belt that exists on a horizontal plane and circles from in front of the lower tantien around to the spine and mingmen, and then continues back around to its point of origination in front of the lower tantien. The dai mai connects all the vertical acupuncture meridians of the body.

Dissolving: A subtle energy technique for releasing bound energy from both within the human body and the etheric body. See Inner Dissolving and Outer Dissolving.

Dragon Cooling Breath: Taoist breathing practice to cool down the practitioner's physical body or qi.

Dragon Heating Breath: Taoist breathing practice to heat up the practitioner's physical body or qi.

Dual cultivation: Practices where two or more people or entities interact to develop their qi. This includes sex, talking, tai chi push hands, sharing energy with trees or other living things in the immediate environment or even interacting with distant objects such as the moon, planets or stars.

E

Earth element: In Chinese cosmology, one of the five basic energies or elements from which all manifested phenomena are created.

Eight energy bodies: In Taoist philosophy, eight clear vibratory frequencies of energy that comprise a human being. Each is called a "body." These are identified as the physical body, etheric or qi body, emotional body, mental body, psychic energy body, karmic or causal body, body of individuality or essence, and body of the Tao.

Eight extraordinary or special meridians: The eight meridians that have special uses in acupuncture above and beyond the normal vertical and horizontal meridians.

Emotional energy body: The third energy body that powers the emotions.

Emptiness: A profound state of spiritual, mental, and psychic equilibrium that is a major goal of many Asian meditation practices and that lies at the heart of the higher levels of achievement in qigong and the internal martial arts.

Energy anatomy: The channels and points within the human body and the field around it through which qi flows.

Energy channels of the body: All the subtle energetic channels of the body through which qi travels.

Energy gates: Major energy relay stations of the body, where the strength of the qi moving through the human body system is regulated.

Enlightenment: According to Taoism, it takes 10,000 lives to reach enlightenment, where a practitioner realizes the body of Tao. The number 10,000 is used in Chinese culture as a metaphor meaning "more than you can realistically easily think about with ordinary consciousness."

Etheric body (qi body): The second of the eight energy bodies of a human being. The bioelectric field that extends anywhere from a few inches to a few hundred feet from a person's body. Commonly called the aura in the West.

Essence: The seventh energy body, also known as the body of individuality. This governs a person's true nature beyond their personality and all that shaped it. Cultivation of this energy body allows awareness of that which enables the actual birth of a full but still evolving spiritual being.

F

Fa jin (fa jing, fa chin): To issue or discharge power. This internal martial arts technique can be used to issue power so it passes through an opponent (without physical harm), moving him in space just as a gust of wind blows dust away.

Fa shen: Projecting spirit. In spiritual push hands, a yang offensive technique that causes moving into or exploding into emptiness.

Fire element: In Chinese cosmology, one of the five basic energies or elements from which all manifested phenomena are created.

Fire tradition: Taoist meditation and energetic methods that emphasize visualizations, pushing one's limits and commonly using full effort to one hundred percent of one's capacity. The Fire Tradition emerged 1,500 years after the Water tradition of Laozi and was influenced by Buddhist thought, yoga and Tantra. Like classical Tantra, the sexual practices of the Fire tradition of Taoism are based on transforming blocked energy, whereas the methods of the Water tradition are based on dissolving blocked energy. The Fire tradition is sometimes referred to as Neo-Taoism.

Five Elements: The five primal elements or energies—Metal, Water, Wood, Fire and Earth—from which all manifested phenomena and dynamics are created.

Frenulum: A band of tissue under the head of the penis. The frenulum is the most sensitive part of the penis, stimulation of which tends to lead to ejaculation.

G

G-spot (Grafenberg spot): An erogenous zone in the vagina which when stimulated can cause intense sexual arousal and orgasms.

Gao Chao: A Chinese term that means "high tide," referring to a female orgasm.

Glans: Erectile tissue at the end of the penis and the clitoris, known as the glans penis and the glans clitoridis.

Governing and conception vessels (du mai and ren mai): Two of the eight extraordinary meridians, the governing and conception vessels activate and balance all the acupuncture channels of the body. The governing vessel goes from the perineum up the spine, over the crown of the head to the mouth. The conception vessel goes down the front of the body from the mouth to the perineum. Together they form a qi pathway known as the Microcosmic Orbit, or Small Heavenly Orbit. The Macrocosmic Orbit, or Large Heavenly Orbit, also includes the arms and legs.

Great meridian: See Dai mai.

H

Heart-mind: The undifferentiated source from where a person's intent and cognition originates before language and thoughts emerge within his or her conscious awareness. There are many degrees and stages of defining it, including the ultimate source of enlightenment. The heart-mind is discernible in deep states of meditation.

Hsing-i or **hsing-i chuan** (xingyiquan): Mind-form boxing. A hard yang internal martial art created by the Chinese general Yue Fei in the thirteenth century. Hsing-i emphasizes all aspects of the mind to create its forms and fighting movements.

I

Internal Martial Arts: The three Chinese martial arts of tai chi, hsing-i and bagua, which use qi for power rather than muscular strength. Aikido in Japan is also a qi-based martial art influenced by bagua.

I Ching *(yi jing): Book of Changes.* This 5,000-year-old work is considered to be the classic Taoist text about the nature of change and how change occurs. The *I Ching* encompasses eight trigrams, known in Chinese as *ba gua,* that embody the eight primal qi energies of which the universe is composed according to Taoist thought. The eight expand to sixty-four by detailing how each of the individual trigrams impacts, mitigates, and expands the others when they are mixed. Bagua zhang is a mind-body-Spirit practice that seeks to have an individual experience within his or her own being what the *I Ching* communicates intellectually.

Inner Dissolving: A basic Taoist qi (neigong) practice for releasing energy blocked anywhere within a person; used primarily to heal and strengthen an individual's emotional, mental, psychic, karmic and essence aspects.

Inter-dimensional jump-gate: An energetic gateway that allows one to consciously leap between dimensions, travelling non-physically outside the body in space and/or time.

Internal alchemy: See Alchemy.

Internal orgasm: A primarily qi-based phenomenon for having an orgasm internally rather than externally. It involving energetically linking one's genitals to the place where one wishes to have an internal orgasm while keeping the mind relaxed.

J
Jing: Sperm/ovary generative energy, the energy of the physical body.

K
Karmic energy body: The sixth energy body, also known as the causal body, which relates to time, space, cause and effect and karma.

Kaballah: Jewish mystical tradition involving an esoteric interpretation of the Torah.

Kundalini: A meditation method of India that uses energy work to unravel the mysteries of human consciousness and enlightenment.

Kwa (kua): The area on each side of the body extending from the inguinal ligaments through the inside of the pelvis to the top (crest) of the hip bones.

L
Labia: The inner and outer lips or folds of the vulva that protect the urethra, vagina and clitoris.

Lao gong (lao gung/kung): The energetic point in the center of the palm; the easiest place in the body from which to project qi externally.

Laozi (Lao Tse, Lao Tzu): Author of the *Tao Te Ching (Dao De Jing),* one of the three classic texts of Taoism, who lived more than 2,500 years ago.

Law of Return: Taoist doctrine stating that whatever energy you put out eventually comes back to you. Also known within Hindu and Buddhist traditions as karma or "cause and effect."

Left and right channels: Two of the three primary energy lines in the body (on its left and right side), the other being the central channel. The paired opposites of the left and right channels of subtle energy are responsible for all the yin/yang dualistic functions of a human being, including the functioning of the body, emotions, psychic activity, and the manifestation of events in the outer world.

Lineage: In the martial, meditation and qi arts, an unbroken line of teaching that runs from one master through successive generations of disciples, each of whom the previous lineage master has trained and specifically authorized to be a master and pass on the knowledge.

Lineage disciple: A formal disciple who is chosen to learn and carry forth to future generations all the intact knowledge of any specific martial, meditation or qi arts lineage.

Liang yi (liang i): The interplay of yin and yang.

Ling: Chinese word for "soul." The primary spiritual purpose for the beginning and intermediate stage of Taoist meditation involves gathering all the energies of an individual into one integrated consciousness. The unified energy creates a ling, which enables an individual after death to reincarnate intact rather than split apart and join with other split entities and reincarnate as a composite soul.

Listening: A primary technique of push hands whereby the practitioner learns to hear and interpret a partner's energy to sense what he or she is doing or about to do.

Liturgy: See Taoist liturgies.

Longevity Breathing: See Taoist Longevity Breathing.

Lower burner (xia jiao): The area of the body between the lower tantien and feet, including the internal organs therein.

Lower tantien (dantian): Located below the navel in the center of the body, this energetic center is primarily responsible for the health of the human body. It is the only energy center where all the energy channels that affect the physical body intersect. Also known in Japanese as the hara and in English as the elixir or cinnabar field.

M

Macrocosmic Orbit (Large Heavenly Orbit): Extends the Microcosmic or Small Heavenly Orbit to the arms and legs. See Governing and Conception Vessels.

Medical qigong: Exercises that work with the qi of the body to specifically help heal health problems.

Mental energy body: The fourth energy body that fuels concrete thought.

Metal element: In Chinese cosmology, one of the five basic energies or elements from which all manifested phenomena are created.

Microcosmic Orbit (Small Heavenly Orbit): See Governing and conception vessels.

Middle burner (zhong jiao): Located in the torso between the solar plexus and the lower tantien, including the internal organs therein. The energy that exists in this middle area of the body coordinates and harmonizes the qi of the upper and lower burners, which lie above and below the middle burner.

Middle tantien (dantian): One of the three major energy centers in the body. Two separate places are considered to be the middle tantien. They are located near each other, each governing different energetic functions. The point located at the solar plexus just below the sternum is responsible for the physical functions of the middle internal organs of the body (liver, spleen, and kidneys), as well as the will to persevere. The point located near the heart on the central channel governs physical, emotional, mental, psychic, or karmic relationships.

Mind of Man: External fixations and conditioning. In the *I Ching*, a concept contrasted with the Mind of Tao. The Mind of Man is driven by short-term satisfactions and worldly pleasures that don't touch the hunger of the soul.

Mind of Tao: In the *I Ching*, a concept contrasted with the Mind of Man. The Mind of Tao leads to a natural, open state of mind that moves from an inner source of love and pure awareness to achieve ongoing spiritual evolution.

Mindstream: The deep subtle stream that underlies one's awareness, usually hidden unless explicitly sought. The Mindstream is the contact point that eventually leads to Universal Consciousness.

Mingmen: Also known as the "Door of Life," this energy center is located on the spine, between the kidneys, directly opposite the lower tantien on the dai mai.

Mudra (seal): A hand/finger/body position or mind state that automatically activates a person's energy channels in a specific fashion or creates a particular mind or psychic state in the practitioner.

N

Natural Breath: When two lovers have developed sufficient connection, they are able to spontaneously reset each other's qi pathways. This is called natural breath. It enables their energy channels to open naturally and easily, without any conscious attempt. Natural breath does not necessarily mean that lovers are breathing in synch.

Nei dan: Literally, "inner cosmic egg/pill." Also known as Ball of Light. A term for the internal alchemy methods of the Fire tradition of Taoism. See Alchemy.

Neigong: Internal power. The original qi cultivation (qigong) system in China invented by the Taoists. It involves sixteen specific components and is the art and science of how to consciously move energy through the body. Taoist neigong forms the foundation for the internal martial arts of tai chi, hsing-i and bagua, as well as for healing and sexual qigong and sexual meditation.

Neo-Taoism: See Fire tradition.

Neo-central Channel: In advanced sexual meditation practices, the neo-central channel is formed when a couple's two central channels link and then merge into one to create a new third channel that exists between the man and the woman.

O

Open/close (kai/he): The Chinese yin/yang paired opposites concept of growing/shrinking, expanding/contracting, and lengthening/shortening, and so on. This universal pulsing occurs at the subatomic level, cellular level, and cosmological level. See Pulsing.

Outer Dissolving: A basic Taoist qi (neigong) practice for releasing blocked internal energy within the body and projecting it externally. Used primarily to heal and strengthen the energies related to the physical body.

P

Peng Zu (Peng Tsu): Known as the Chinese Taoist Methuselah who purportedly lived for eight hundred years.

Perineum: The area between the anus and the scrotum in a male, and between the anus and vulva in a female.

Physical energy body: The first of the eight energy bodies. This powers the physical body.

Prostate: This gland is located just underneath and around the neck of the bladder, in front of the rectum and behind the pubic bone. Part of the male reproductive system, the prostate produces the fluid component of semen.

Psychic energy body: The fifth energy body through which one finds hidden internal capacities, such as perception of the spirit world.

Pulsing (kai-he): Opening and closing the joints, muscles, soft tissues, internal organs, glands, blood vessels and cerebrospinal system, as well as the body's subtle energy anatomy. Pulsing is one of the sixteen components of neigong. See Open/close.

Q

Qi (chi, ki in Japanese): Energy, subtle life force, internal energy, internal power. Invisible energy that empowers something to manifest, work and function. This concept underlies Chinese, Japanese, and Korean culture, in which the world is perceived not purely in terms of physical matter but also in terms of invisible energy.

Qigong (chi gung, chi kung): Energy work/power. The ancient Chinese art and science of developing and cultivating qi. Qigong techniques may be done standing, moving, sitting, lying down, and during sex. These exercises balance, regulate, and strengthen energy channels, centers, and points of the body.

Qigong tui na (Chi gung tweina): Therapeutic bodywork with qi. A specialty of Chinese medicine, where the healer directly emits and rebalances the qi in the patient's body to bring about a therapeutic result. Its diagnostic techniques are based on reading the energy of the external aura, as well as the subtle energy of the internal tantiens of the body.

R

Red dust: The Taoist term for in the transitory desires, attachments, illusions and fixations that consume a person's life force and obscure his or her true nature. Samsara is the parallel word in Buddhism.

Rules of Heaven: This refers to the Taoist view that the material world is organized and animated by a higher, unseen order within the context of the universal laws of yin and yang.

S

Sexual qigong: Intentional engagement with the subtle energy dimension of sexuality. Most of the energetic sexual meditation practices that Westerners have come to know as "Tantra" in Taoism falls under the category of energy sex or sexual qigong, rather than sexual meditation.

Sexual meditation: Taoist sexual practices involving the Inner Dissolving process to access, activate and release blockages in all eight energy bodies. The goal is to achieve full spiritual awakening and realize one's full human potential.

Shang jiao: See Upper burner.

Shen: Spirit or psychic, karmic and essence energy.

Shengong: Literally, "spirit work." In terms of Taoist meditation. Shengong is the spiritual side of qigong. Shengong is the fusion of qigong with the emotional, mental, psychic and karmic energy bodies to the level of one's essence.

Spirit: The word "Spirit" with an initial capital denotes what is known in Chinese as *shen,* one of the three treasures of Taoism. *Shen* encompasses psychic, karmic and essence energy.

Spiritual Immortal: Within the Taoist tradition, someone who has actualized all eight energy bodies. An Immortal's consciousness has merged with the Tao.

Sticking: In tai chi push hands, a technique where partners maintain continuous physical or energetic contact with one another.

T

Tai chi chuan (tai ji quan, taijiquan): Supreme ultimate martial arts fist. One of the three internal martial arts of China, most known for its emphasis on softness, slow-motion movement, and its sophisticated qigong methodology based on whole-body physical coordination. Done by the majority of its practitioners primarily for health, not combat. As a martial art, tai chi emphasizes softness, yielding techniques and counterattack strategies, and a blending of soft (yin) and hard (yang) internal power.

Tai chi push hands (tui shou): The continuous two-person hand-touching practice of the internal martial art of tai chi chuan, which forms the bridge between the form movements of tai chi and its self-defense techniques. It also develops a foundation in sensitivity training useful for Taoist sexual practices.

Tantien (dandian): According to Taoism and traditional Chinese medicine, the three primary centers in the human body, sometimes called "elixir fields," where qi collects and from which it is dispersed and circulated throughout the human body, mind and spirit.

Tantra: Ancient Sanskrit word meaning continuity coming from the root "to expand." Tantra includes a variety of spiritual practices involving, for example, sex, movement, breathing, energy work and meditation, generally with the aim of achieving bliss and enlightenment. It has strongly influenced Tibetan Buddhism and Hinduism.

Tao/Taoism (dao): The Way. The practical, mystical religion of China that formed the original underpinnings of classical Chinese culture, including the yin-yang play of opposites, Chinese medicine, and the art of strategy and war.

Tao te: Within Taoism, a universal view of morality.

Tao jia (dao jia, tao chia): The mystical inner esoteric practices of Taoism. Includes the beginning stage of Taoist meditation that involves methods for completely stilling the mind and an advanced stage, which involves internal alchemy, or transformation of inner energies for realizing and becoming one with the Tao, the nature of the universe itself.

Tao jiao (dao jiao, tao chiao): The outer aspects of Taoism, including religious ceremonies, mediums, idol worship and fortune-telling.

Tao shi (dao shi, dao shr): The Taoist word for priest, meaning spiritual teacher.

Tao Te Ching *(Dao De Jing):* Translated as "The Way and Its Power," this is one of the three seminal texts of Taoism, written by Laozi (LaoTse, Lao Tzu) more than 2,500 years ago. The other two texts are the *I Ching* and the *Book of Zhuangzi*.

Taoist Immortal: See Spiritual Immortal.

Taoist Liturgies: Chants in ancient Chinese whose frequencies are used in very specific ways, first to work with the energies of the eight energy bodies of human beings and finally to enable the practitioner to realize the vibratory quality of the entire universe. Not to be confused with the common practice of "toning."

Taoist Longevity Breathing: The author has developed this method to teach authentic Taoist breathing in systematic stages. Breathing with the whole body has been used for millennia to enhance the ability to dissolve and release energy blockages in the mind and body, enhancing well-being and spiritual awareness. Incorporating these breathing techniques into any other Taoist energy practice will help bring out its full potential.

Taoist Neigong Yoga: Taoist yoga is ancient China's soft yet powerful alternative to what is popularly known today as Hatha yoga. Taoist Neigong Yoga is the system that the author has developed to teach this. Combining gentle postures, neigong

neigong and Taoist Longevity Breathing techniques systematically opens the body's energy channels, thereby activating and stimulating qi flow. Postures, held from two to five minutes, require virtually no muscular effort.

Three Treasures: These are jing (sperm/ovary generative energy), qi (vital energy, including thoughts, emotions and psychic energy), and shen (Spirit or karmic and essence energy).

Transmission: A direct transfer, mind-to-mind, energy to energy and body-to-body, of the totality of a learning experience from a master to a student.

U

Universal Consciousness: Also known as the Tao. The unchanging source of the universe.

Universal Morality: According to Taoism, that which furthers everything sooner or later. This is taken from a universal perspective rather than merely that of the human perspective on the earth.

Upper burner (shang jiao): Located in the upper body above the chest, including the arms and head, this burner is related to psychic energy.

Upper tantien (dantian): Located in the brain, this tantien controls human perceptual mechanisms and psychic functions.

V

Vulva: A woman's external genitalia.

W

Water element: In Chinese cosmology, one of the five basic energies or elements from which all manifested phenomena are created.

Water tradition: Taoist meditation and energetic methods that emphasize using full effort without strain or force. More than 2,500 years old, this is the original tradition of Taoism that was passed down through Laozi and Zhuangzi.

Wei qi (wei chi): The layer of energy between a person's skin and muscle that protects against disease entering the body from the external environment. It is the connecting medium between the etheric body and the acupuncture channels in the body.

Wood element: In Chinese cosmology, one of the five basic energies or elements from which all manifested phenomena are created.

Wu de: Martial arts morals. This refers to using martial arts to build a sound moral character, based on ordinary Confucian and Buddhist values.

Wu chi (wu ji): Literally, limitless or infinite. The great emptiness from which all manifestation flows, also known as the Tao.

Wu wei: Doing without doing or the action of non-action. This is a fundamental Taoist concept of having action arise from an empty mind without preconception or agenda—action that operates by spontaneously following the natural course of universal energy as it manifests itself without strain or ego involvement.

X

Xia jiao: See Lower burner.

Xing-yi, xingyiquan: See Hsing-i.

Y

Yang: Male projecting energy. See Yin-yang.

Yin: Female absorbing energy. See Yin-yang.

Yin-yang: The classic Taoist concept that the universe is composed of opposites (such as sun-moon, active-passive, work-rest, happiness-sadness) that are not antagonistic but complementary and necessary to fulfill each other. It is through the yin-yang play of opposites that all manifestation, obvious or subtle, occurs.

Z

Zhong jiao: See Middle burner.

Zhuangzi (Chuang Tse, Chuang Tzu): Author of the *Book of Zhuangzi,* one of the three classic texts of Taoism. The best known "crazy wisdom" teacher of Taoism. See Crazy wisdom teachers.

Zi ran: Nature or naturalness, a key Taoist concept.

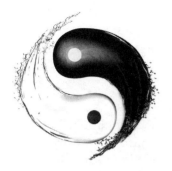

APPENDIX F

Frantzis Energy Arts System

Bruce Frantzis, drawing on more than a decade of Taoist training in China and over forty years of training instructors, has developed the Frantzis Energy Arts System, a practical, comprehensive series of programs that can enable people of all ages and fitness levels to increase their core energy and attain vibrant health. He is the founder of Energy Arts, Inc., which offers a continually expanding list of books, DVDs, CDs, online training programs and events in North America and Europe. Find out the latest details and sign up for the Energy Arts email list to receive free product downloads at www.EnergyArts.com.

Taoist methods for developing qi—energy arts—fall into the following broad categories and all are included in the Frantzis Energy Arts System:

- Tai Chi, Bagua and Hsing-i
- Qigong/Neigong
- Taoist Neigong Yoga
- Healing others with Qigong Tui Na
- Taoist Meditation
- Taoist Sexual Practices

TAI CHI, BAGUA AND HSING-I

Historically in China, the three primary internal martial arts of tai chi chuan, bagua zhang and hsing-i chuan have been practiced for health, martial power and as moving meditation. In addition to teaching these practices at instructor trainings and other courses worldwide, lineage holder Bruce Frantzis has created three separate mastery programs for home and online study: the *Tai Chi Mastery*

Program, the *Bagua Mastery Program,* and the *Hsing-i Mastery Program.* These programs contain some of the most comprehensive material ever recorded on the internal workings of these arts.

TAI CHI CHUAN

Most Westerners learn tai chi purely as a health exercise, although it was traditionally learned as a martial art. Tai chi relaxes and regulates the central nervous system, releases physical and emotional stress and promotes mental and emotional well-being. Tai chi's gentle, non-jarring movements are ideal for people of any age and body type and can cultivate a high degree of relaxation, balance and physical coordination in the practitioner.

Tai chi is commonly referred to as a form of moving meditation. Tai chi's slow, graceful movements provide relaxed focus, quiet down your internal dialogue and engender a deep sense of relaxation that helps release inner tensions. Frantzis trained extensively in the traditional Wu, Yang and Chen styles of tai chi chuan, including short and long forms, push hands, self-defense techniques and traditional weapons such as sticks and swords.

Related Products:

- *Tai Chi Mastery Program* [50+ DVDs, written and online material]
- *The Power of Internal Martial Arts and Chi: Combat and Energy Secrets of Ba Gua, Tai Chi and Hsing-i* [Book]
- *Tai Chi and Bagua* [Book]
- *Tai Chi: Health for Life* [Book]
- *Yang Style Tai Chi Fighting Applications* [DVD—Archive footage]

BAGUA ZHANG

Even more ancient than tai chi, bagua circle walking was developed more than 4,000 years ago in Taoist monasteries as a health and meditation art. The aim of its techniques is to develop the potential of the mind and achieve stillness and clarity; to generate a strong, healthy, disease-free body; and, perhaps most importantly, to maintain internal balance while one's external or inner world rapidly changes.

Bagua is first and foremost a qi art embodying the eight primal energies that are encompassed by the eight trigrams of the *I Ching.* Its basic internal power training consists of learning eight palm changes and combining them with walking, spiraling and twisting arm movements and constant changes of direction.

Bagua was designed to fight up to eight opponents at once. Virtually no other martial art system or style, internal or external, has combined and seamlessly integrated the whole pantheon of martial arts fighting techniques into one package as effectively as bagua.

Internal martial arts such as bagua and tai chi teach you to use relaxation, qi, and stillness of mind to accomplish the pragmatic goal of winning in a violent confrontation, rather than using muscular tension, strength or anger to gain or project power.

Related Products:

- *Bagua Mastery Program* [45+ DVD/CDs, 1,000-page training manual and online material]
- *Tai Chi and Bagua* [Book]
- *The Power of Internal Martial Arts and Chi: Combat and Energy Secrets of Ba Gua, Tai Chi and Hsing-i* [Book]

HSING-I CHUAN

Hsing-i (also transliterated as xingyi) emphasizes all aspects of the mind to create its forms and fighting movements. This art is an equally potent healing practice because it makes people healthy and then very strong. The five primal elements or phases of energy—Metal, Water, Wood, Fire and Earth—upon which Chinese medicine is based and from which all manifested phenomena are created—govern hsing-i's five basic movements. Hsing-i's training is based on a linear, militaristic approach: marching in straight lines, with a powerful emphasis at the end of every technique on mentally or physically taking an enemy down.

Related Products:

- *Hsing-i Chuan Mastery Program* [30+ DVDs]
- *I Chuan Standing Postures* [4-DVD set]
- *The Power of Internal Martial Arts and Chi: Combat and Energy Secrets of Ba Gua, Tai Chi and Hsing-i* [Book]

QIGONG/NEIGONG PRACTICES

The Frantzis Energy Arts System includes six primary qigong courses that, together with the Taoist Longevity Breathing® program, progressively and safely incorporate all aspects of neigong—the original qi cultivation (qigong) system in China that originated from the Taoists. Although the qigong techniques are very old, Bruce Frantzis' system of teaching them is unique and is specifically tailored to Westerners and the needs of modern life.

The core practices consist of:

- Taoist Longevity Breathing
- Dragon and Tiger Medical Qigong
- Opening the Energy Gates of Your Body Qigong
- The Marriage of Heaven and Earth Qigong
- Bend the Bow Spinal Qigong
- Spiraling Energy Body Qigong
- Gods Playing in the Clouds Qigong

These core qigong programs were deliberately chosen because they are among the most effective and treasured of Taoist energy practices. They are ideal for clearly and progressively learning the sixteen components of neigong.

TAOIST LONGEVITY BREATHING

Frantzis has developed the method of Taoist Longevity Breathing to teach authentic Taoist breathing in systematic stages. Whole-body breathing has been used for millennia to enhance the ability to dissolve and release energy blockages in the mind-body, enhancing well-being and spiritual awareness. Incorporating these breathing techniques into any other Taoist energy practice will help bring out its full potential.

Related Products:

- *Taoist Breathing for Tai Chi and Meditation* [2-CD Set]
- *Longevity Breathing* [DVD]

DRAGON AND TIGER MEDICAL QIGONG

This is one of the most direct and accessible low-impact qigong healing methods that China has produced. This 1,500-year-old form of medical qigong affects the human body in a manner similar to acupuncture. Its seven simple movements can be done by virtually anyone, whatever their age or state of health.

Related Products:

- *Dragon and Tiger Medical Qigong: Health and Energy in Seven Simple Movements* [2 Books, 2-DVD Set and Poster]
- *Dragon and Tiger Medical Qigong Online Training Program* [6 hours of instruction in over 50 separate videos]
- *Chi Revolution,* which describes how chi or qi is the power behind spirituality, meditation, sexual vitality, acupuncture, internal martial arts and the divination methods of the *I Ching,* and includes a mini qi workout [Book]

OPENING THE ENERGY GATES OF YOUR BODY QIGONG

This program introduces 3,000-year-old qigong techniques that are fundamental to advancing any energy arts practice. This form covers basic body alignments, developing and increasing internal awareness of qi in the body and Outer Dissolving to release blocked energy.

Related Products:

- *Opening the Energy Gates of Your Body: Qigong for Lifelong Health* [Book, 2-CD Set and Poster]

THE MARRIAGE OF HEAVEN AND EARTH QIGONG

This qigong set incorporates techniques widely used in China to help heal back, neck, spine and joint problems. It is especially effective for helping to mitigate repetitive stress injury and carpal tunnel problems. This program teaches some important neigong components, including opening and closing (pulsing), more complex breathing techniques and how to move qi through the energy channels of the body.

BEND THE BOW SPINAL QIGONG

Bend the Bow Spinal Qigong continues the work of strengthening and regenerating the spine that is introduced in Marriage of Heaven and Earth Qigong. This program incorporates neigong components for awakening and controlling the energies of the spine.

SPIRALING ENERGY BODY QIGONG

This advanced program dramatically raises one's energy level and allows the practitioner to master how qi moves in circles and spirals throughout the body. It incorporates neigong components for: directing the upward flow of energy; projecting qi along the body's spiraling pathways; delivering or projecting energy at will to or from any part of the body; and activating the body's left, right and central channels, as well as the Microcosmic Orbit.

GODS PLAYING IN THE CLOUDS QIGONG

This qigong set incorporates some of the oldest and most powerful Taoist rejuvenation techniques. This program amplifies all the physical, breathing and energetic components learned in all the earlier qigong programs and completes the process of integrating all the components of neigong. It is also the final stage of learning to strengthen and balance the energies of the three tantiens, central energy channel and spine. Gods Playing in the Clouds Qigong serves as a spiritual bridge from qigong to Taoist meditation.

SHENGONG

Where qigong/neigong and meditation meet is shengong or spiritual qigong. The beginning stage of qigong focuses mostly on the first two energy bodies (the physical and etheric). Shengong goes further and works with the higher energy bodies—emotional, mental, psychic and karmic energy bodies up to the level of a person's essence. Over the years, Frantzis has been progressively incorporating more shengong within the qi practices that he teaches.

TAOIST NEIGONG YOGA

Taoist Yoga is ancient China's soft yet powerful alternative to what is popularly known today as Hatha yoga. Frantzis learned this during his Taoist priesthood training. The system he has developed to teach this is called Taoist Neigong Yoga. Its primary emphasis is to stimulate the flow of qi and free up any blocked energy. Neigong Yoga combines gentle postures with neigong components and Longevity Breathing techniques to systematically open the body's energy channels, thereby activating and stimulating qi flow. Postures are held from two to five minutes and require virtually no muscular effort, enabling you to easily focus on what is internal so you can feel where the qi is blocked and gently free it up.

Related Product: *Taoist Yoga* [Kindle E-Book]

HEALING OTHERS WITH QIGONG TUI NA

Part of Frantzis' Taoist training in China was to become a doctor of Chinese medicine, primarily using the qigong healing techniques known as *qigong tui na*. During this training period, he worked with more than 10,000 patients. Frantzis no longer works as a qigong doctor, either privately or in clinics, but occasionally offers trainings in therapeutic healing techniques.

Qigong tui na is a special branch of Chinese medicine that is designed to unblock, free and balance qi in others. You learn to project energy from your hands, voice and eyes to facilitate healing using 200 different hand techniques. You also learn how to avoid burnout from your therapeutic practice. To heal others, you must first learn to unblock and free your own qi and to control the specific pathways through which it flows.

TAOIST MEDITATION

Frantzis is a lineage holder in the gentle Water method of Taoist meditation passed down from the teachings of Laozi over 2,500 years ago. Taoist meditation enables you to use qi to help you release anxieties, expectations, and negative emotions— referred to as blockages—that prevent you from feeling truly alive and joyful. Taoist meditation uses two primary methods, Outer and Inner Dissolving, to release blockages with a person's eight energy bodies.

There are three primary goals in practicing Taoist meditation. The first goal is to address spiritual responsibility for yourself, helping you become a relaxed, spontaneous, fully mature and open human being. A second goal is awakening the great human potential inside you, fostering compassion and balance. The third is reaching inner stillness— a place deep inside you that is absolutely permanent and stable. As your practice deepens, the sixteen-part neigong system is brought into play to accelerate the evolutionary spiritual process.

Related Products:

- *Taoist Meditation Circle* is an online program and group that includes various techniques and guided practice sessions. It teaches core meditation skills such as concentration, focus and awareness training. This is a foundation program and leads to the more advanced Taoist meditation practices such as Inner Dissolving. Taoist Meditation Circle members are given a step-by-step meditation program, monthly meditation practices and access to a private online meditation community to ask questions and share experiences. [Online Program]

- *Tao Te Ching: A Practitioners Guide* presents the *Tao Te Ching* experientially, from an insider's view, for those who want to both read the text and who are ready to apply the practices from Taoism to their life. The *Tao Te Ching* was written by Laozi in approximately 600 B.C.E. and contains 81 chapters in total. Each month members receive an adapted translation plus audio commentary and practice session on one or more chapters of the *Tao Te Ching*, the text that is the philosophical and religious underpinning for Taoism. [Online Program]

- *Relaxing into Your Being: Chi, Breathing and Dissolving Inner Pain* [Book]

- *The Great Stillness: Body Awareness, Moving Meditation and Sex Qigong* [Book]

- *Tao of Letting Go: Meditation for Modern Living* reveals how the Inner Dissolving method of Taoist meditation can help you let go of tension, fear, anger and pain [Book and 6-CD Set]

- *Ancient Songs of the Tao,* a collection of never-before-recorded chants in ancient Chinese that balance and transform the energetic frequencies within a human being [3-CD Set]

- *Strings of the Tao,* in which Frantzis chants powerful liturgies accompanied by former Kitaro violinist, Steve Kindler [CD]

TAOIST SEXUAL PRACTICES

Taoist sexual practices can add a whole new dimension to lovemaking, making it much more satisfying and fulfilling than normally possible. The Taoists have an extensive repertoire of techniques for

- Improving ordinary sex
- Incorporating qigong into lovemaking
- Sexual meditation as a vehicle for spiritual awakening

Sexual qigong involves the sixteen neigong components, beginning with Taoist Outer Dissolving, opening and closing (pulsing) and working with the etheric body, all of which are best learned as solo practices before being incorporated into sexual activity.

Inner Dissolving is a key component of both Taoist sitting meditation and sexual meditation. The ultimate goal of sexual meditation is to achieve a true merging with one's partner, and then together merge with Universal Consciousness itself.

Interactive practices with a partner can accelerate the progress of development in both sexual qigong and sexual meditation, allowing each partner to gain up to four times the energy than he or she would have access to in solo practices.

Related Products:
- *Taoist Sexual Meditation: Connecting to Love, Energy and Spirit* [Book]
- *Chi Revolution,* which describes how chi or qi is the power behind, for example, spirituality and sexual vitality. The Chi Rev Workout included covers basic qigong that is used in sexual qigong, such as Longevity Breathing, beginning Outer Dissolving, working with the heart center and tracing the etheric body. [Book]

TRAINING OPPORTUNITIES AND EVENTS

Bruce Frantzis is the founder of Energy Arts, Inc. Energy Arts offers instructor certification programs, retreats, corporate and public workshops, and lectures worldwide. Frantzis teaches Energy Arts courses in qigong; Longevity Breathing; the internal martial arts of bagua, tai chi and hsing-i; Neigong Yoga; the healing techniques of qigong tui na; and the Water method of Taoist meditation.

Comprehensive multimedia training courses may also be available from time to time. Topics may include meditation, bagua, tai chi and qigong. See *EnergyArts.com* for current programs.

INSTRUCTOR CERTIFICATION

Prior training in Frantzis Energy Arts programs is a requirement for most instructor courses. The certification process is rigorous to ensure that instructors teach the authentic traditions inherent in these arts.

TRAIN WITH A FRANTZIS ENERGY ARTS CERTIFIED INSTRUCTOR

The Energy Arts website, *EnergyArts.com,* contains a directory of all the certified instructors worldwide. Since Bruce Frantzis no longer offers regular ongoing classes, he recommends locating an instructor in your area for regular training and for building on or preparing for his teachings.

ENERGY ARTS EMAIL LIST

Please visit EnergyArts.com to:
- Join our list to get free articles and audio material by Bruce Frantzis.
- Receive the latest details on events and training materials.
- See video clips of qigong and martial arts forms.
- Find a Certified Energy Arts Instructor near you or learn how to become one.
- Inquire about hosting a workshop or speaking engagement.
- Request media appearances, interviews and articles

CONTACT INFORMATION

Energy Arts, Inc.
P.O. Box 99
Fairfax, CA 94978-0099
USA
Phone: (415) 454-5243
www.EnergyArts.com

Bibliography

Anand, Margot, *The Art of Sexual Ecstasy: The path of Sacred Sexuality for Western Lovers*. Los Angeles: Jeremy P. Tarcher, Inc. 1989.

Capra, Fritjof, *The Tao of Physics*. Boston: Shambhala, 1999.

Chang, Stephen, *The Tao of Sexology*. San Francisco: Tao Publishing, 1986.

Cleary, Thomas, *The Taoist Classics: Volume Three*. Boston: Shambhala, 1991.

Comfort, Alex, *The New Joy of Sex*. New York: Pocket Books, 1991.

Daedone, Nicole, *Slow Sex: The Art and Craft of the Female Orgasm*. New York: Grand Central Life and Style, 2011.

Dale, Cyndi, *The Subtle Body: An Encyclopedia of Your Energetic Anatomy*. Boulder: Sounds True, 2009.

Deida, David, *Finding God through Sex*. Boulder, Colorado: Sounds True, 2005.

Foucault, Michel, *The History of Sexuality, Vol. 1: An Introduction*. New York: Vintage Books, 1978.

Fromm, Erich, *The Art of Loving*. New York: Perennial Classics. 1956, 2000.

Gladwell, Malcolm, *Outliers*. New York: Little, Brown and Company. 2008.

Huang Di Nei Jing Su Wen (Basic Questions from the Yellow Emperor's Inner Canon), various English translations available.

Kerner, Ian, *She Comes First*. New York: Harper, 2004.

Lama Yeshe, *Introduction to Tantra: A Vision of Totality*. Boston: Wisdom Publications, 1987.

Lao-Tzu (Laozi, Lao Tse), *Tao Te Ching (Dao De Jing)*. Translated by Robert G. Henricks. USA: Ballantine Books, 1989. Various English translations available.

Liedloff, Jean, *The Continuum Concept*. Cambridge: Perseus, 1975.

Needham, Joseph, ed., *Science and Civilisation in China*. Cambridge: Cambridge University Press, 1954, 2008.

Norbu, Namkhai, *The Crystal and the Way of Light.* New York: Routledge and Kegan Paul, 1986.

Reid, Daniel, *The Tao of Health, Sex and Longevity.* London: Simon & Schuster, 1989.

Ritsema, Rudolf, and Shantena Augusto Sabbadini, trans., *The Original I Ching Oracle.* London: Watkins Publishing, 2005. Various other translations of the *I Ching* available.

Roach, Mary, *Bonk: The Curious Coupling of Science and Sex.* New York: W. W. Norton, 2008.

Ryan, Christopher, and Jetha, Cacilda, *Sex at Dawn: How We Mate, Why We Stray, and What It Means for Modern Relationships.* New York: Harper Perennial, 2010.

Saxon, Lynn, *Sex at Dusk.* 2012.

Shaw, Miranda, *Passionate Enlightenment: Women in Tantric Buddhism.* Princeton, New Jersey: Princeton University Press, 1994.

Snellgrove, David, *The Hevajra Tantra: A Critical Study.* London: Oxford University Press, 1959.

Sogyal Rinpoche, *The Tibetan Book of Living and Dying.* New York: HarperSanFrancisco, 1994.

Sun Simiao, ed., *Beiji Qian Jin Yao Fang (One Thousand Golden Important Prescriptions).* Various English translations available.

Wrangham, Richard, and Peterson, Dale, *Demonic Males.* New York: Houghton Mifflin, 1996.

Zhuangzi (Chuang Tzu), *The Way of Chuang Tzu,* translated by Thomas Merton. Boston: Shambhala Publications, 2004.

Zhuangzi (Chuang Tzu), *Zhuangzi: Basic Writings,* translated by Burton Watson. New York: Columbia University Press, 2003.

Index